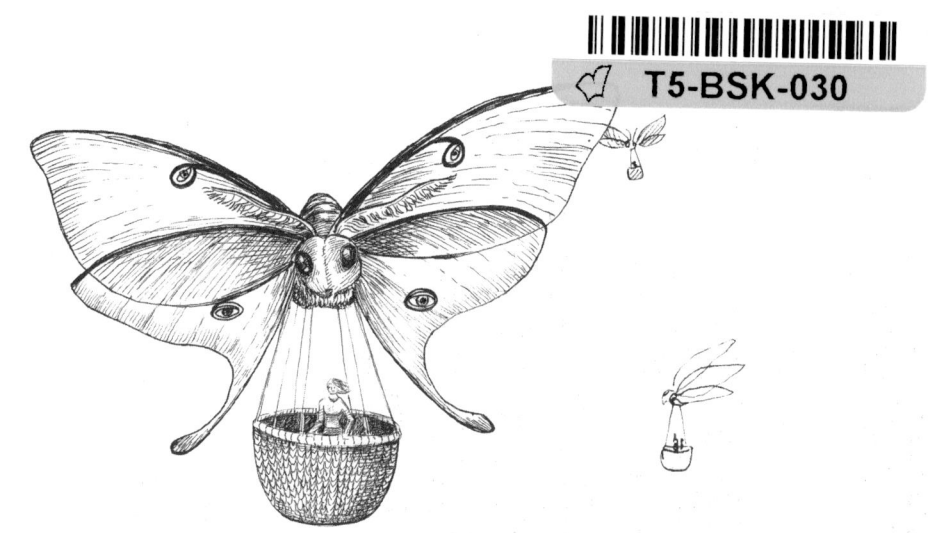

sleepless planet

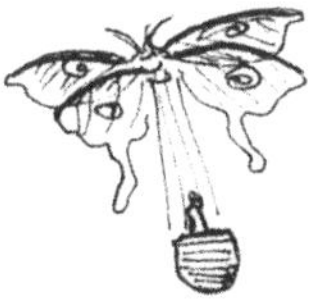

a graphic guide to healing from insomnia

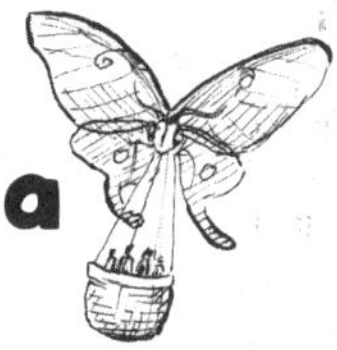

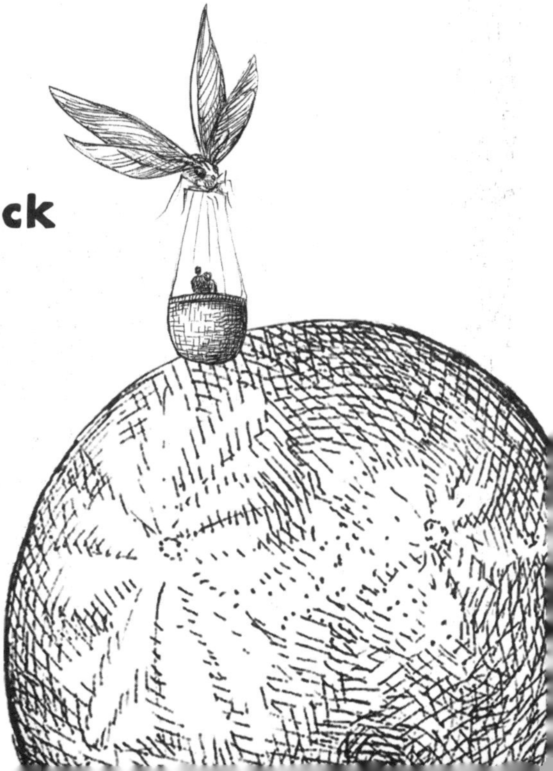

Maureen Burdock

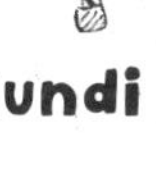

Graphic Mundi

The information and advice presented in this book are not meant to substitute for the advice and services of a trained health professional. Please consult your healthcare professional with regard to all matters pertaining to your health and well-being, especially those that may require diagnosis or medical attention.

Library of Congress Cataloging-in-Publication Data

Names: Burdock, Maureen, 1970- author.
Title: Sleepless planet : a graphic guide to healing from insomnia / Maureen Burdock.
Description: University Park, PA : Graphic Mundi, [2025]
Summary: "Explores the cultural and historical contexts of insomnia while documenting one individual's journey to overcome chronic sleep difficulties. This graphic narrative follows consultations with specialists, experiments with therapies, and efforts to build healthier habits, offering an accessible account of strategies for addressing a widespread sleep disorder"—Provided by publisher.
Identifiers: LCCN 2025023684 | ISBN 9781637790939 paperback
Subjects: LCSH: Insomnia—Comic books, strips, etc. | Insomnia—Treatment—Comic books, strips, etc. | LCGFT: Nonfiction comics | Graphic novels | Graphic medicine (Comics)
Classification: LCC RC548 .B87 2025
LC record available at https://lccn.loc.gov/2025023684

Copyright © 2025 Maureen Burdock
All rights reserved
Printed in China
Published by The Pennsylvania State University Press,
University Park, PA 16802-1003

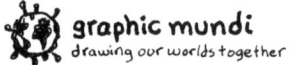

Graphic Mundi is an imprint of
The Pennsylvania State University Press.

The Pennsylvania State University Press is a member of the Association of University Presses.

It is the policy of The Pennsylvania State University Press to use acid-free paper. Publications on uncoated stock satisfy the minimum requirements of American National Standard for Information Sciences—Permanence of Paper for Printed Library Material, ANSI Z39.48-1992.

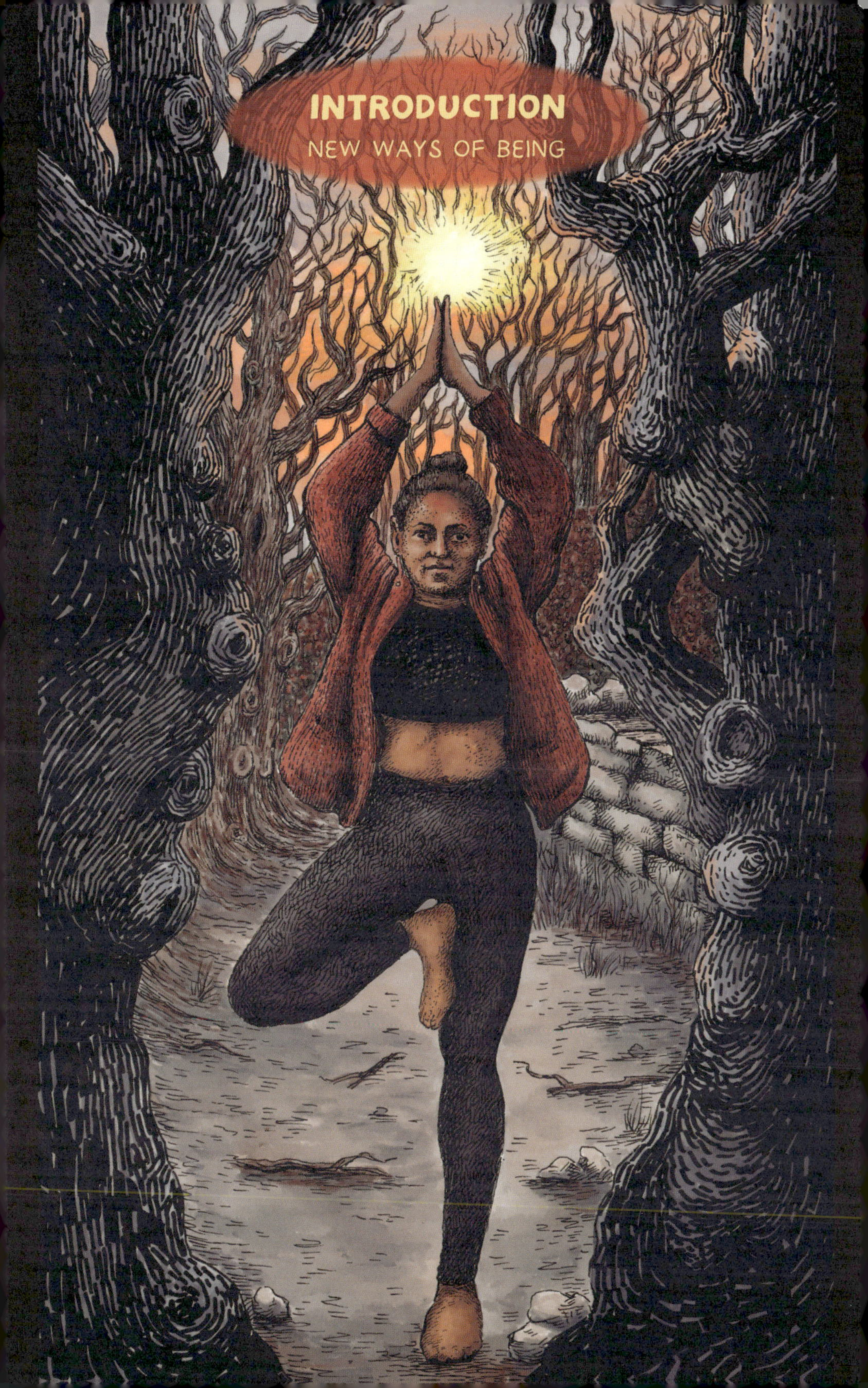
INTRODUCTION
NEW WAYS OF BEING

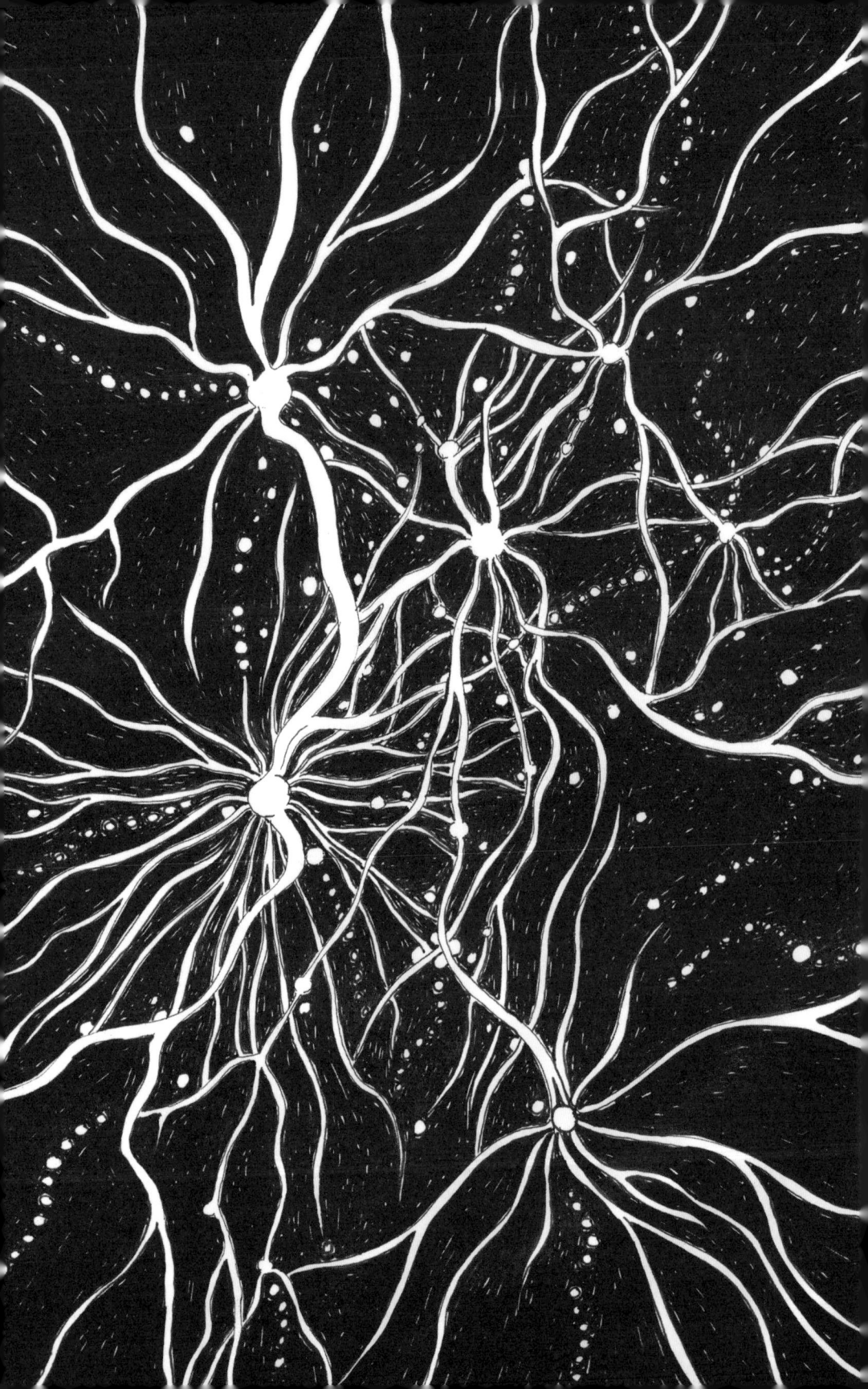

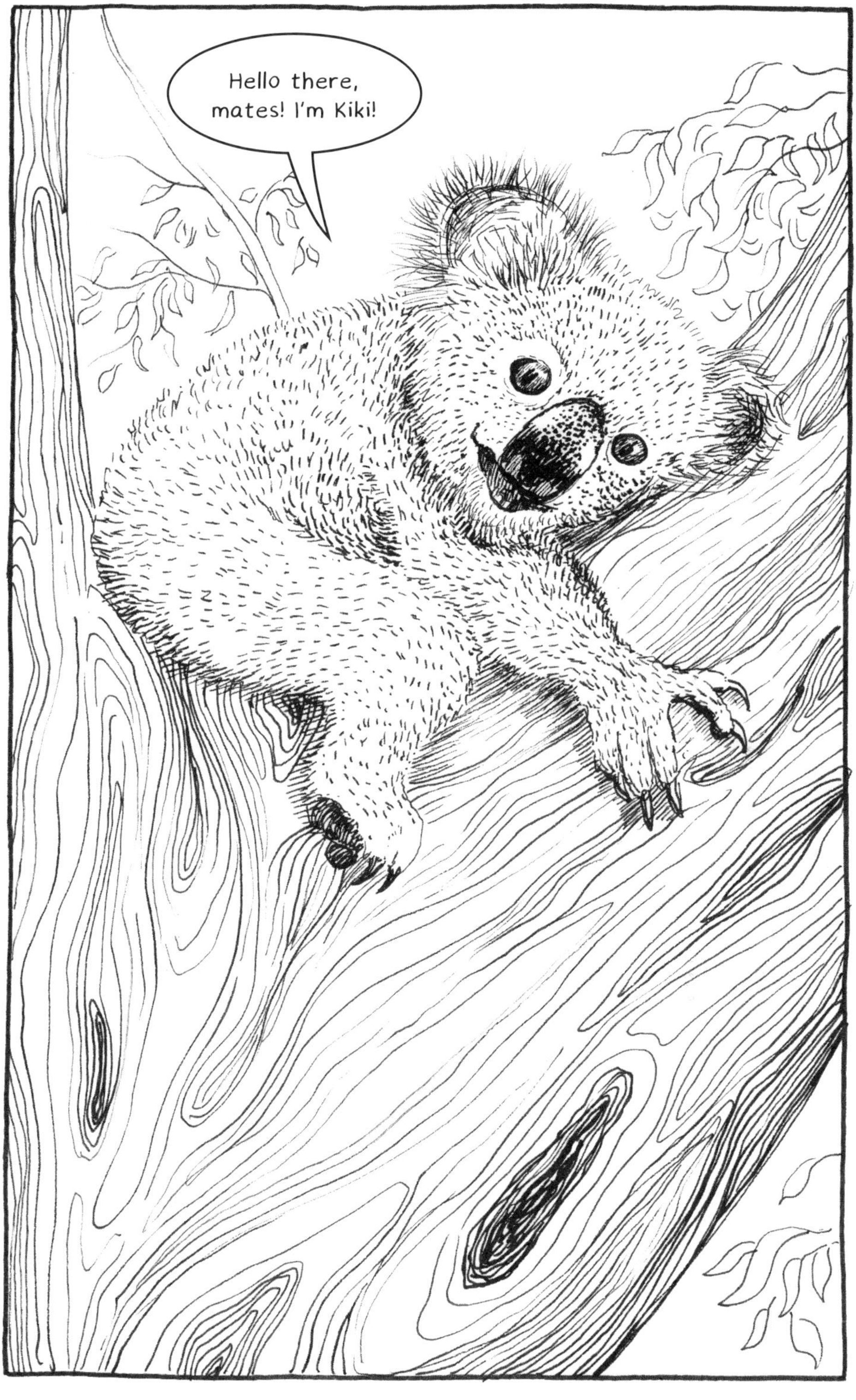
Hello there, mates! I'm Kiki!

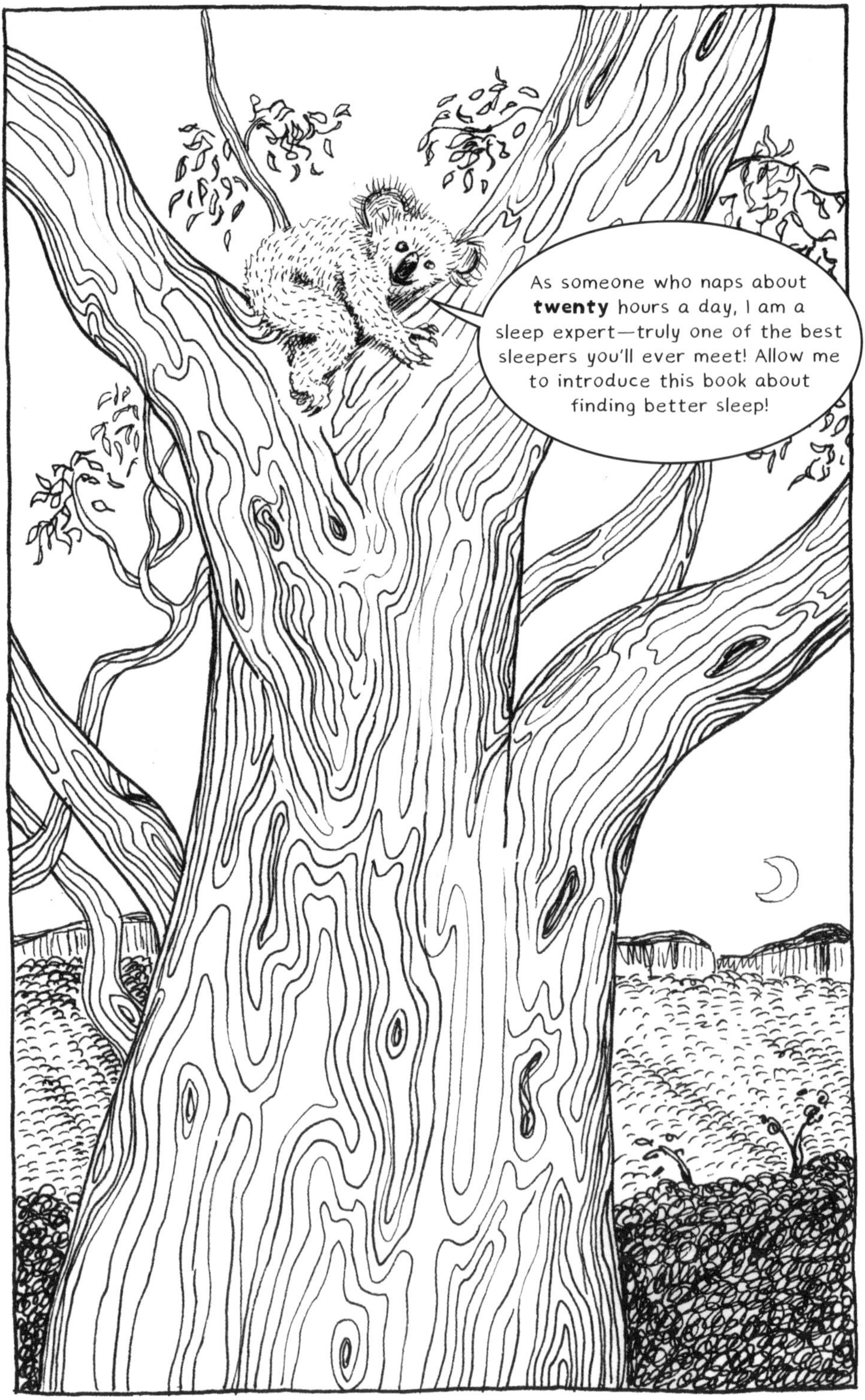
As someone who naps about **twenty** hours a day, I am a sleep expert—truly one of the best sleepers you'll ever meet! Allow me to introduce this book about finding better sleep!

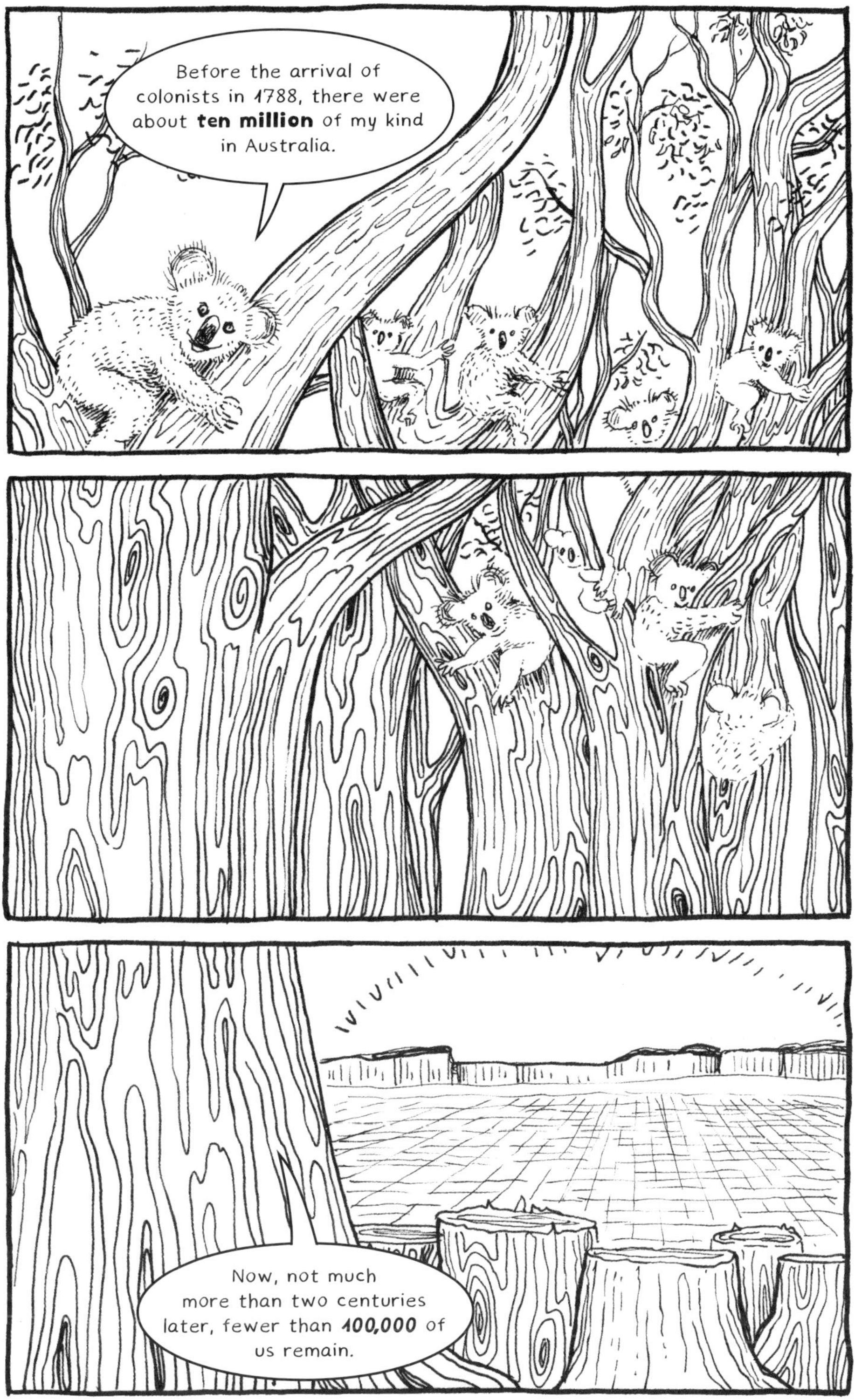
Before the arrival of colonists in 1788, there were about **ten million** of my kind in Australia.
Now, not much more than two centuries later, fewer than **100,000** of us remain.

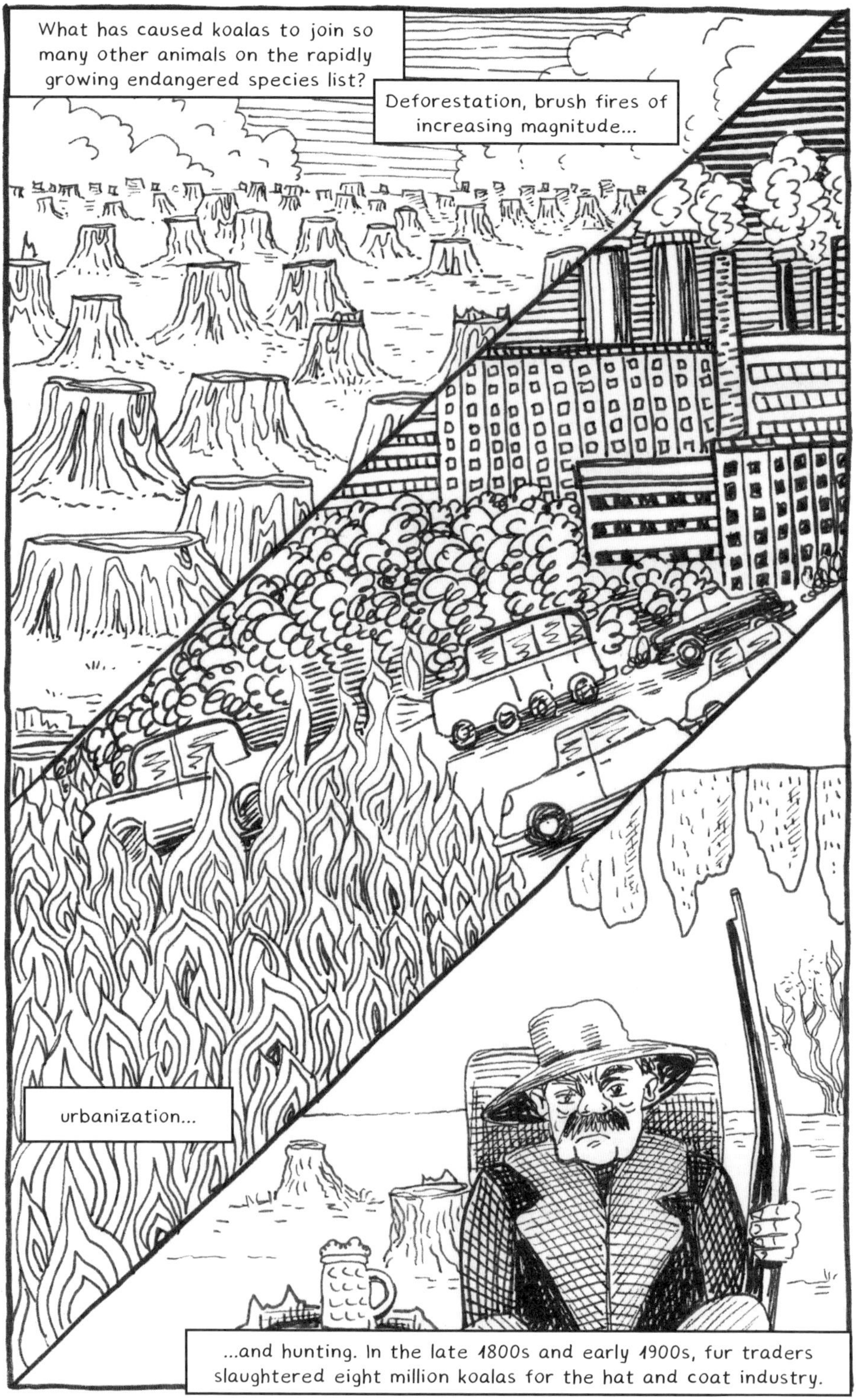
What has caused koalas to join so many other animals on the rapidly growing endangered species list?
Deforestation, brush fires of increasing magnitude...
urbanization...
...and hunting. In the late 1800s and early 1900s, fur traders slaughtered eight million koalas for the hat and coat industry.

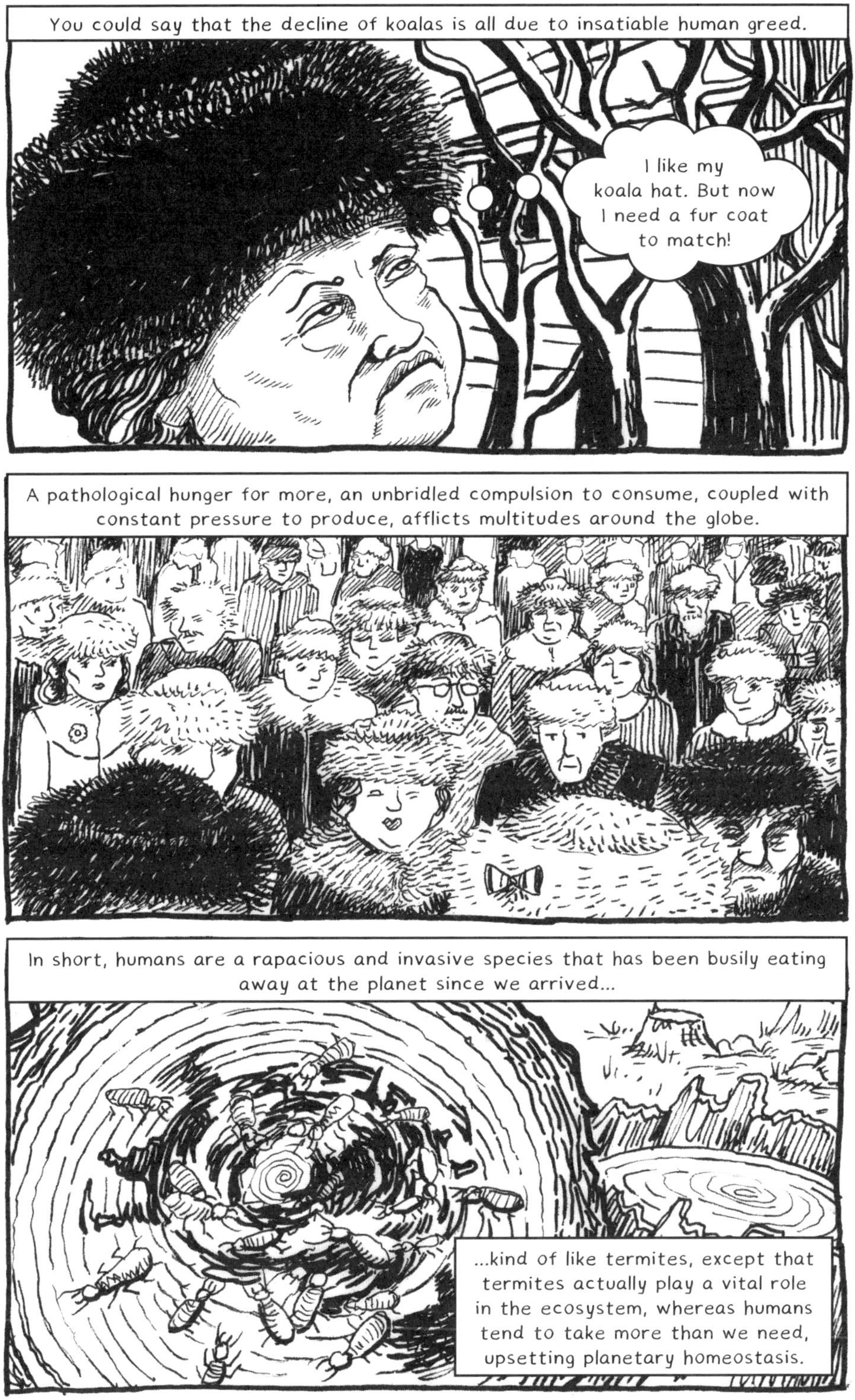
You could say that the decline of koalas is all due to insatiable human greed.
I like my koala hat. But now I need a fur coat to match!
A pathological hunger for more, an unbridled compulsion to consume, coupled with constant pressure to produce, afflicts multitudes around the globe.
In short, humans are a rapacious and invasive species that has been busily eating away at the planet since we arrived...
...kind of like termites, except that termites actually play a vital role in the ecosystem, whereas humans tend to take more than we need, upsetting planetary homeostasis.

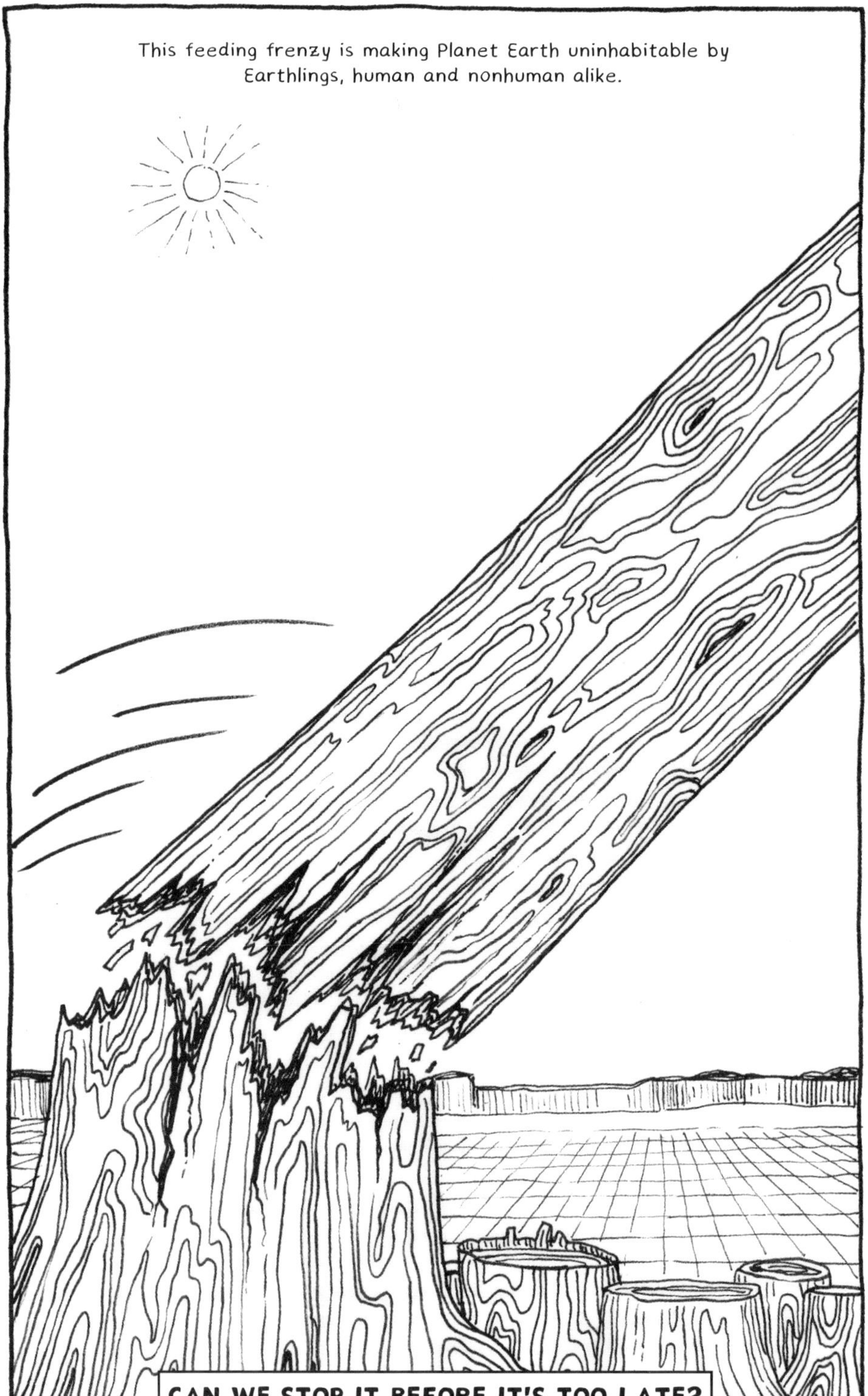
This feeding frenzy is making Planet Earth uninhabitable by Earthlings, human and nonhuman alike.
CAN WE STOP IT BEFORE IT'S TOO LATE?

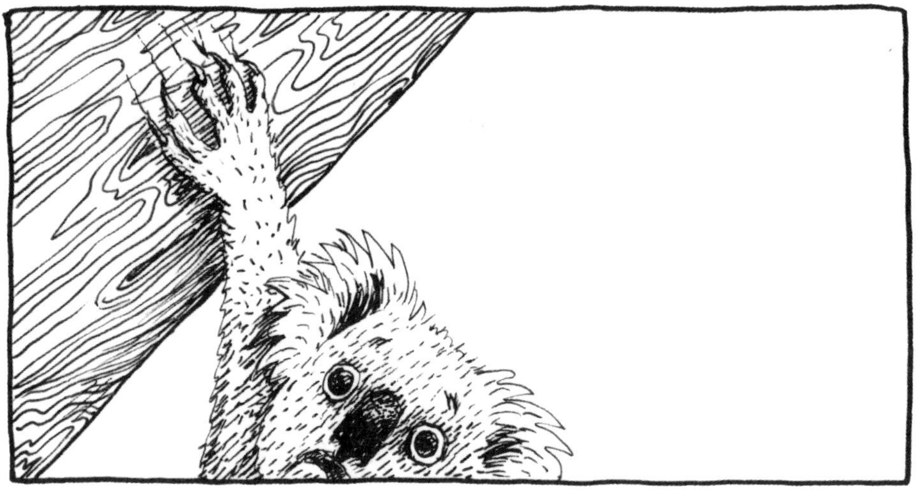

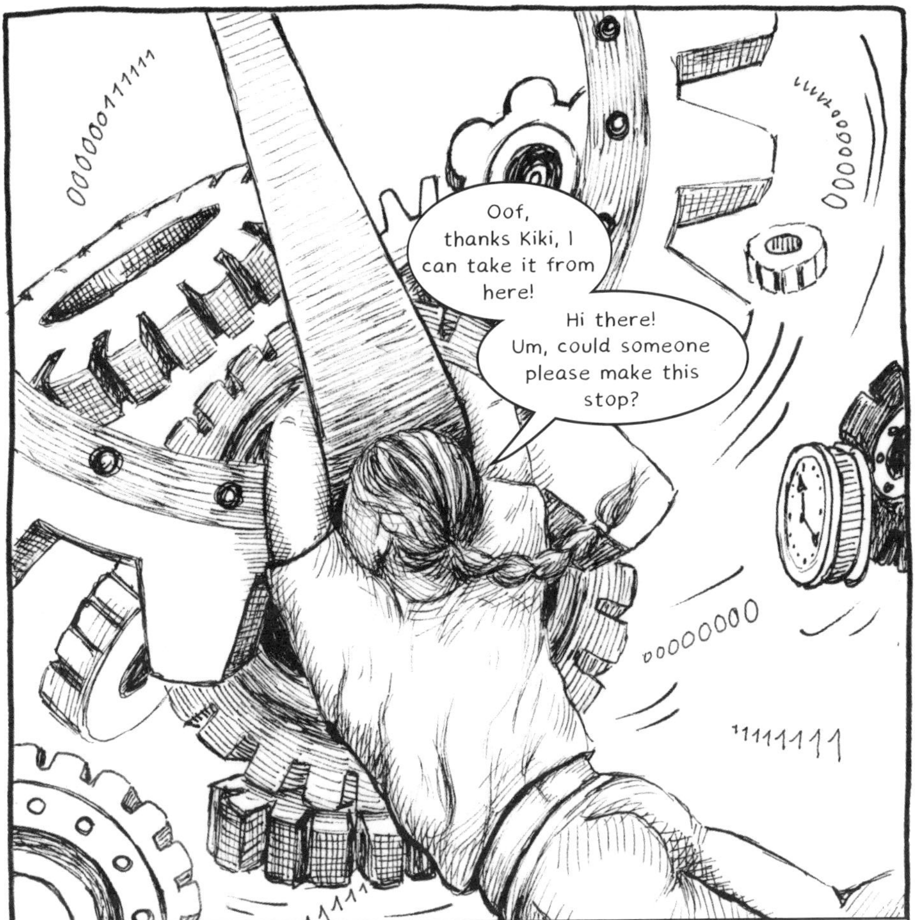
000000111111
Oof, thanks Kiki, I can take it from here!
Hi there! Um, could someone please make this stop?

Without being fully aware of it, I, too, had been swept along by this culture of perpetual "progress."

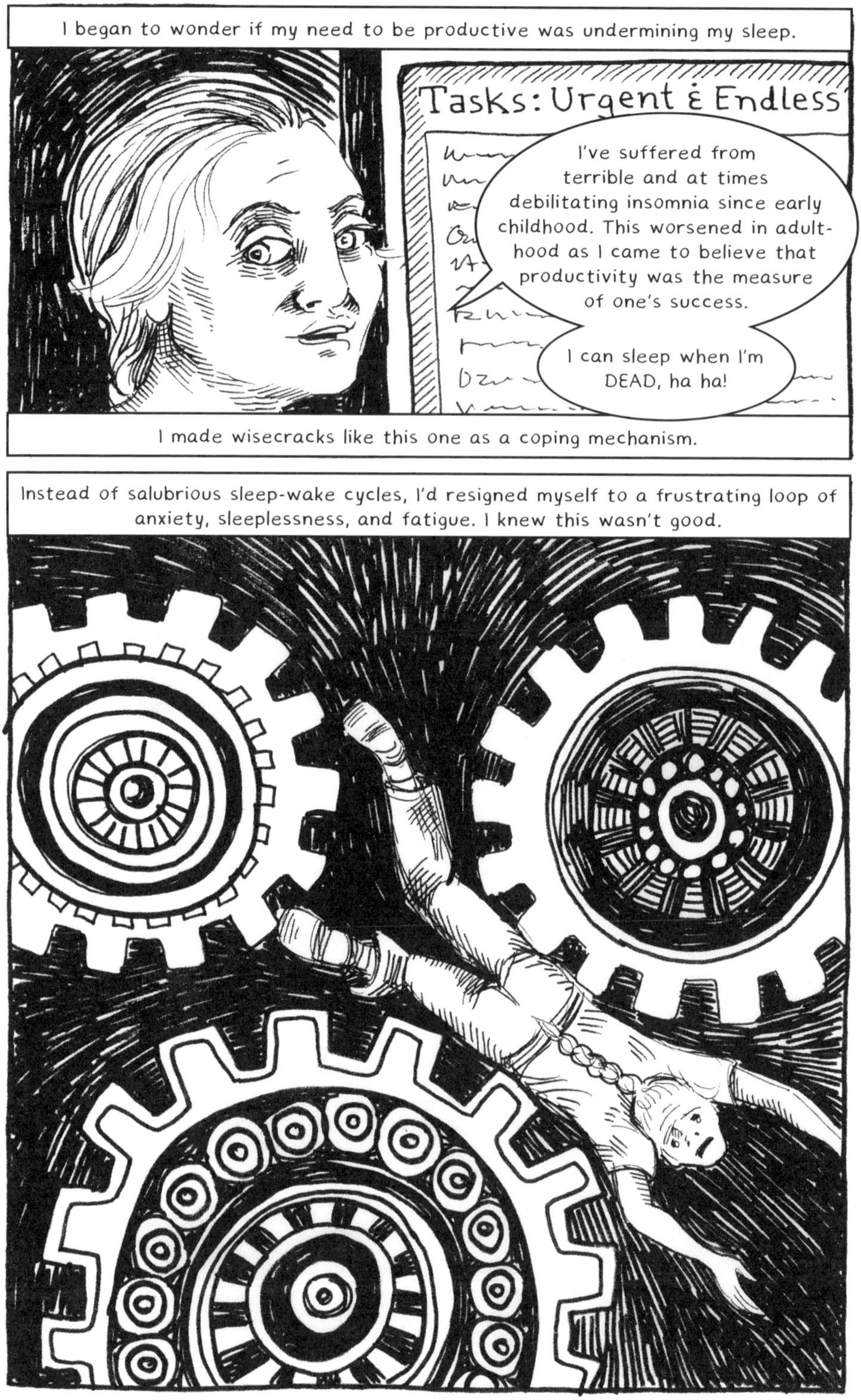
I began to wonder if my need to be productive was undermining my sleep.
Tasks: Urgent & Endless
I've suffered from terrible and at times debilitating insomnia since early childhood. This worsened in adulthood as I came to believe that productivity was the measure of one's success.
I can sleep when I'm DEAD, ha ha!
I made wisecracks like this one as a coping mechanism.
Instead of salubrious sleep-wake cycles, I'd resigned myself to a frustrating loop of anxiety, sleeplessness, and fatigue. I knew this wasn't good.

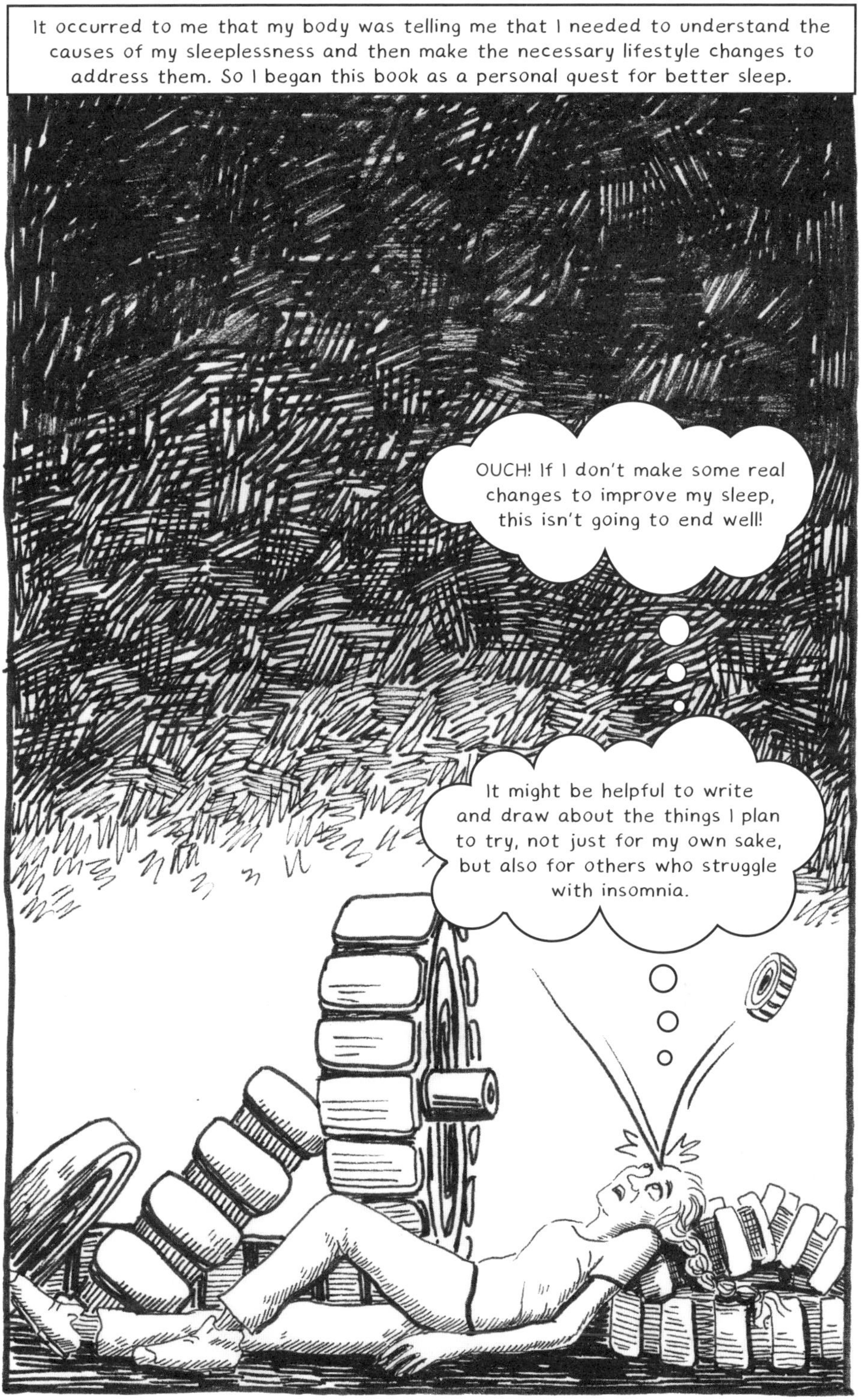
It occurred to me that my body was telling me that I needed to understand the causes of my sleeplessness and then make the necessary lifestyle changes to address them. So I began this book as a personal quest for better sleep.
OUCH! If I don't make some real changes to improve my sleep, this isn't going to end well!
It might be helpful to write and draw about the things I plan to try, not just for my own sake, but also for others who struggle with insomnia.

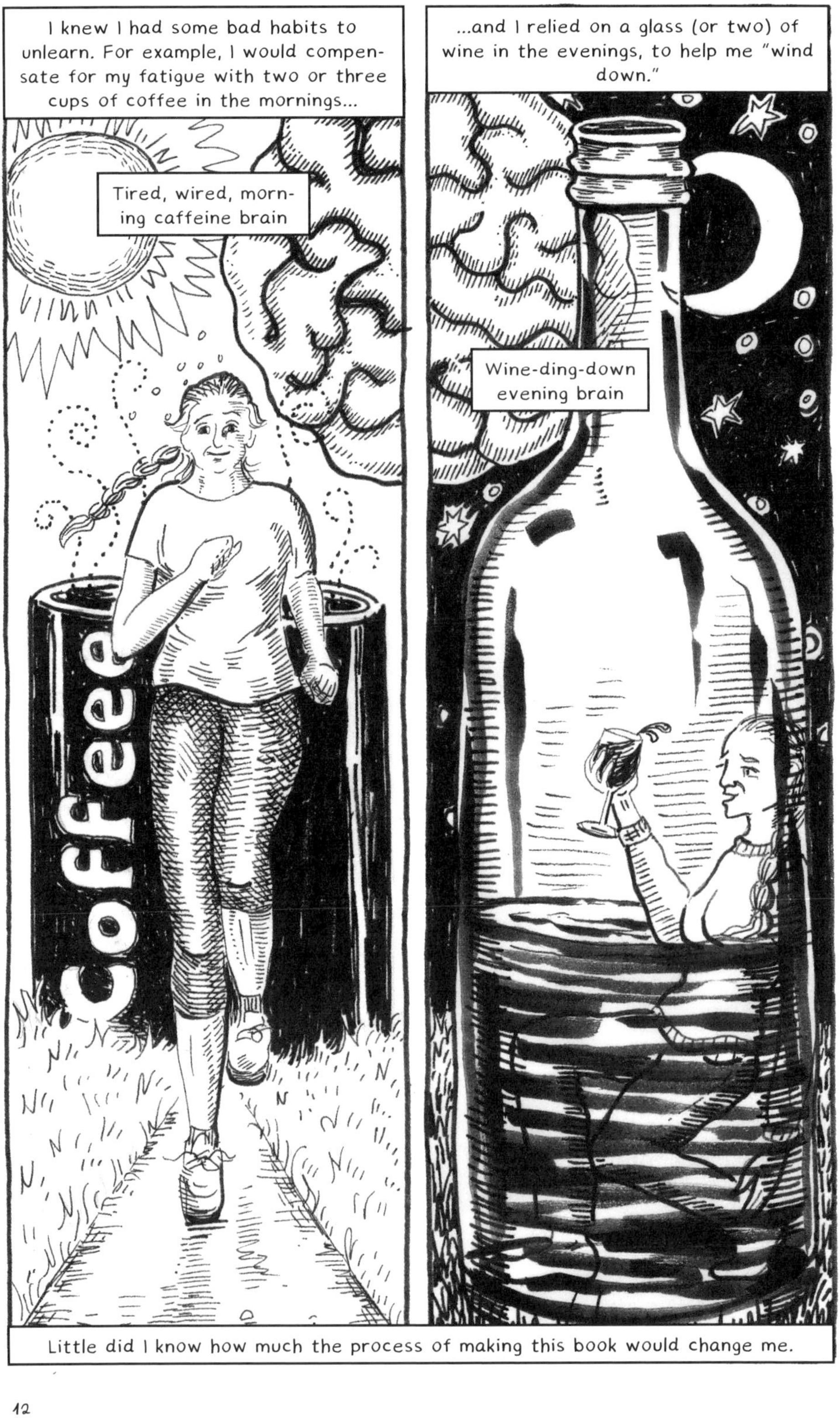

I knew I had some bad habits to unlearn. For example, I would compensate for my fatigue with two or three cups of coffee in the mornings...
Tired, wired, morning caffeine brain
Coffee
...and I relied on a glass (or two) of wine in the evenings, to help me "wind down."
Wine-ding-down evening brain
Little did I know how much the process of making this book would change me.

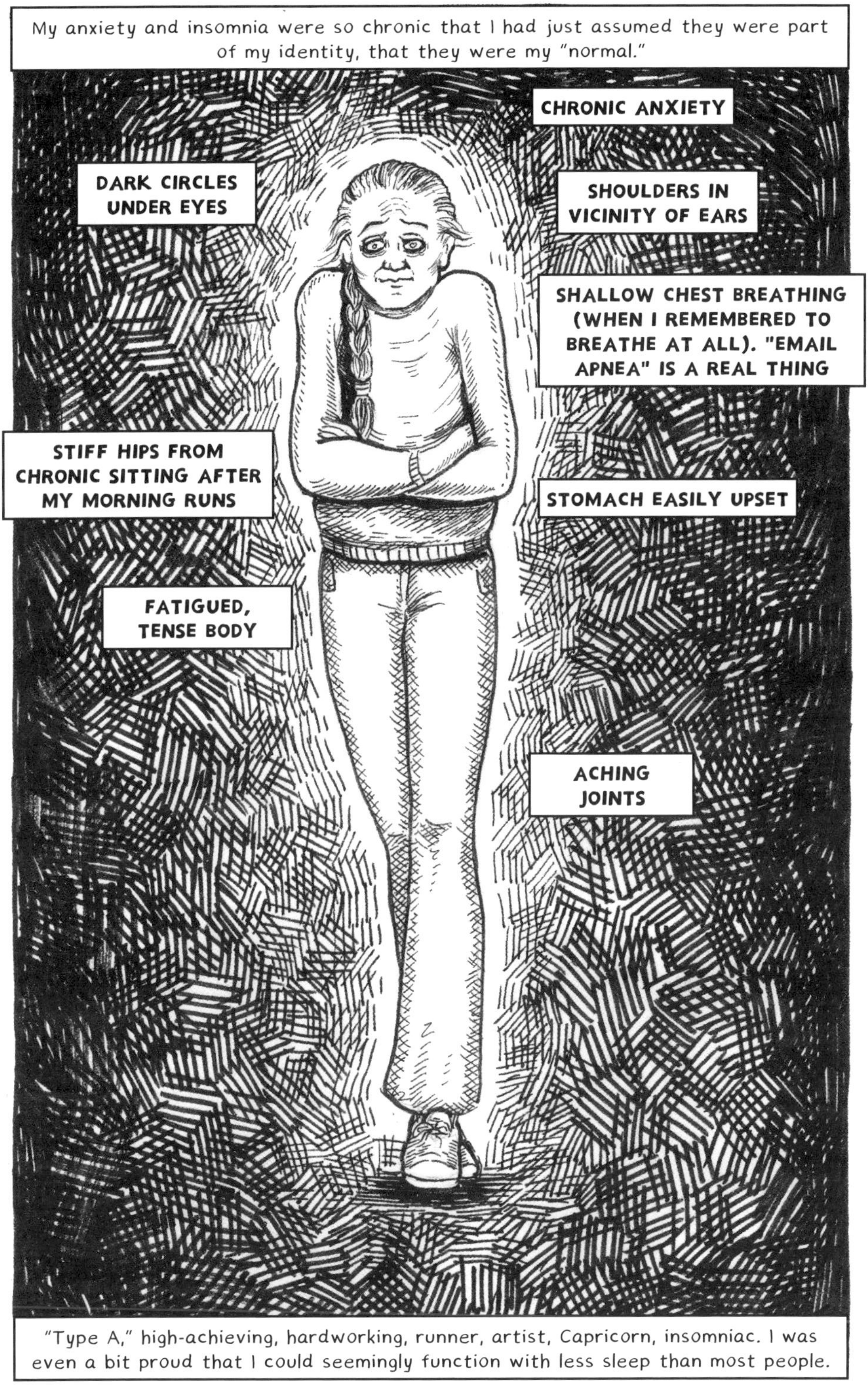
My anxiety and insomnia were so chronic that I had just assumed they were part of my identity, that they were my "normal."
CHRONIC ANXIETY
DARK CIRCLES UNDER EYES
SHOULDERS IN VICINITY OF EARS
SHALLOW CHEST BREATHING (WHEN I REMEMBERED TO BREATHE AT ALL). "EMAIL APNEA" IS A REAL THING
STIFF HIPS FROM CHRONIC SITTING AFTER MY MORNING RUNS
STOMACH EASILY UPSET
FATIGUED, TENSE BODY
ACHING JOINTS
"Type A," high-achieving, hardworking, runner, artist, Capricorn, insomniac. I was even a bit proud that I could seemingly function with less sleep than most people.

My resolution to work intensively on my insomnia and to create this book about it made me stop and take a closer look at myself. It was humbling to realize how some of my thinking and behaviors mirrored industrial capitalist beliefs that are devastating on a social and planetary scale. I had this compulsion to be productive for a set number of hours daily, coupled with the fear of being considered lazy if those productivity targets weren't met; a constant fear of falling short; the belief that simply being kind and helpful in the world wasn't enough; the propensity to want to "escape" via mindless entertainment and less-than-optimal health habits...

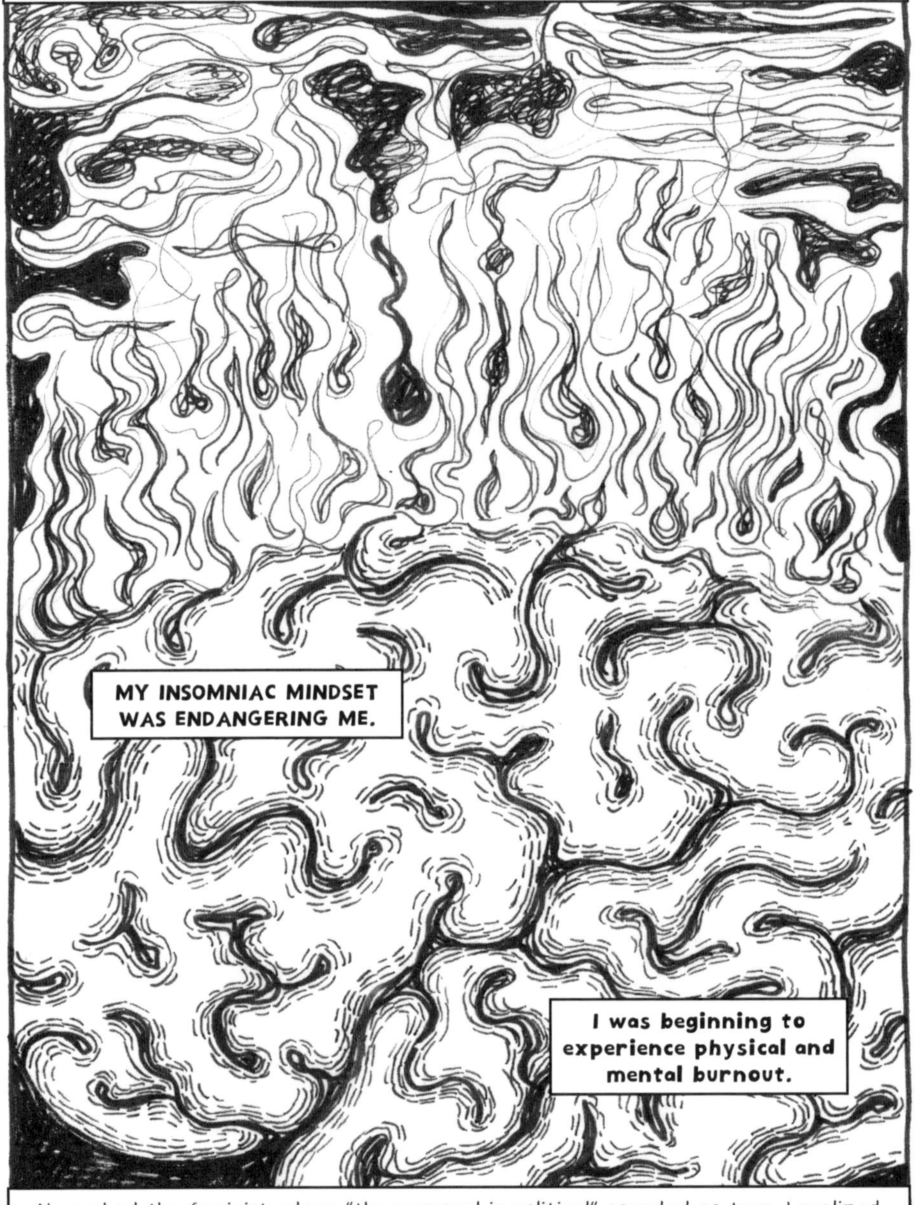
MY INSOMNIAC MINDSET WAS ENDANGERING ME.
I was beginning to experience physical and mental burnout.

Never had the feminist adage "the personal is political" sounded so true. I realized that the motto "I'll sleep when I'm dead," however tongue-in-cheek, really **was** deadly.

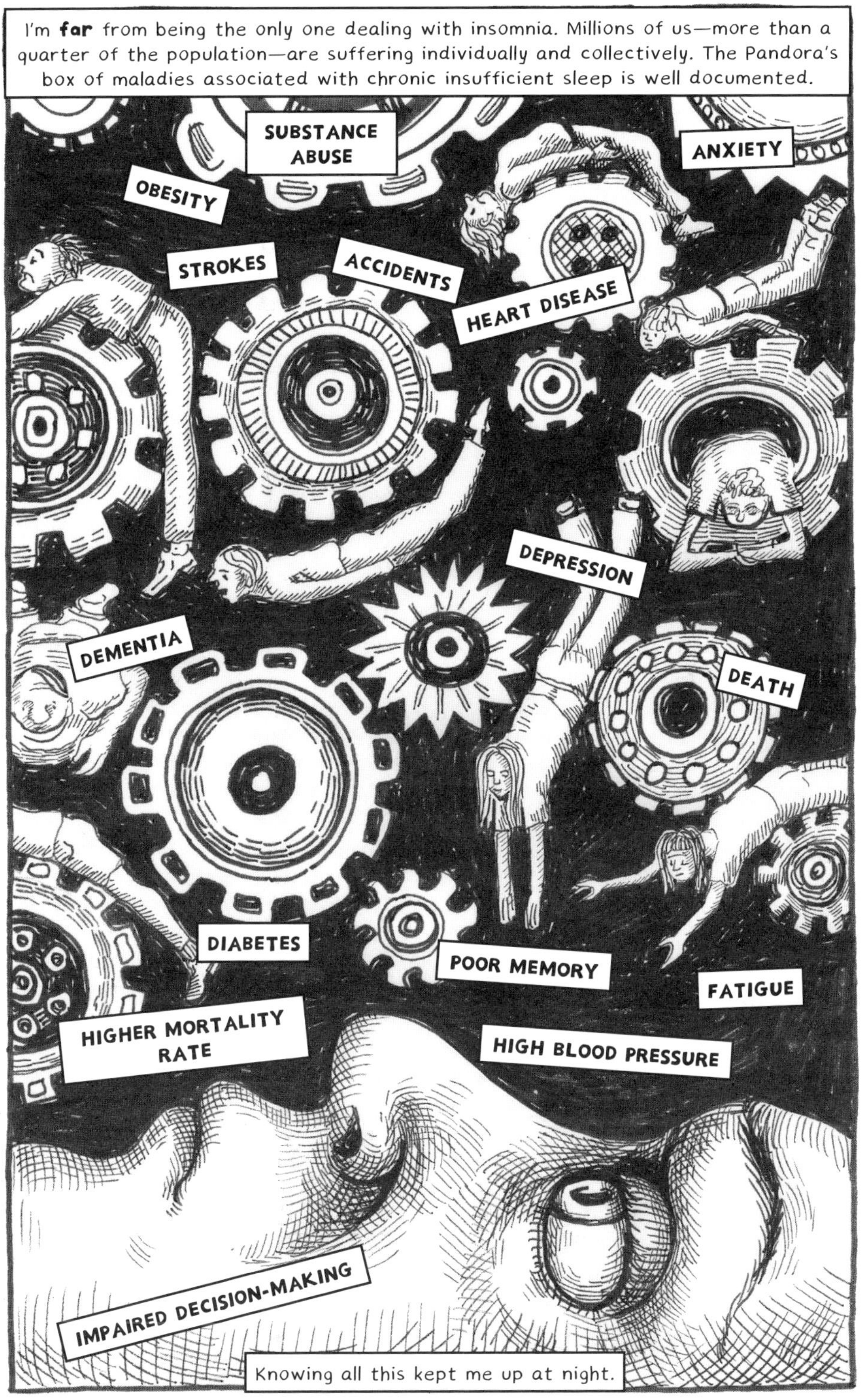
I'm **far** from being the only one dealing with insomnia. Millions of us—more than a quarter of the population—are suffering individually and collectively. The Pandora's box of maladies associated with chronic insufficient sleep is well documented.
SUBSTANCE ABUSE
ANXIETY
OBESITY
STROKES
ACCIDENTS
HEART DISEASE
DEPRESSION
DEMENTIA
DEATH
DIABETES
POOR MEMORY
FATIGUE
HIGHER MORTALITY RATE
HIGH BLOOD PRESSURE
IMPAIRED DECISION-MAKING
Knowing all this kept me up at night.

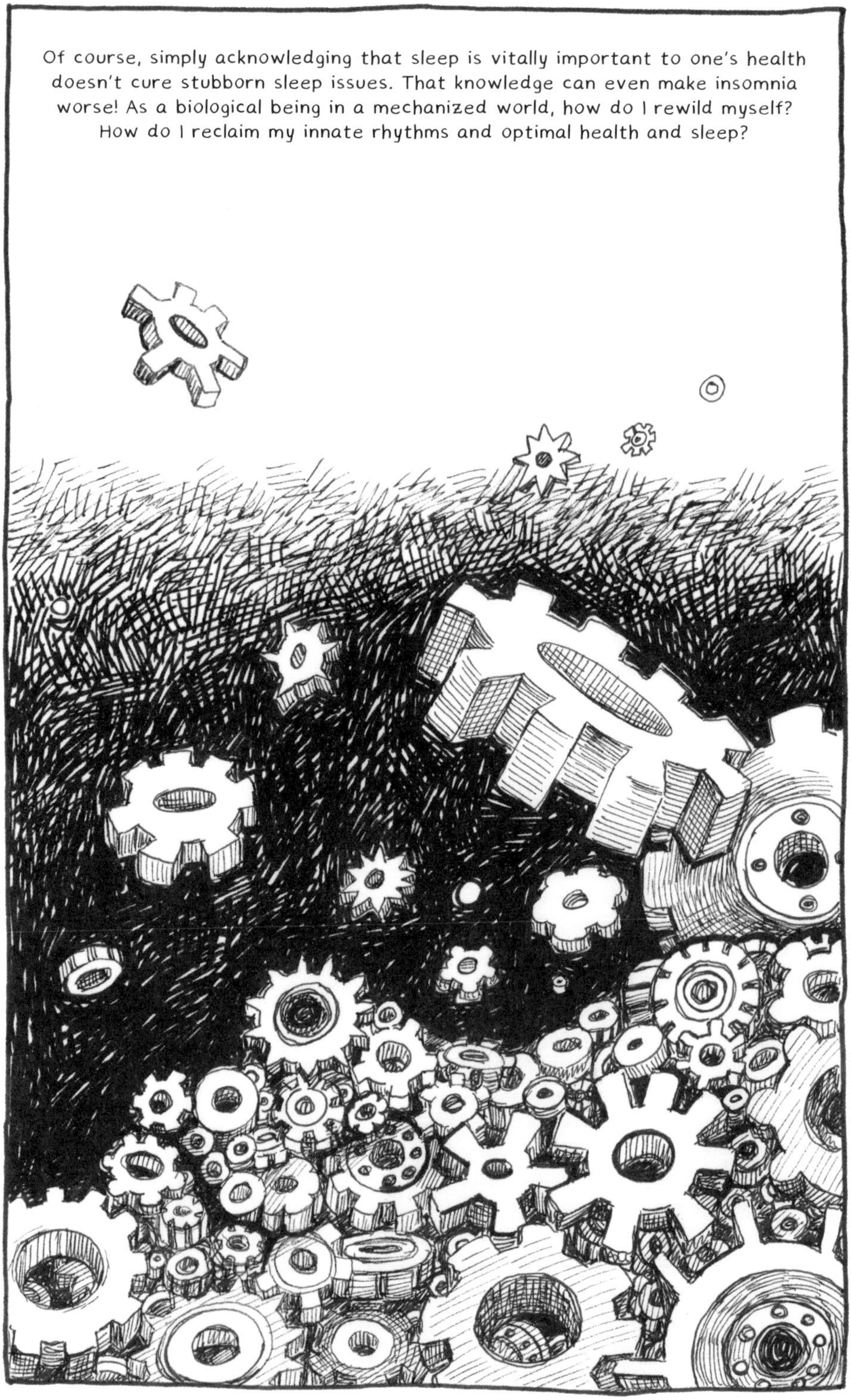
Of course, simply acknowledging that sleep is vitally important to one's health doesn't cure stubborn sleep issues. That knowledge can even make insomnia worse! As a biological being in a mechanized world, how do I rewild myself? How do I reclaim my innate rhythms and optimal health and sleep?

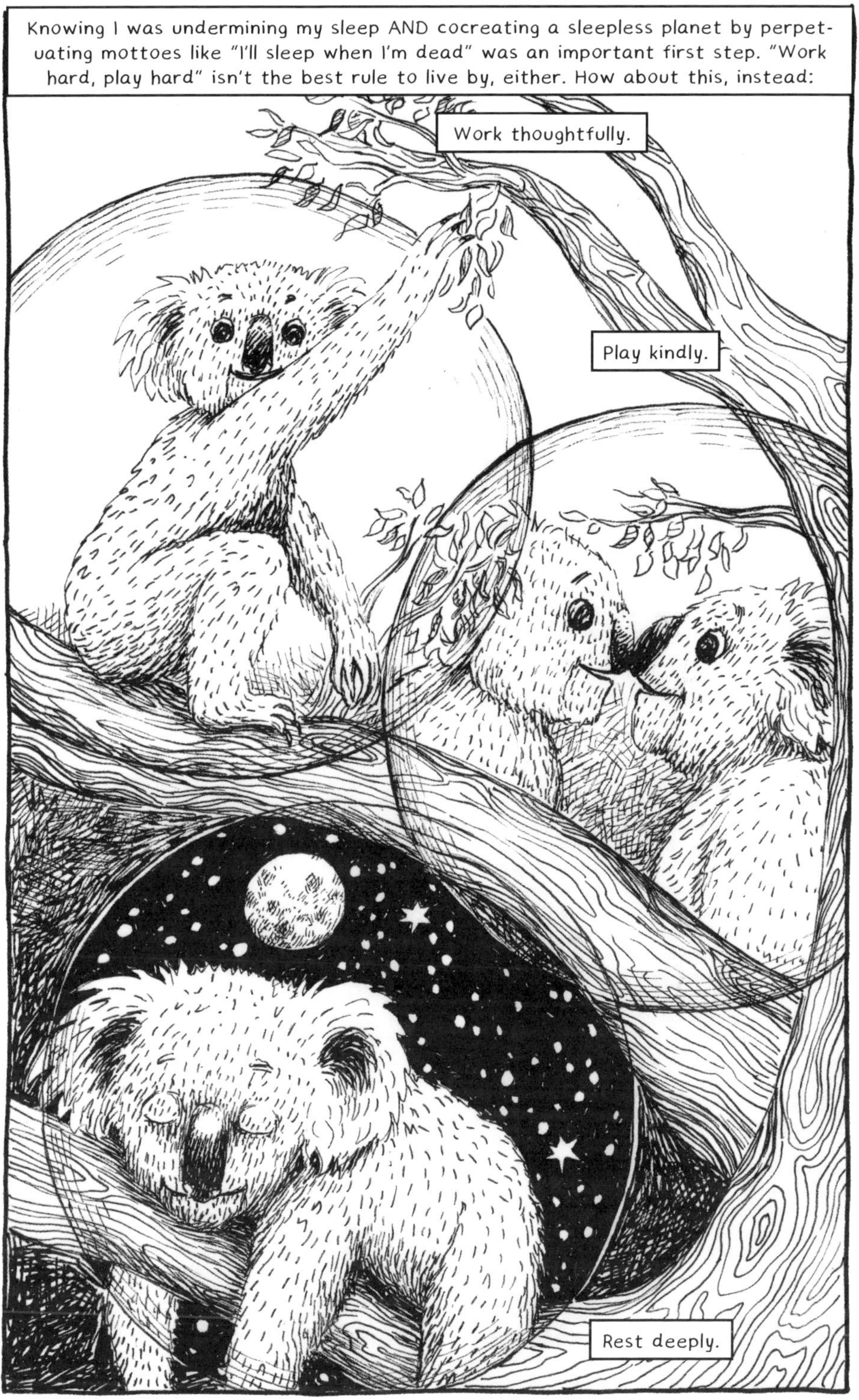
Knowing I was undermining my sleep AND cocreating a sleepless planet by perpetuating mottoes like "I'll sleep when I'm dead" was an important first step. "Work hard, play hard" isn't the best rule to live by, either. How about this, instead:
Work thoughtfully.
Play kindly.
Rest deeply.

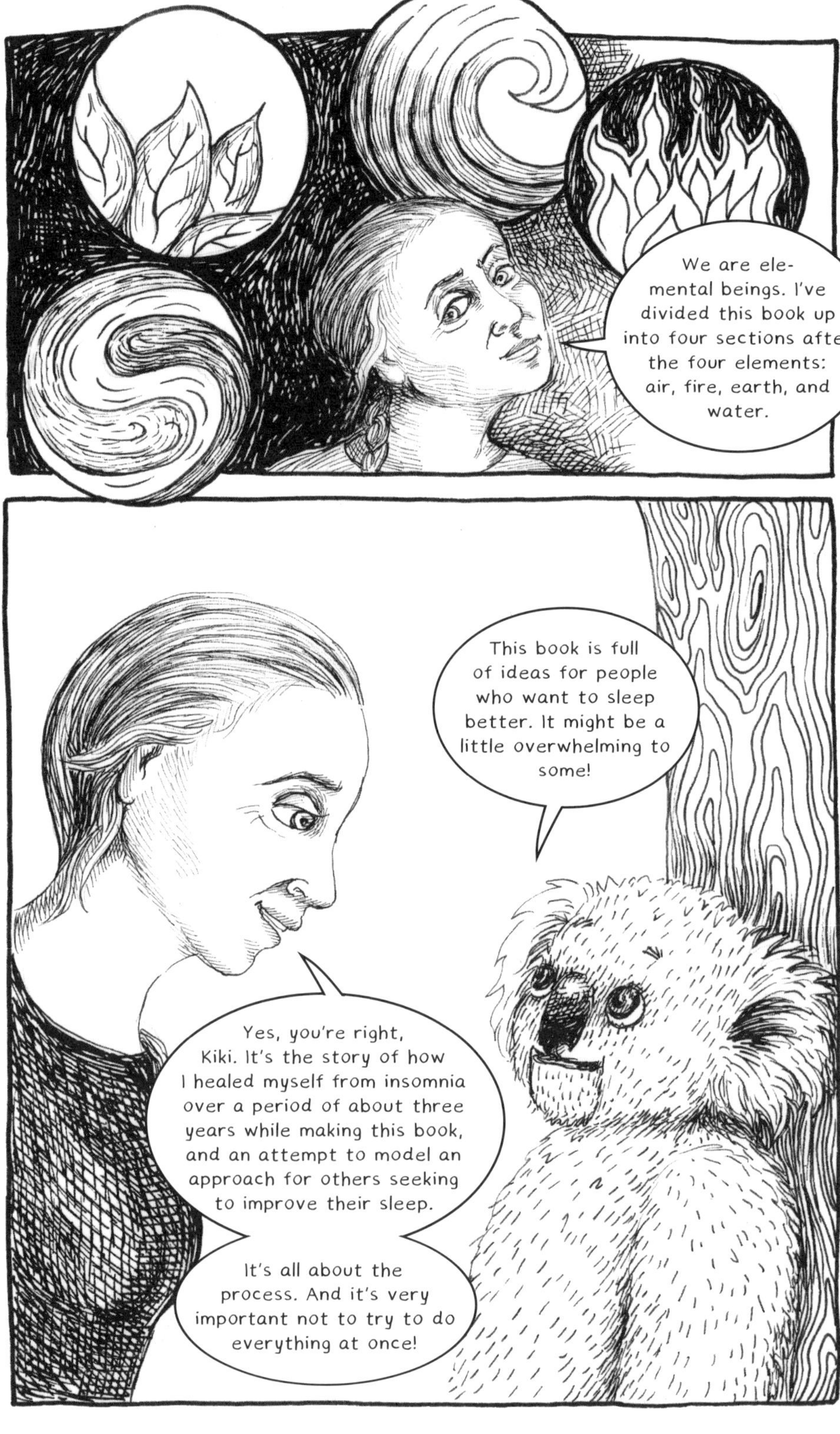
We are elemental beings. I've divided this book up into four sections after the four elements: air, fire, earth, and water.
This book is full of ideas for people who want to sleep better. It might be a little overwhelming to some!
Yes, you're right, Kiki. It's the story of how I healed myself from insomnia over a period of about three years while making this book, and an attempt to model an approach for others seeking to improve their sleep.
It's all about the process. And it's very important not to try to do everything at once!

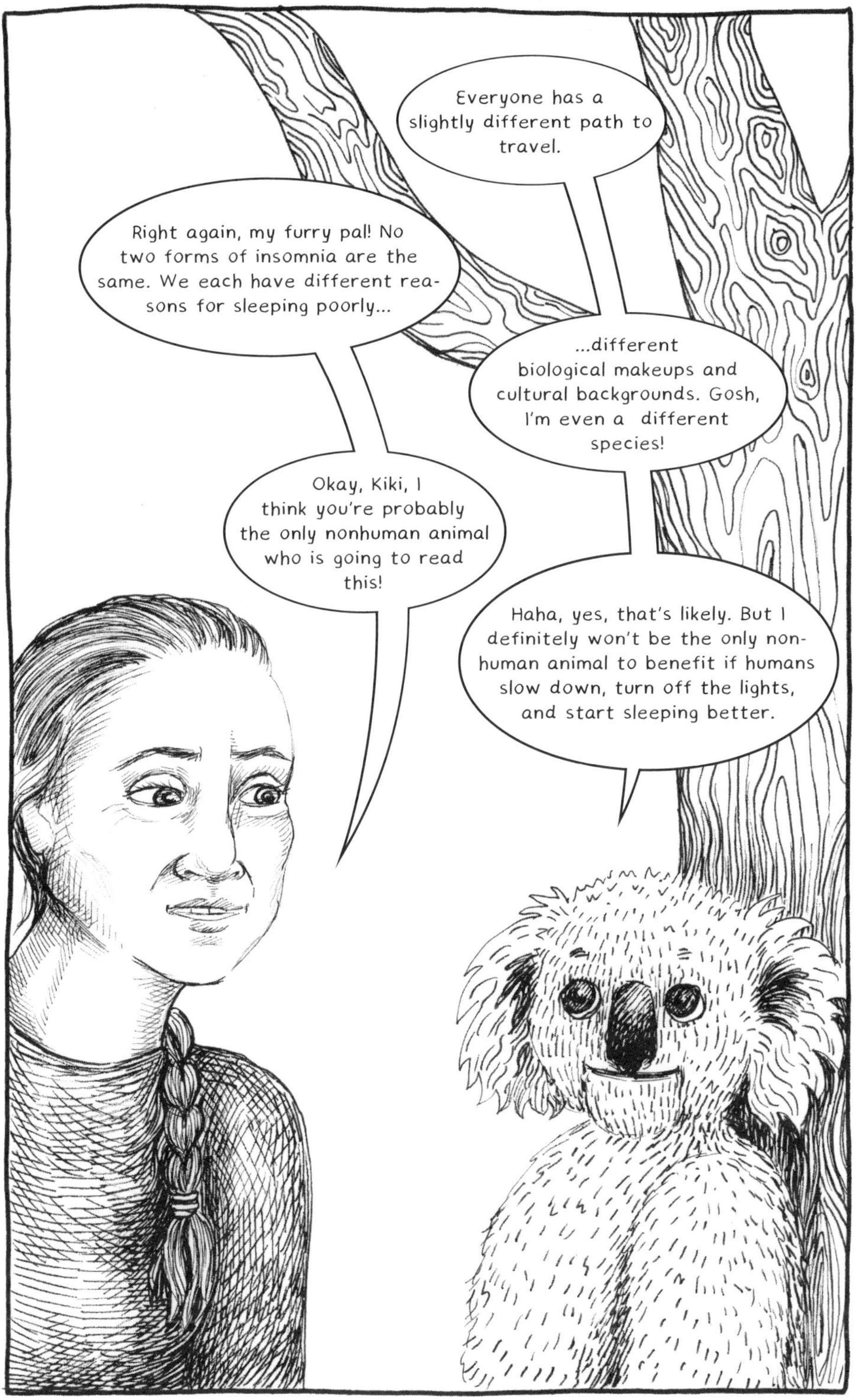
Everyone has a slightly different path to travel.
Right again, my furry pal! No two forms of insomnia are the same. We each have different reasons for sleeping poorly...
...different biological makeups and cultural backgrounds. Gosh, I'm even a different species!
Okay, Kiki, I think you're probably the only nonhuman animal who is going to read this!
Haha, yes, that's likely. But I definitely won't be the only nonhuman animal to benefit if humans slow down, turn off the lights, and start sleeping better.

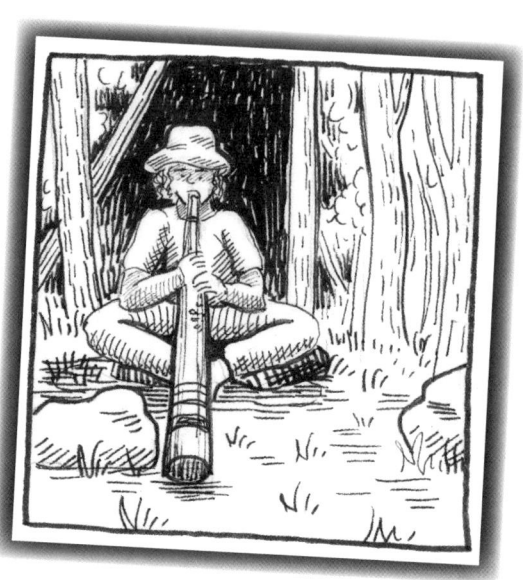

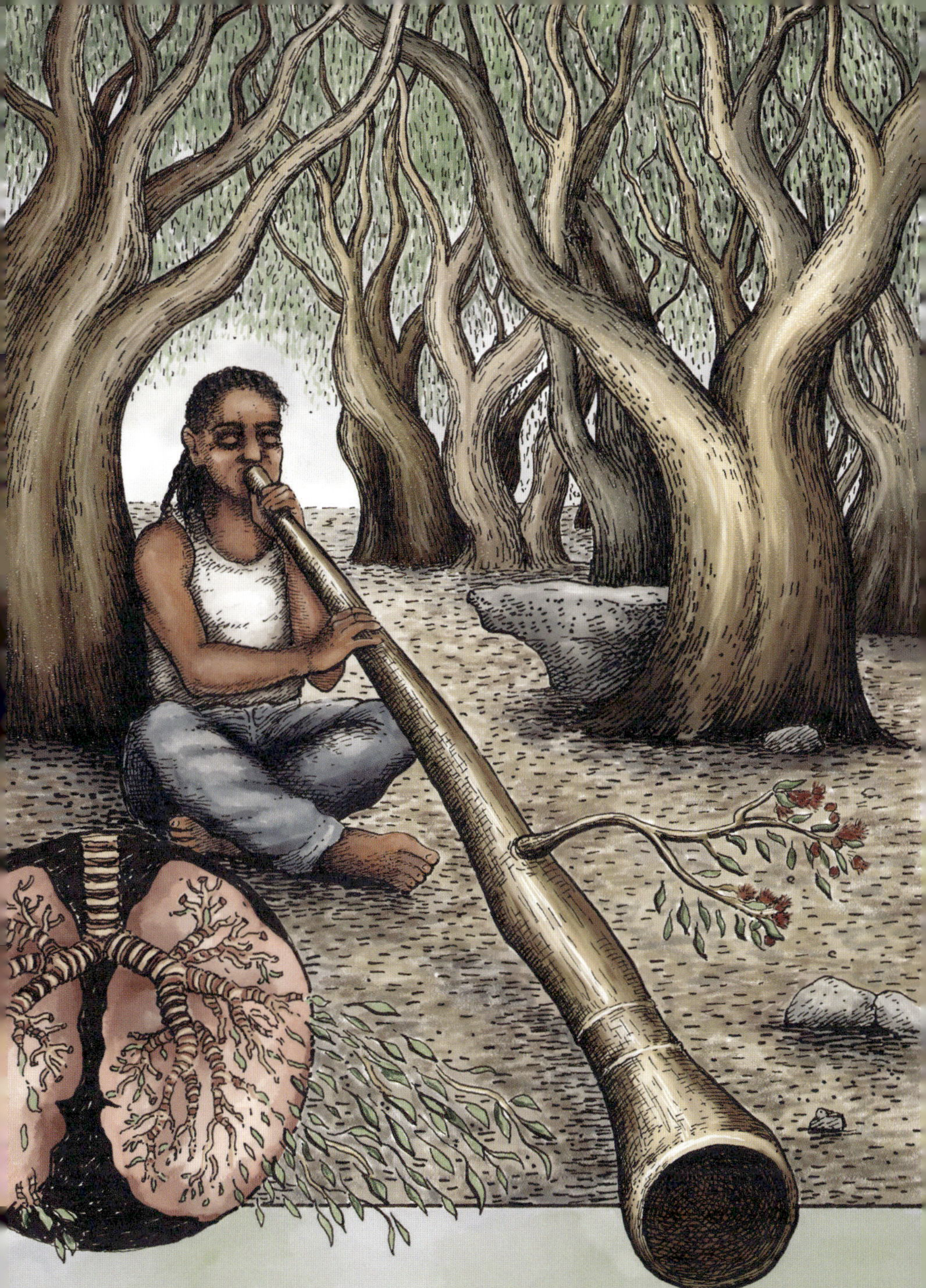

PART ONE: AIR

Just Breathe

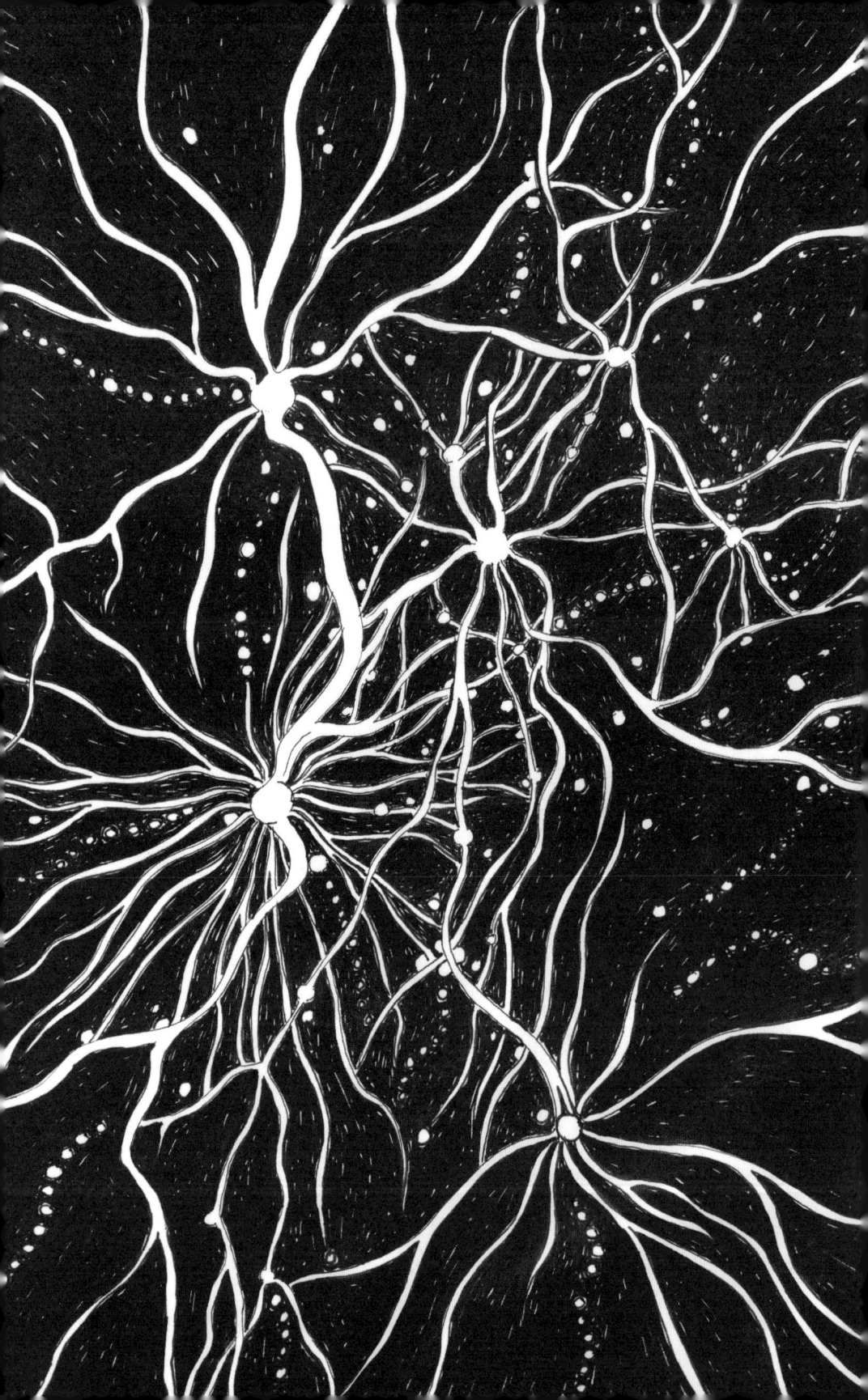

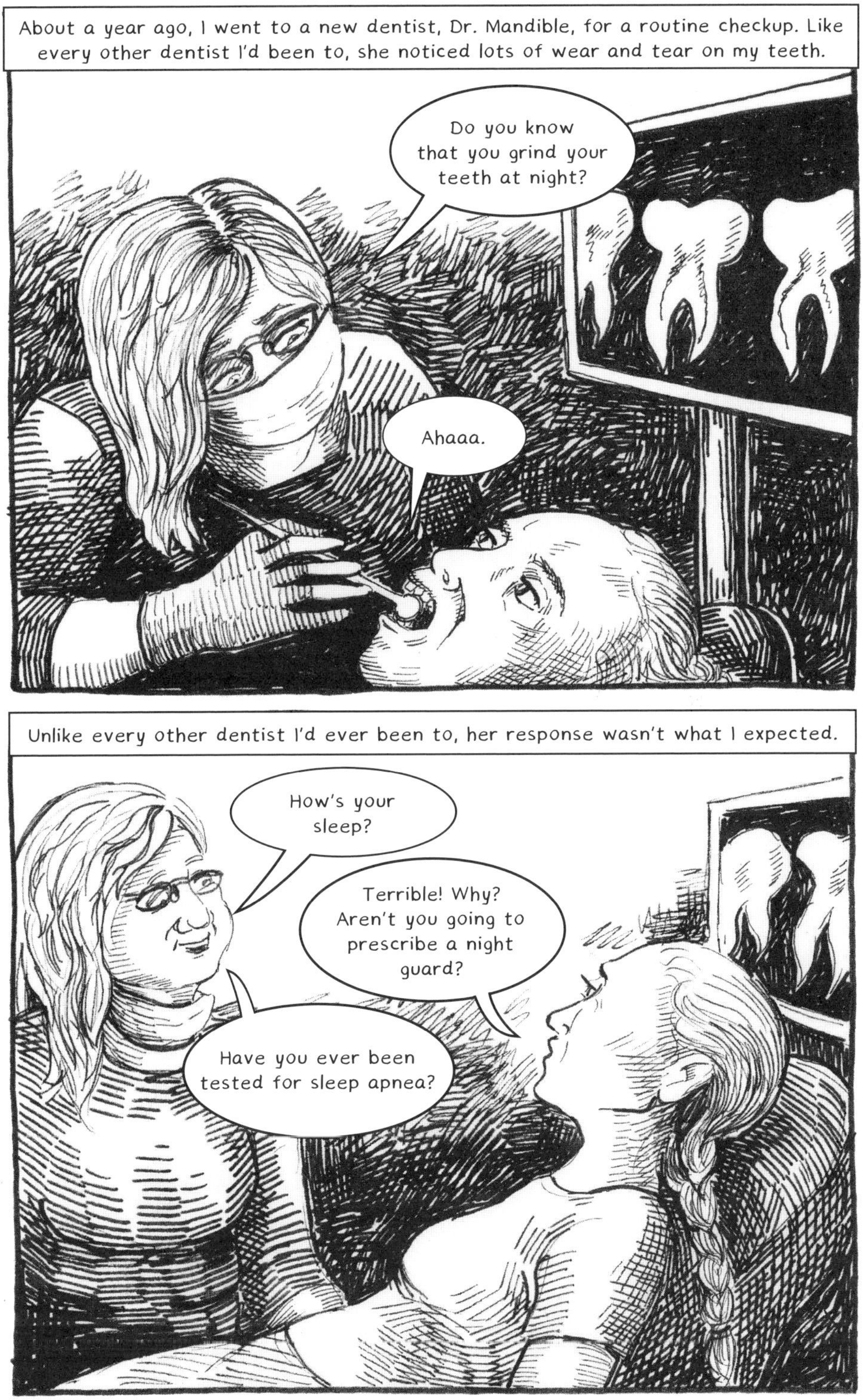
About a year ago, I went to a new dentist, Dr. Mandible, for a routine checkup. Like every other dentist I'd been to, she noticed lots of wear and tear on my teeth.
Do you know that you grind your teeth at night?
Ahaaa.
Unlike every other dentist I'd ever been to, her response wasn't what I expected.
How's your sleep?
Terrible! Why? Aren't you going to prescribe a night guard?
Have you ever been tested for sleep apnea?

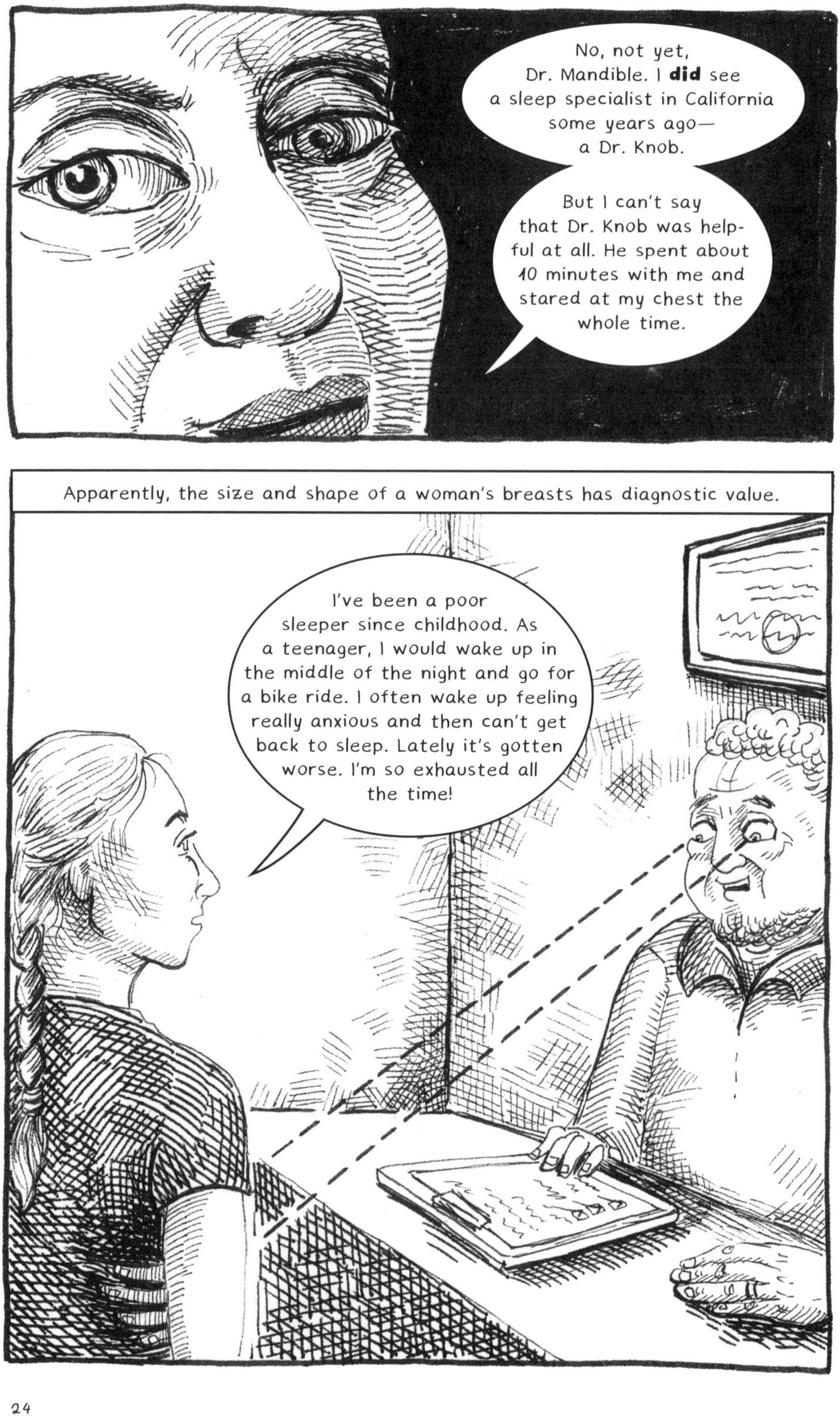
No, not yet, Dr. Mandible. I **did** see a sleep specialist in California some years ago— a Dr. Knob.
But I can't say that Dr. Knob was help-ful at all. He spent about 10 minutes with me and stared at my chest the whole time.
Apparently, the size and shape of a woman's breasts has diagnostic value.
I've been a poor sleeper since childhood. As a teenager, I would wake up in the middle of the night and go for a bike ride. I often wake up feeling really anxious and then can't get back to sleep. Lately it's gotten worse. I'm so exhausted all the time!

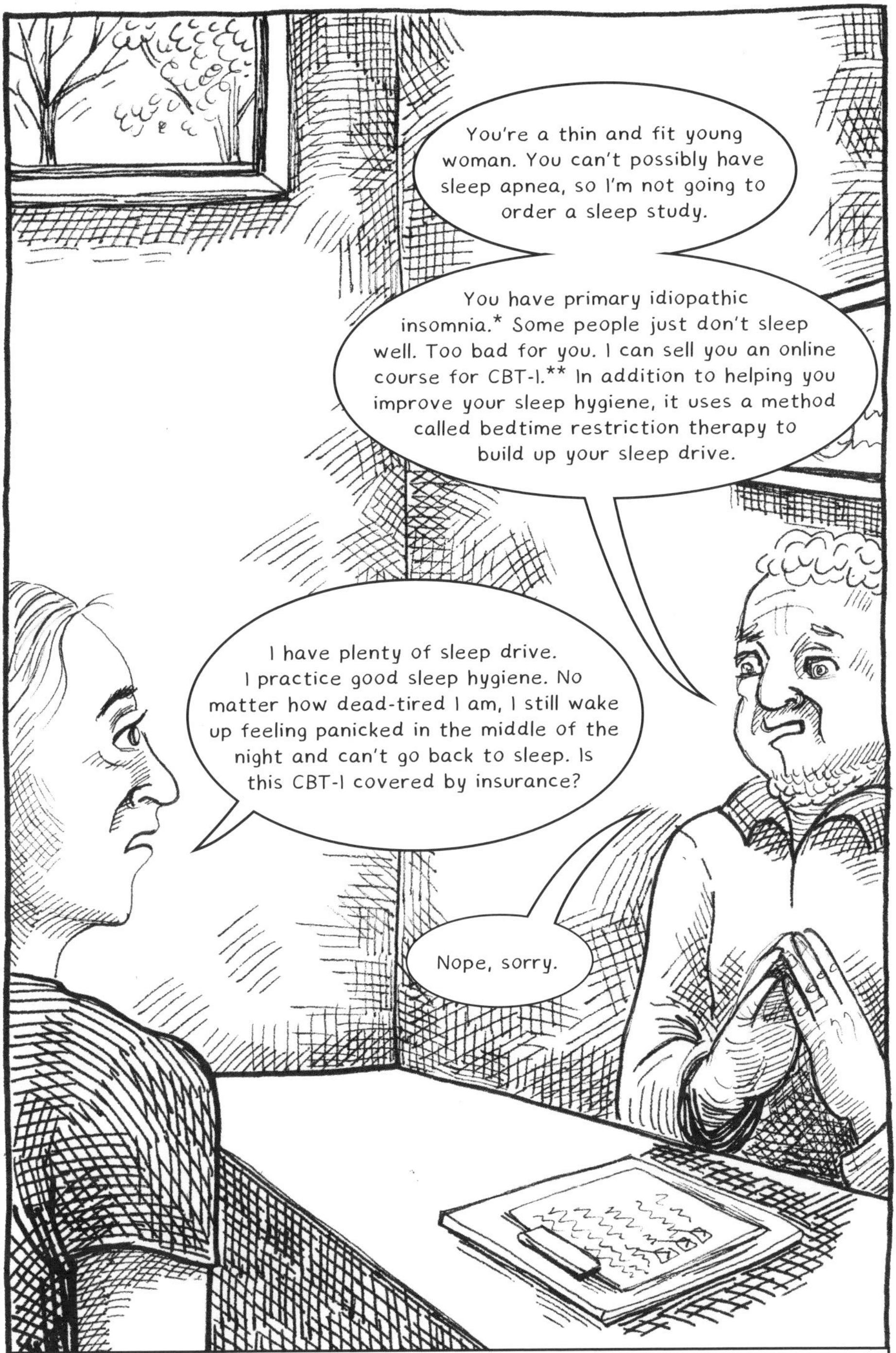
You're a thin and fit young woman. You can't possibly have sleep apnea, so I'm not going to order a sleep study.
You have primary idiopathic insomnia.* Some people just don't sleep well. Too bad for you. I can sell you an online course for CBT-I.** In addition to helping you improve your sleep hygiene, it uses a method called bedtime restriction therapy to build up your sleep drive.
I have plenty of sleep drive. I practice good sleep hygiene. No matter how dead-tired I am, I still wake up feeling panicked in the middle of the night and can't go back to sleep. Is this CBT-I covered by insurance?
Nope, sorry.

*Primary means there is no known underlying cause such as illness or chronic pain; idiopathic means the cause is unknown (too often because your doctor hasn't spent much time listening to you).

**CBT-I stands for cognitive behavioral therapy for insomnia. See Part III for more!

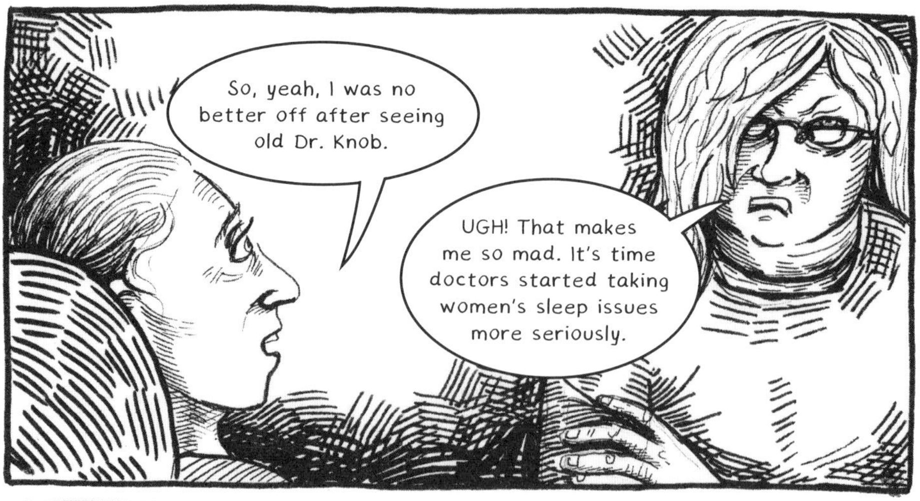
So, yeah, I was no better off after seeing old Dr. Knob.
UGH! That makes me so mad. It's time doctors started taking women's sleep issues more seriously.

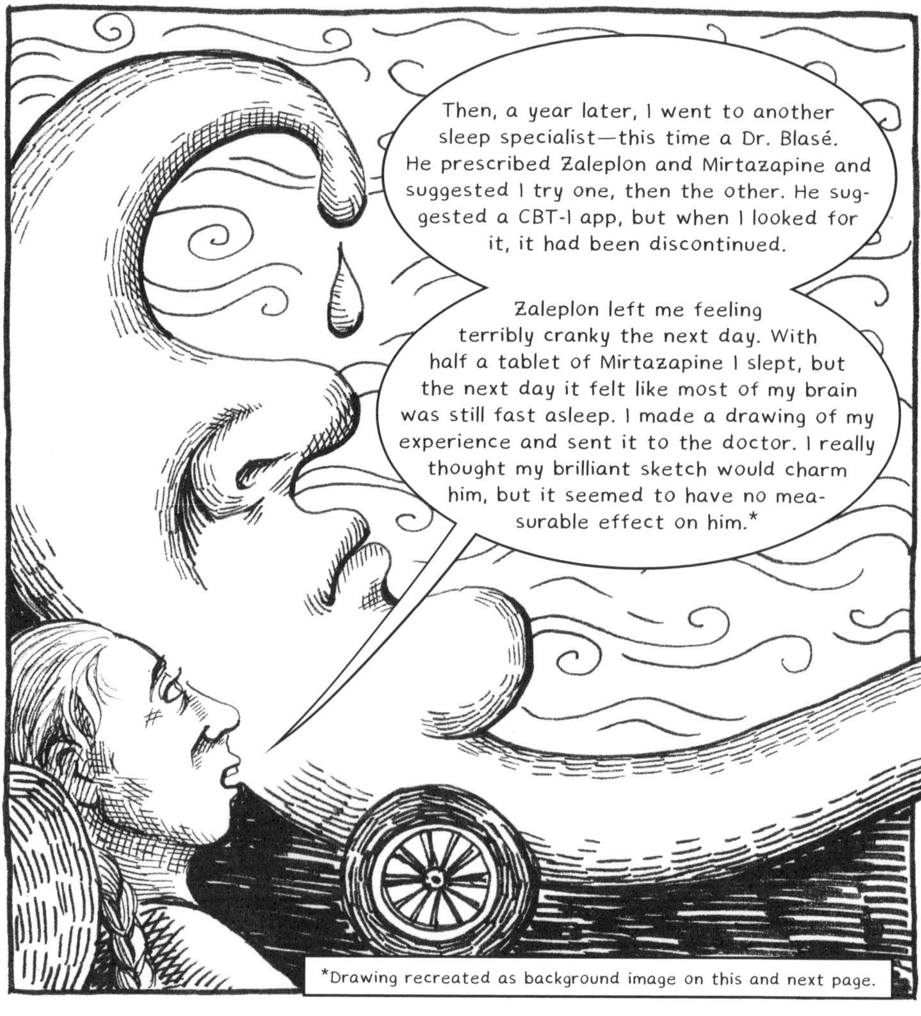
Then, a year later, I went to another sleep specialist—this time a Dr. Blasé. He prescribed Zaleplon and Mirtazapine and suggested I try one, then the other. He suggested a CBT-I app, but when I looked for it, it had been discontinued.
Zaleplon left me feeling terribly cranky the next day. With half a tablet of Mirtazapine I slept, but the next day it felt like most of my brain was still fast asleep. I made a drawing of my experience and sent it to the doctor. I really thought my brilliant sketch would charm him, but it seemed to have no measurable effect on him.*
*Drawing recreated as background image on this and next page.

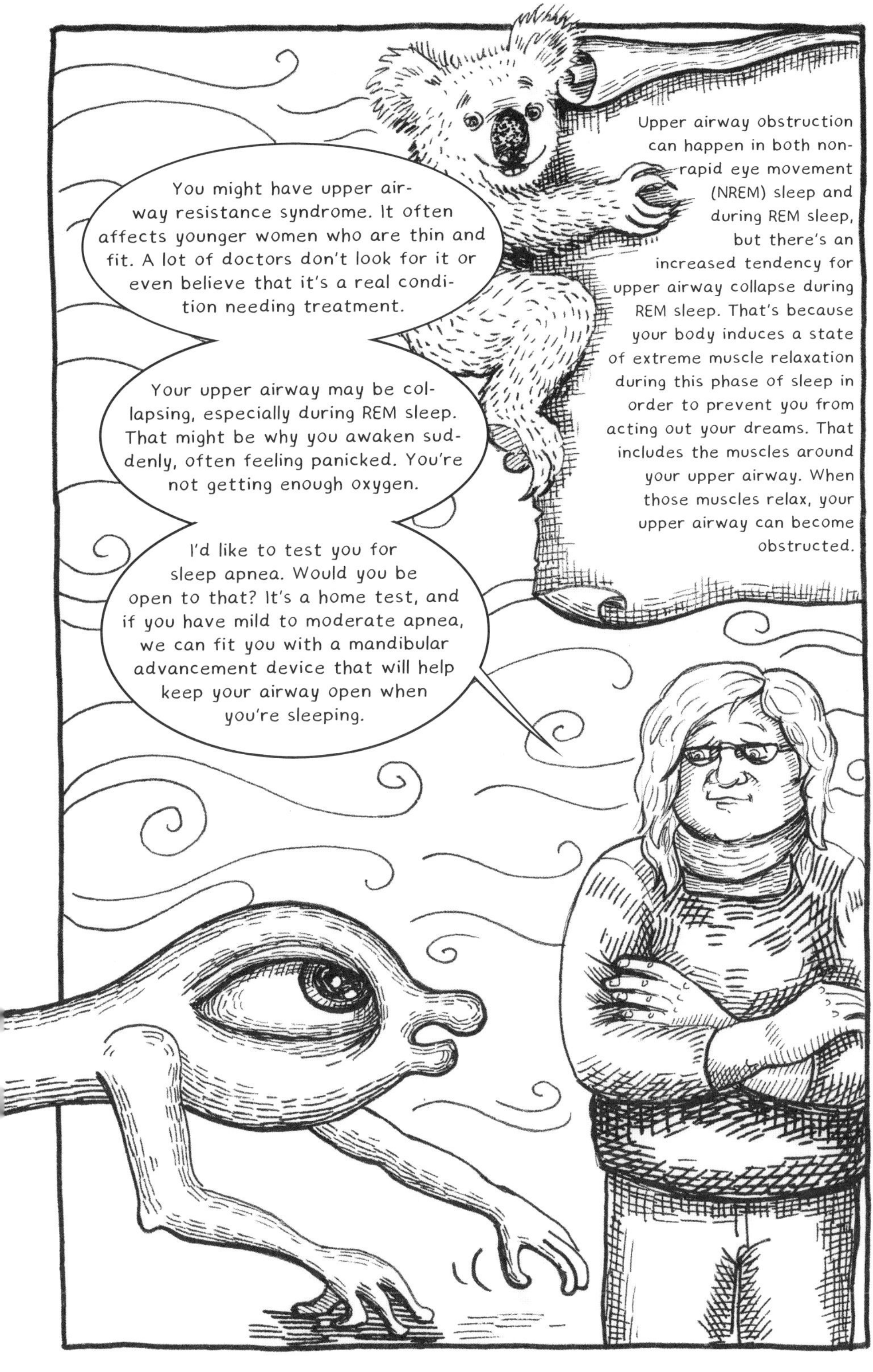
Upper airway obstruction can happen in both non-rapid eye movement (NREM) sleep and during REM sleep, but there's an increased tendency for upper airway collapse during REM sleep. That's because your body induces a state of extreme muscle relaxation during this phase of sleep in order to prevent you from acting out your dreams. That includes the muscles around your upper airway. When those muscles relax, your upper airway can become obstructed.
You might have upper airway resistance syndrome. It often affects younger women who are thin and fit. A lot of doctors don't look for it or even believe that it's a real condition needing treatment.
Your upper airway may be collapsing, especially during REM sleep. That might be why you awaken suddenly, often feeling panicked. You're not getting enough oxygen.
I'd like to test you for sleep apnea. Would you be open to that? It's a home test, and if you have mild to moderate apnea, we can fit you with a mandibular advancement device that will help keep your airway open when you're sleeping.

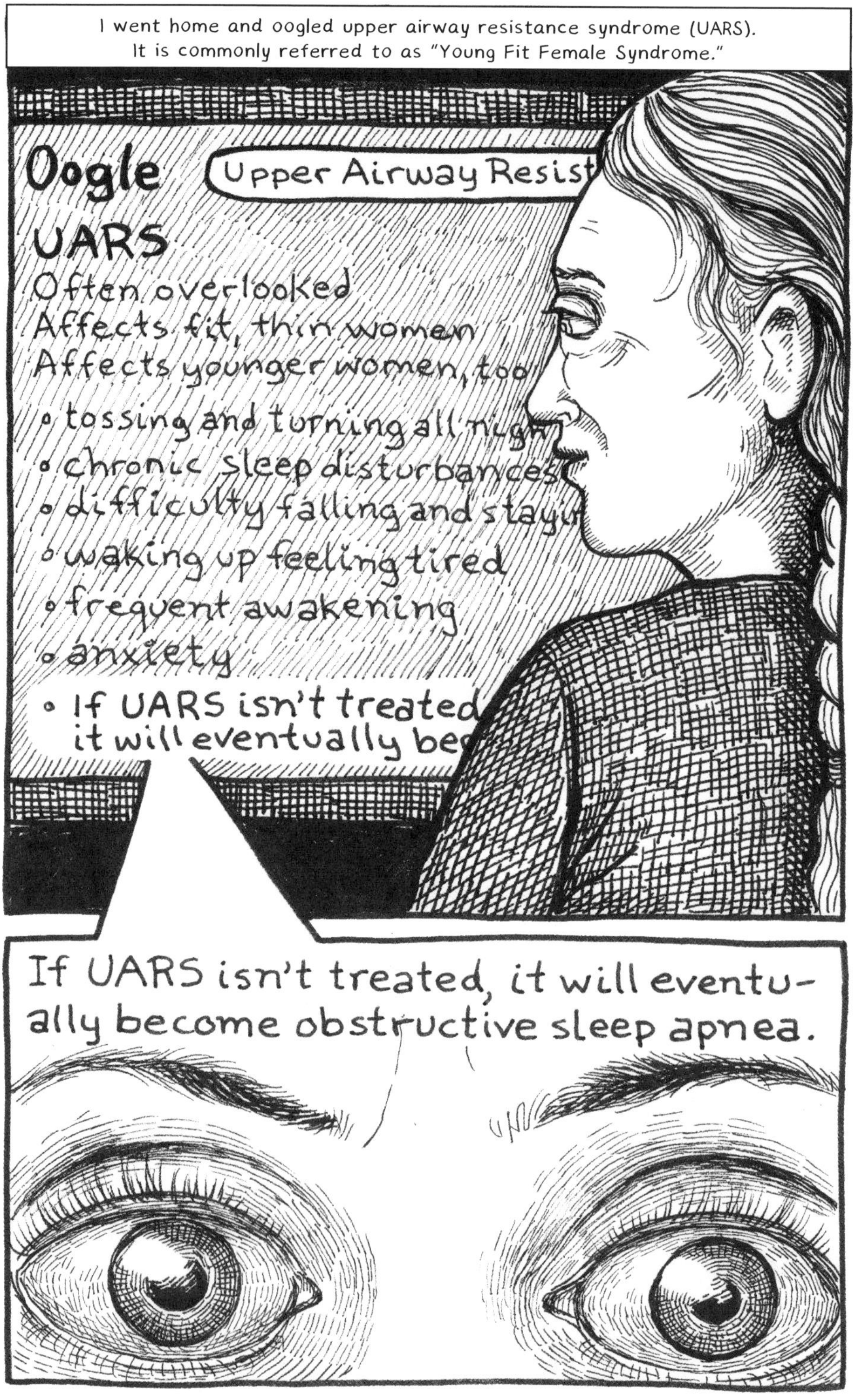
I went home and oogled upper airway resistance syndrome (UARS).
It is commonly referred to as "Young Fit Female Syndrome."
Oogle
Upper Airway Resist
UARS
Often overlooked
Affects fit, thin women
Affects younger women, too
• tossing and turning all nigh
• chronic sleep disturbances
• difficulty falling and stayi
• waking up feeling tired
• frequent awakening
• anxiety
• If UARS isn't treated
it will eventually be
If UARS isn't treated, it will eventu-ally become obstructive sleep apnea.

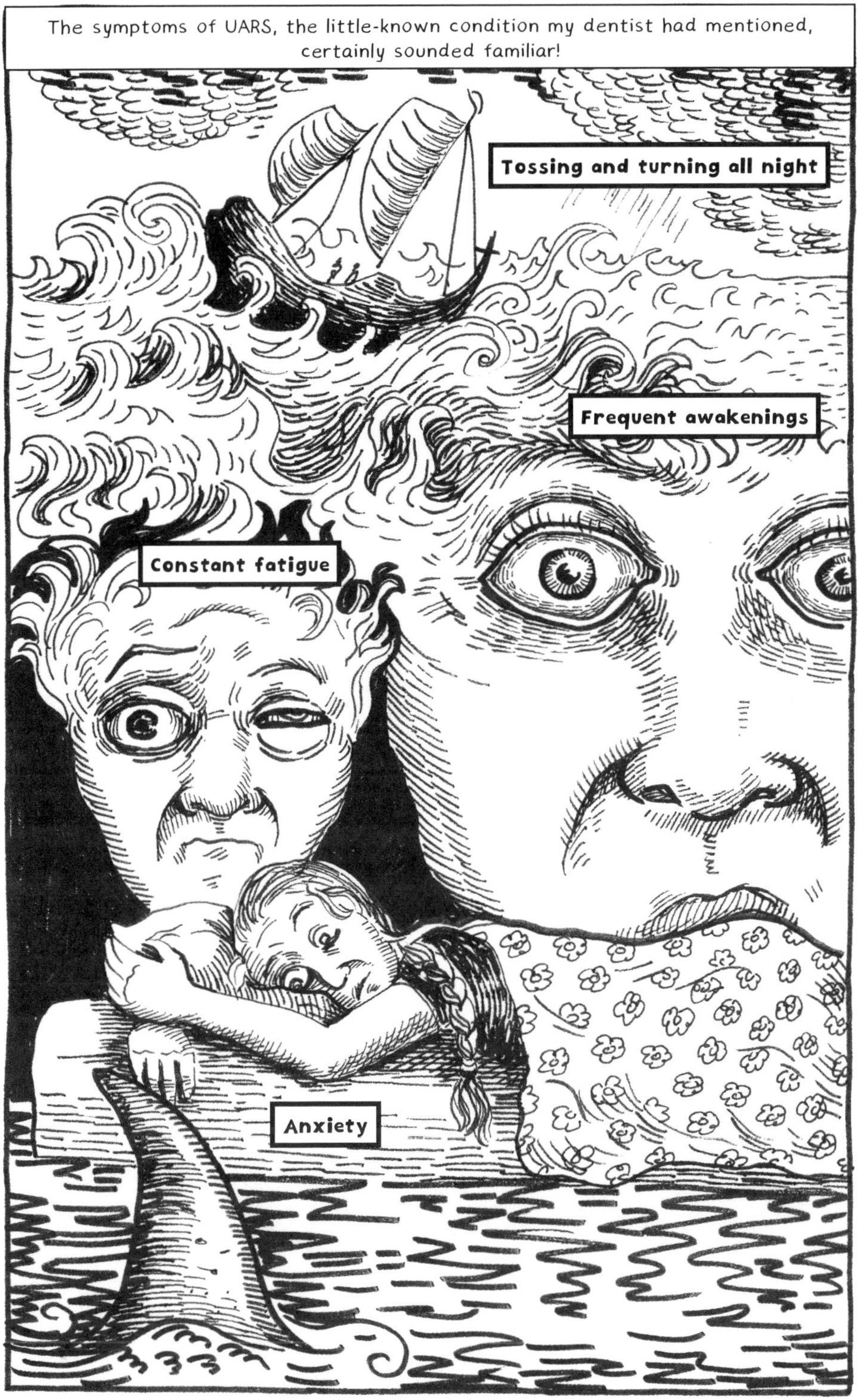
The symptoms of UARS, the little-known condition my dentist had mentioned, certainly sounded familiar!
Tossing and turning all night
Frequent awakenings
Constant fatigue
Anxiety

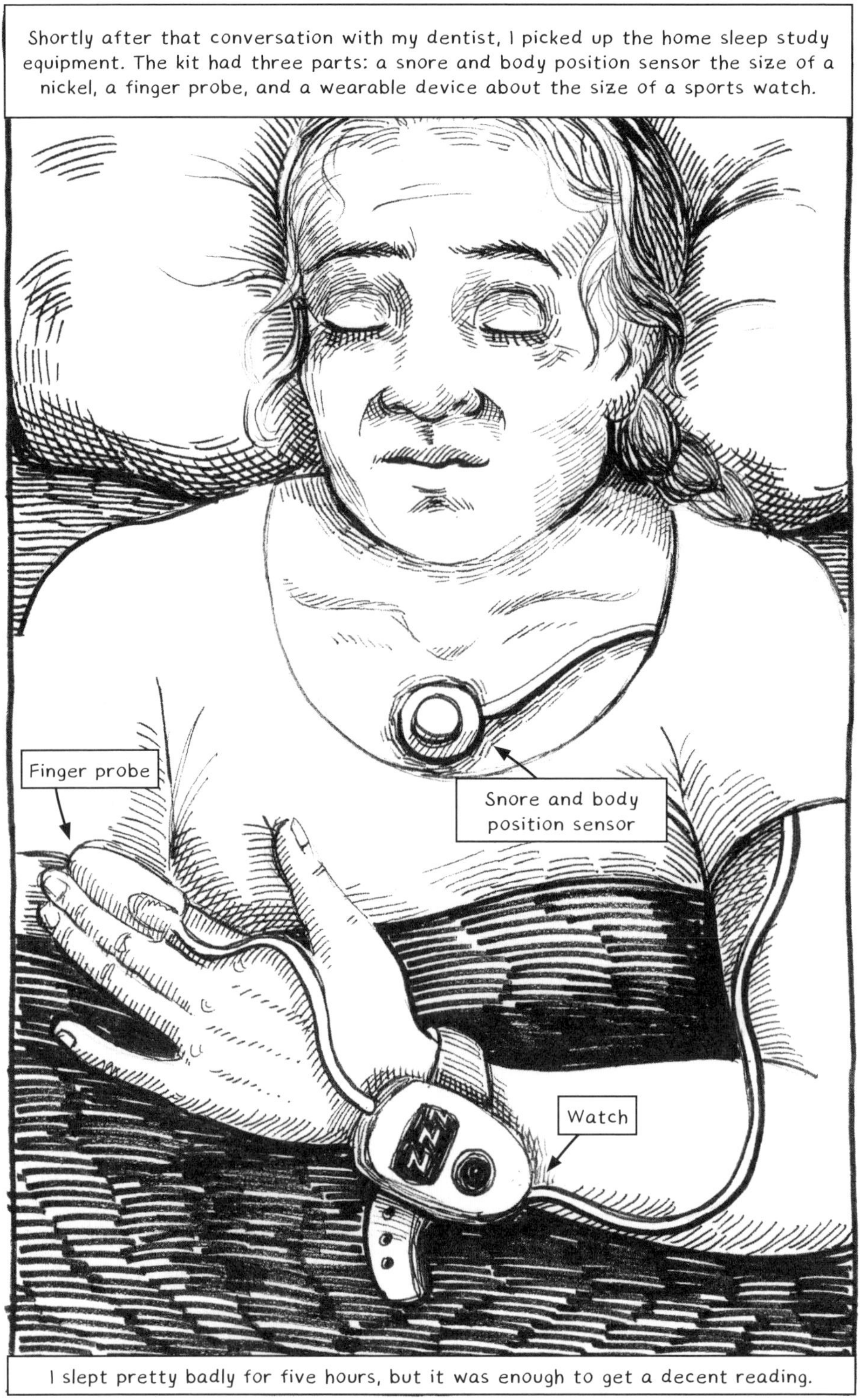
Shortly after that conversation with my dentist, I picked up the home sleep study equipment. The kit had three parts: a snore and body position sensor the size of a nickel, a finger probe, and a wearable device about the size of a sports watch.
Finger probe
Snore and body position sensor
Watch
I slept pretty badly for five hours, but it was enough to get a decent reading.

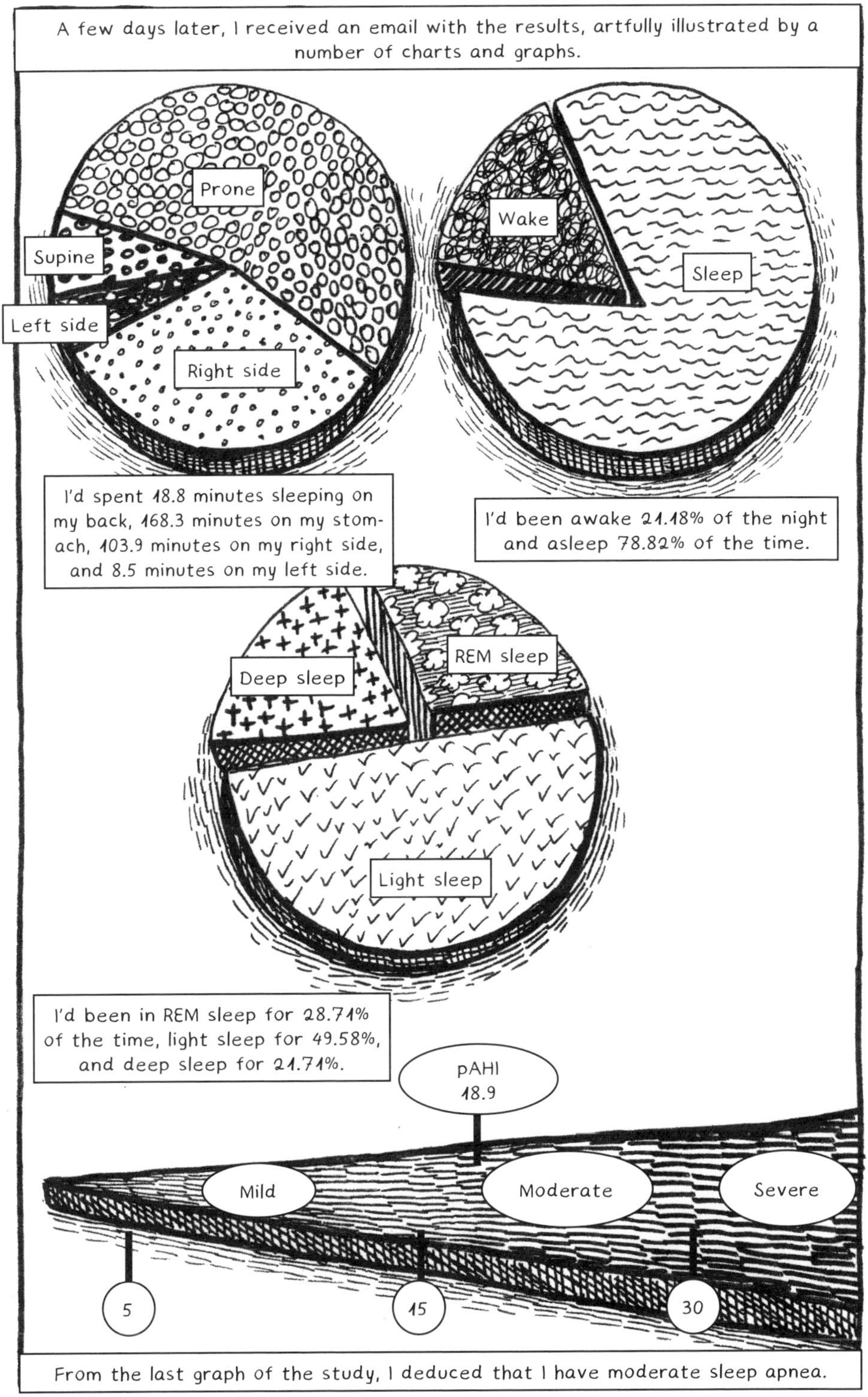
A few days later, I received an email with the results, artfully illustrated by a number of charts and graphs.
Prone
Supine
Left side
Right side
Wake
Sleep
I'd spent 18.8 minutes sleeping on my back, 168.3 minutes on my stomach, 103.9 minutes on my right side, and 8.5 minutes on my left side.
I'd been awake 21.18% of the night and asleep 78.82% of the time.
Deep sleep
REM sleep
Light sleep
I'd been in REM sleep for 28.71% of the time, light sleep for 49.58%, and deep sleep for 21.71%.
pAHI
18.9
Mild
Moderate
Severe
5
15
30
From the last graph of the study, I deduced that I have moderate sleep apnea.

According to the study results, I had a pAHI score of 18.9. But what did this mean? When I oogled pAHI, I was presented with two possible definitions:

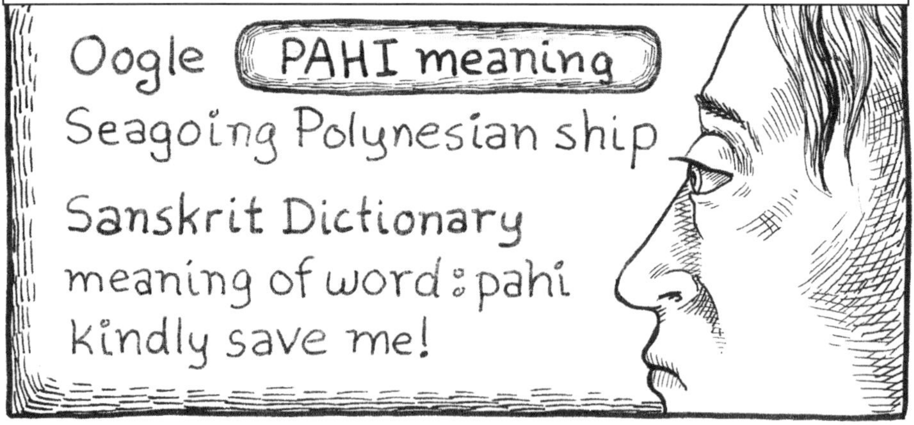
Oogle
PAHI meaning
Seagoing Polynesian ship
Sanskrit Dictionary meaning of word: pahi
Kindly save me!

In combination, these two definitions seemed to summarize my problem really well.

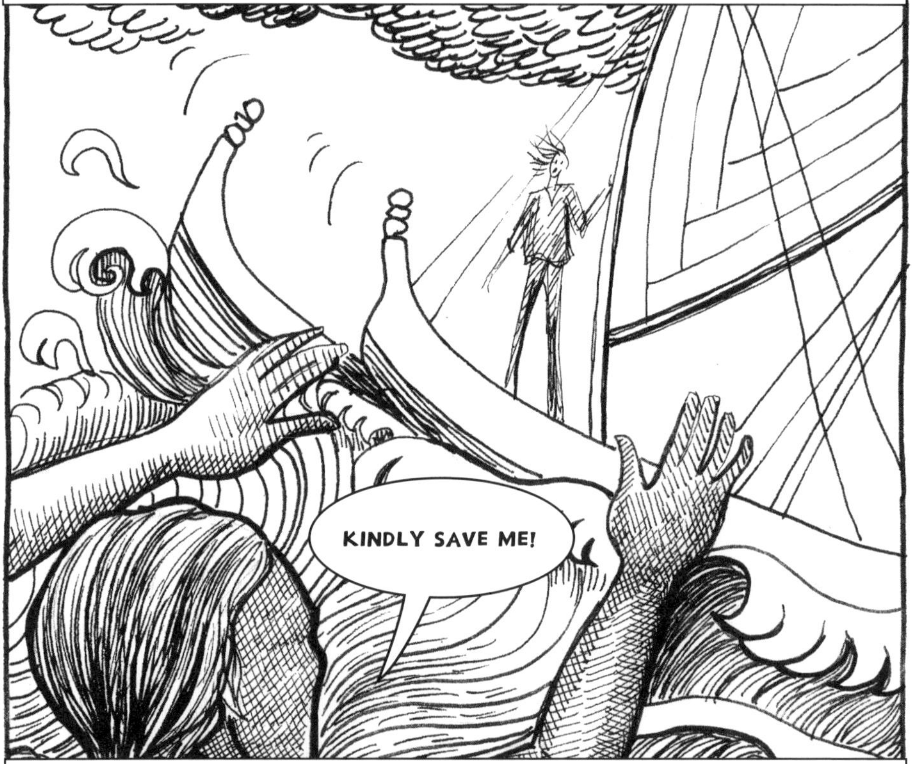
KINDLY SAVE ME!

Eventually I figured out that in the context of a sleep study, pAHI stands for "peripheral arterial tone apnea hypopnea index." Not nearly as colorful as ships and distress cries. AHI is the number of times you have apnea (cessation of breathing) or hypopnea (significant drop in airflow) during one night, divided by the hours of sleep. My number on that graph meant I was having about 19 episodes per hour of sleep. So in a sense, I **was** drowning.

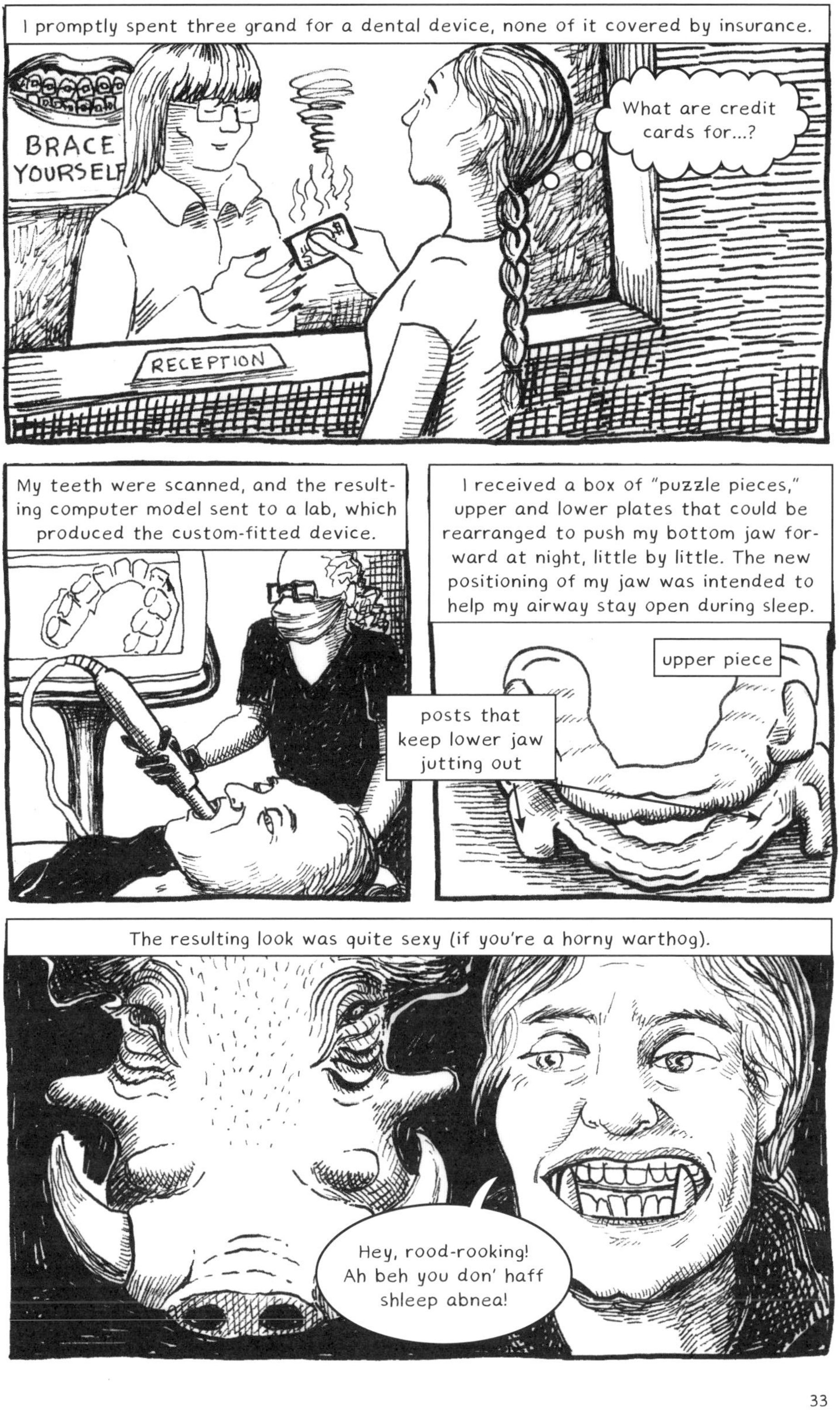
I promptly spent three grand for a dental device, none of it covered by insurance.
BRACE YOURSELF
What are credit cards for...?
RECEPTION
My teeth were scanned, and the resulting computer model sent to a lab, which produced the custom-fitted device.
I received a box of "puzzle pieces," upper and lower plates that could be rearranged to push my bottom jaw forward at night, little by little. The new positioning of my jaw was intended to help my airway stay open during sleep.
upper piece
posts that keep lower jaw jutting out
The resulting look was quite sexy (if you're a horny warthog).
Hey, rood-rooking!
Ah beh you don' haff shleep abnea!

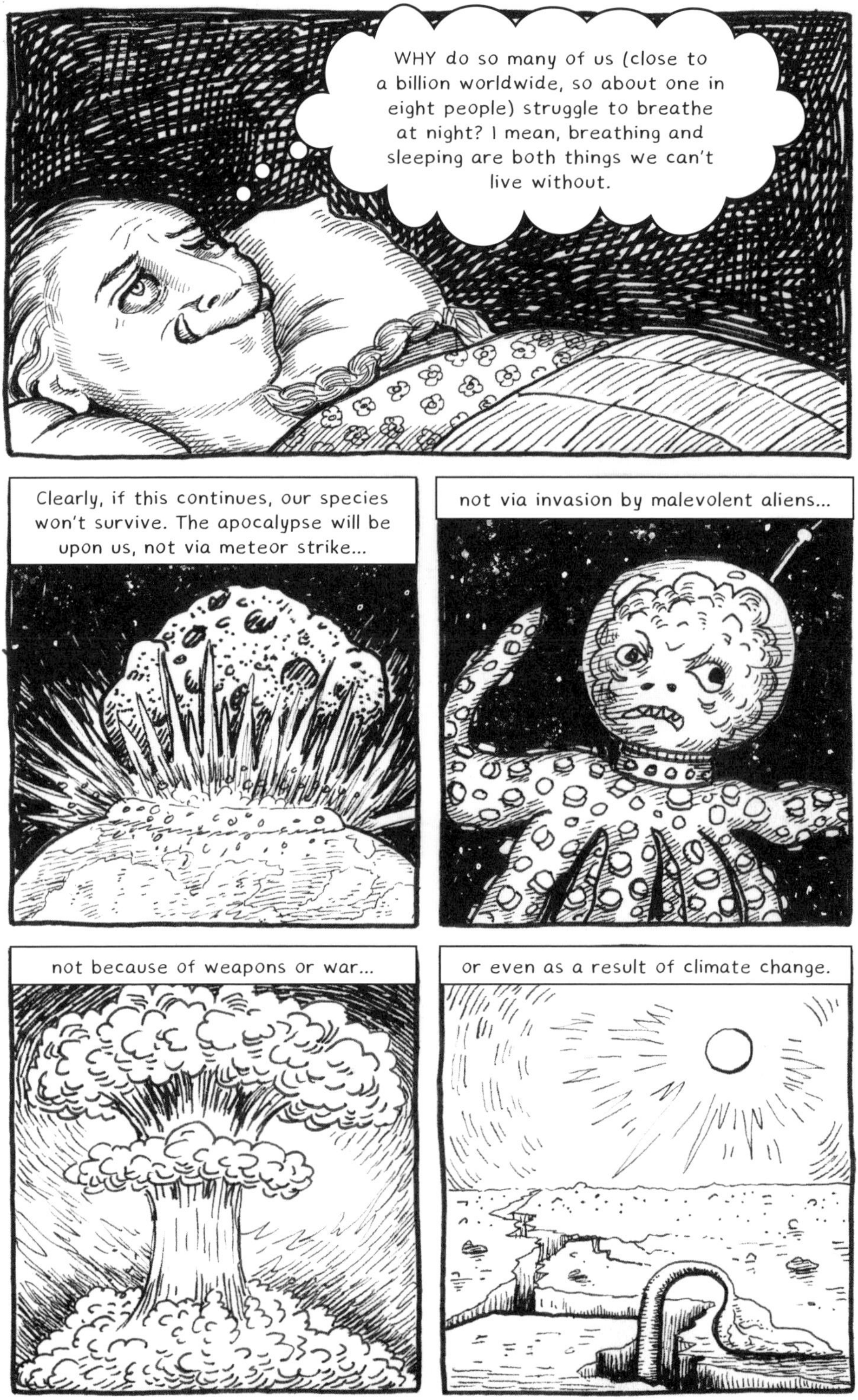
WHY do so many of us (close to a billion worldwide, so about one in eight people) struggle to breathe at night? I mean, breathing and sleeping are both things we can't live without.
Clearly, if this continues, our species won't survive. The apocalypse will be upon us, not via meteor strike...
not via invasion by malevolent aliens...
not because of weapons or war...
or even as a result of climate change.

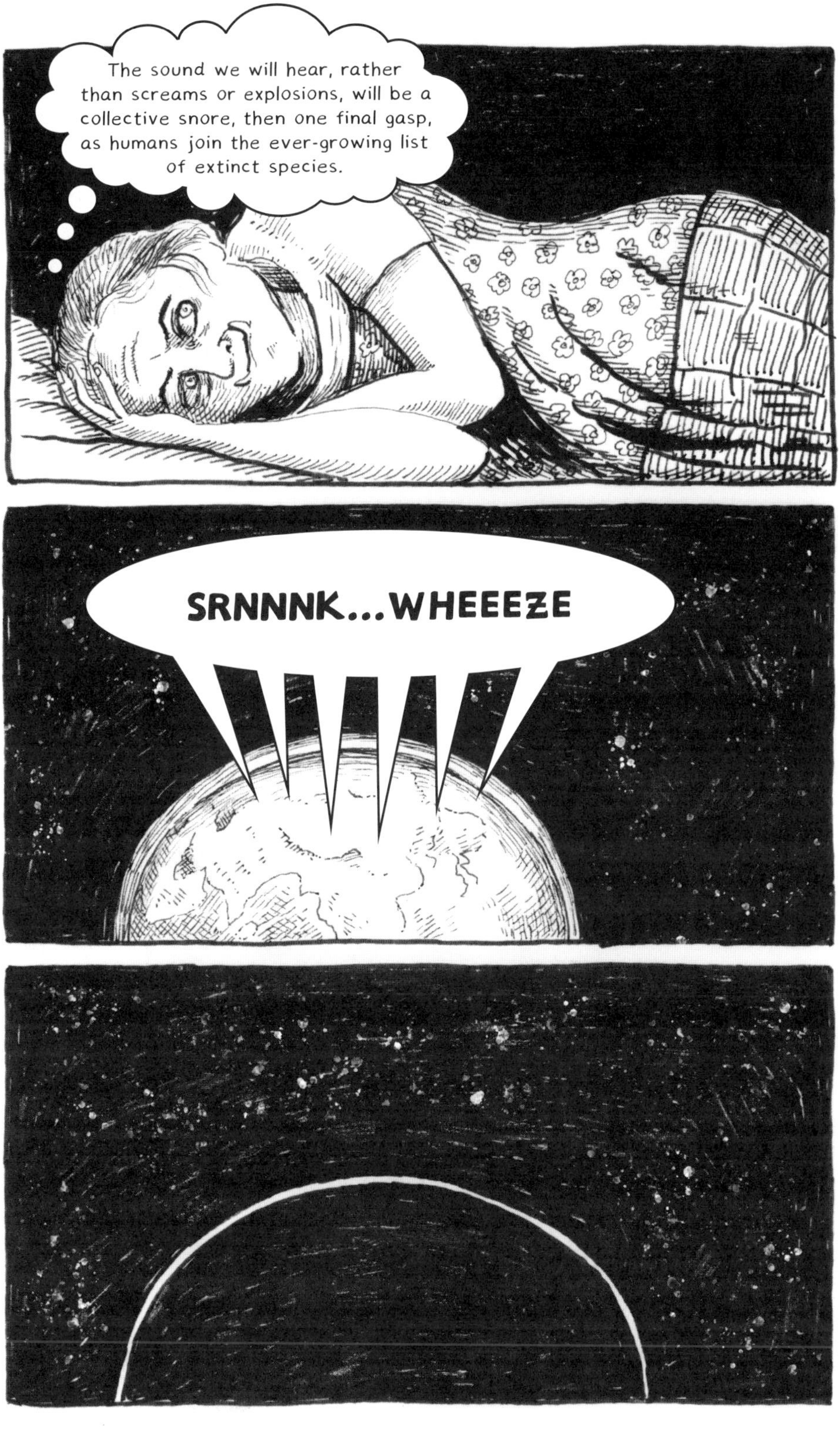
The sound we will hear, rather than screams or explosions, will be a collective snore, then one final gasp, as humans join the ever-growing list of extinct species.
SRNNNK...WHEEEZE

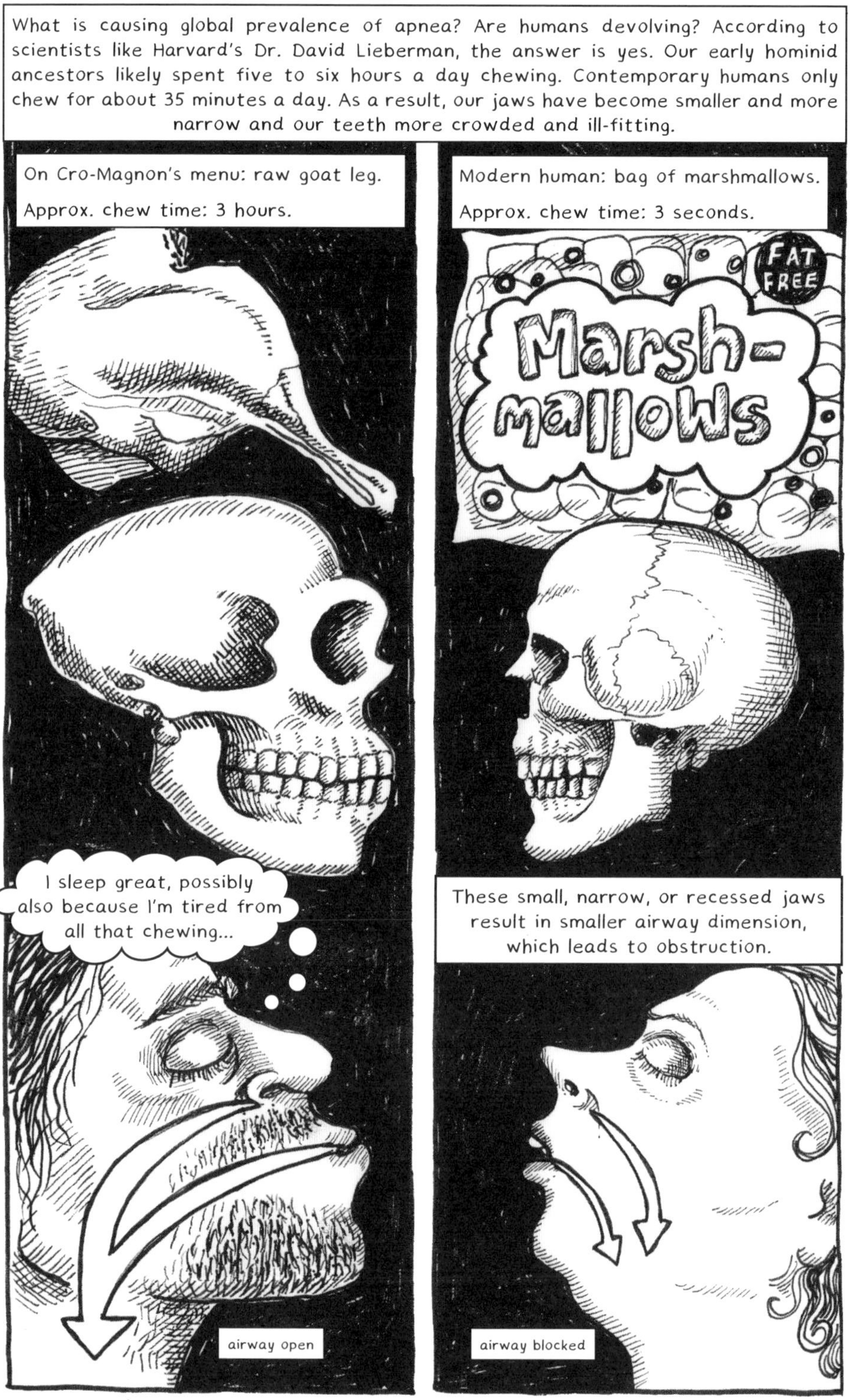
What is causing global prevalence of apnea? Are humans devolving? According to scientists like Harvard's Dr. David Lieberman, the answer is yes. Our early hominid ancestors likely spent five to six hours a day chewing. Contemporary humans only chew for about 35 minutes a day. As a result, our jaws have become smaller and more narrow and our teeth more crowded and ill-fitting.
On Cro-Magnon's menu: raw goat leg.
Approx. chew time: 3 hours.
Modern human: bag of marshmallows.
Approx. chew time: 3 seconds.
FAT FREE
Marsh-mallows
I sleep great, possibly also because I'm tired from all that chewing...
airway open
These small, narrow, or recessed jaws result in smaller airway dimension, which leads to obstruction.
airway blocked

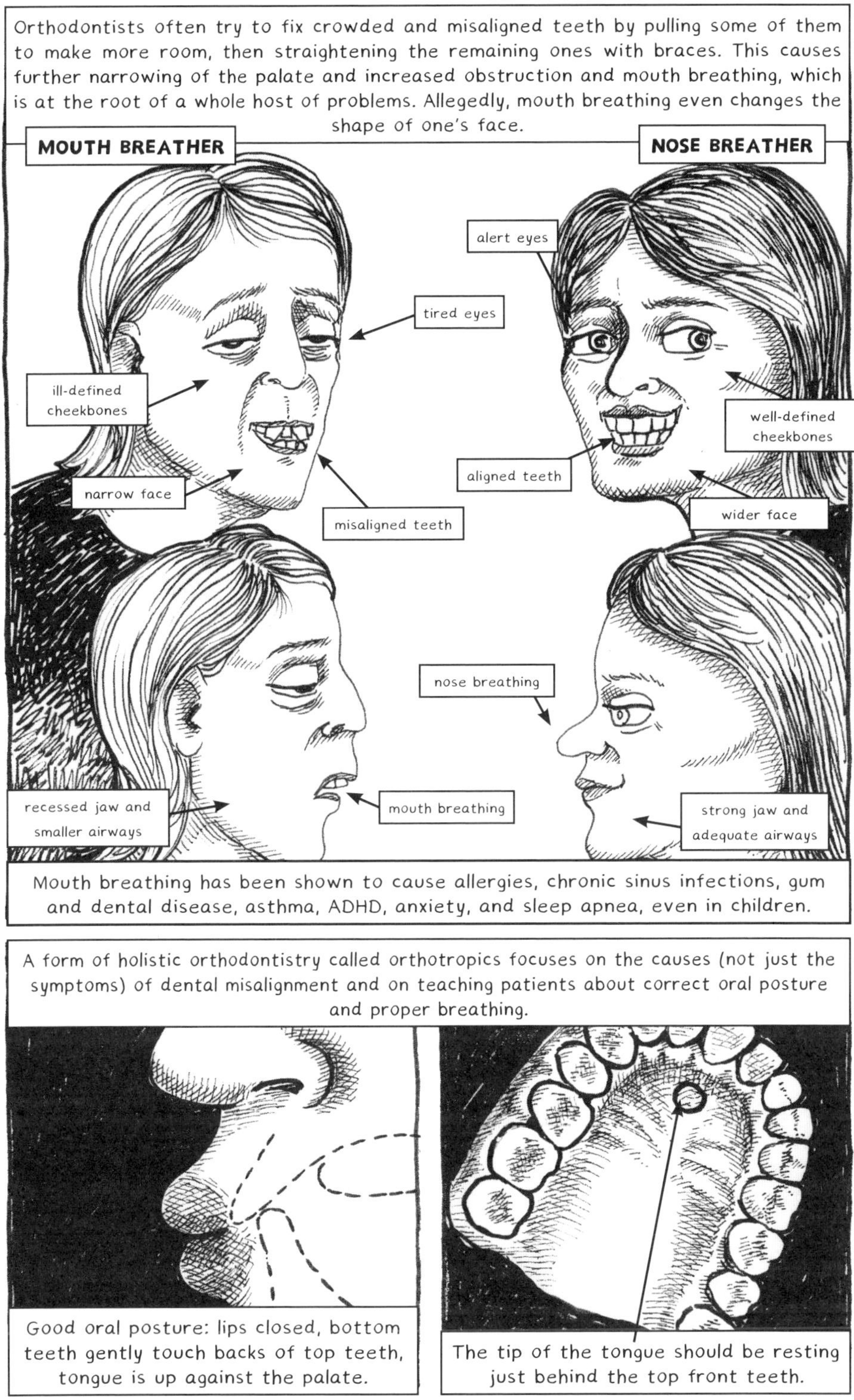

Orthodontists often try to fix crowded and misaligned teeth by pulling some of them to make more room, then straightening the remaining ones with braces. This causes further narrowing of the palate and increased obstruction and mouth breathing, which is at the root of a whole host of problems. Allegedly, mouth breathing even changes the shape of one's face.

MOUTH BREATHER / **NOSE BREATHER**

- alert eyes
- tired eyes
- ill-defined cheekbones
- well-defined cheekbones
- narrow face
- aligned teeth
- misaligned teeth
- wider face
- nose breathing
- recessed jaw and smaller airways
- mouth breathing
- strong jaw and adequate airways

Mouth breathing has been shown to cause allergies, chronic sinus infections, gum and dental disease, asthma, ADHD, anxiety, and sleep apnea, even in children.

A form of holistic orthodontistry called orthotropics focuses on the causes (not just the symptoms) of dental misalignment and on teaching patients about correct oral posture and proper breathing.

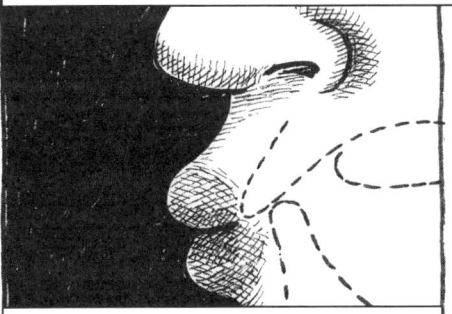

Good oral posture: lips closed, bottom teeth gently touch backs of top teeth, tongue is up against the palate.

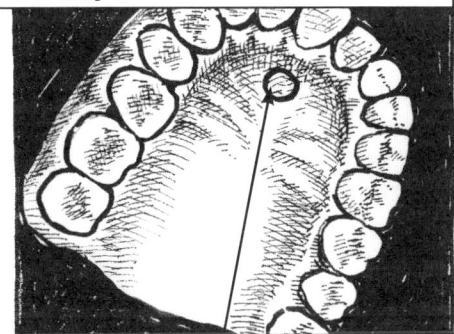

The tip of the tongue should be resting just behind the top front teeth.

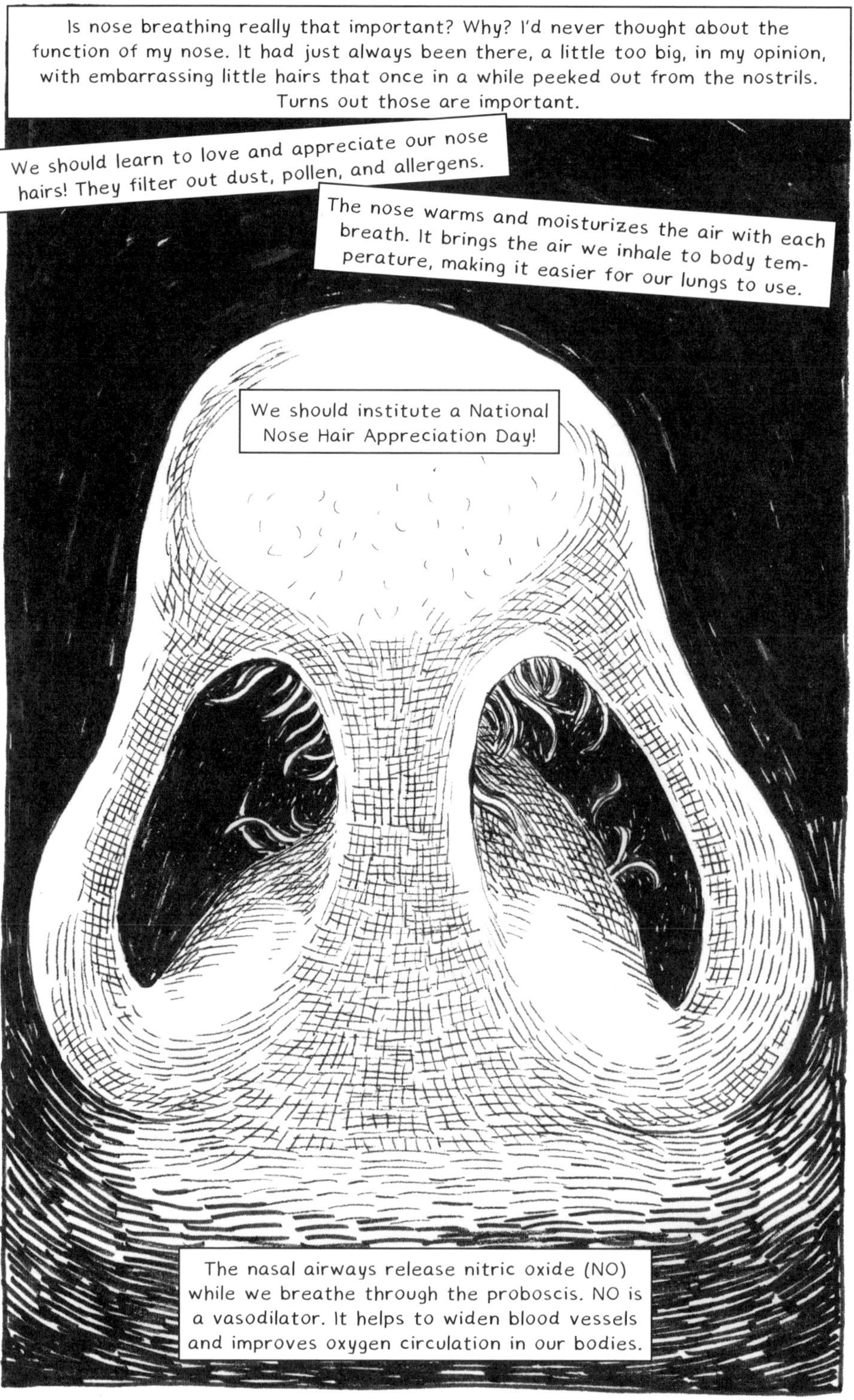
Is nose breathing really that important? Why? I'd never thought about the function of my nose. It had just always been there, a little too big, in my opinion, with embarrassing little hairs that once in a while peeked out from the nostrils. Turns out those are important.
We should learn to love and appreciate our nose hairs! They filter out dust, pollen, and allergens.
The nose warms and moisturizes the air with each breath. It brings the air we inhale to body temperature, making it easier for our lungs to use.
We should institute a National Nose Hair Appreciation Day!
The nasal airways release nitric oxide (NO) while we breathe through the proboscis. NO is a vasodilator. It helps to widen blood vessels and improves oxygen circulation in our bodies.

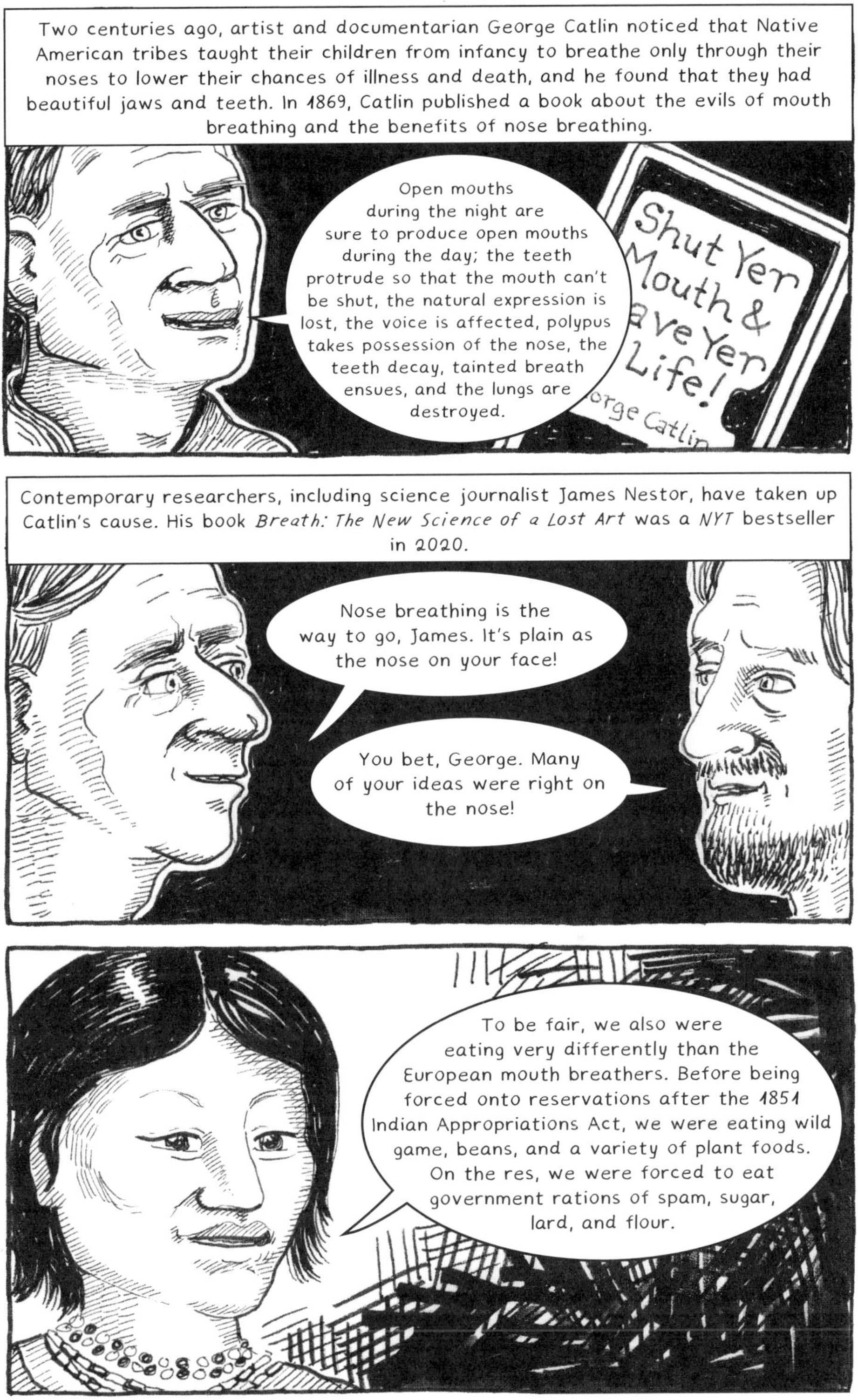
Two centuries ago, artist and documentarian George Catlin noticed that Native American tribes taught their children from infancy to breathe only through their noses to lower their chances of illness and death, and he found that they had beautiful jaws and teeth. In 1869, Catlin published a book about the evils of mouth breathing and the benefits of nose breathing.
Open mouths during the night are sure to produce open mouths during the day; the teeth protrude so that the mouth can't be shut, the natural expression is lost, the voice is affected, polypus takes possession of the nose, the teeth decay, tainted breath ensues, and the lungs are destroyed.
Shut Yer Mouth & ave Yer Life!
orge Catlin
Contemporary researchers, including science journalist James Nestor, have taken up Catlin's cause. His book *Breath: The New Science of a Lost Art* was a *NYT* bestseller in 2020.
Nose breathing is the way to go, James. It's plain as the nose on your face!
You bet, George. Many of your ideas were right on the nose!
To be fair, we also were eating very differently than the European mouth breathers. Before being forced onto reservations after the 1851 Indian Appropriations Act, we were eating wild game, beans, and a variety of plant foods. On the res, we were forced to eat government rations of spam, sugar, lard, and flour.

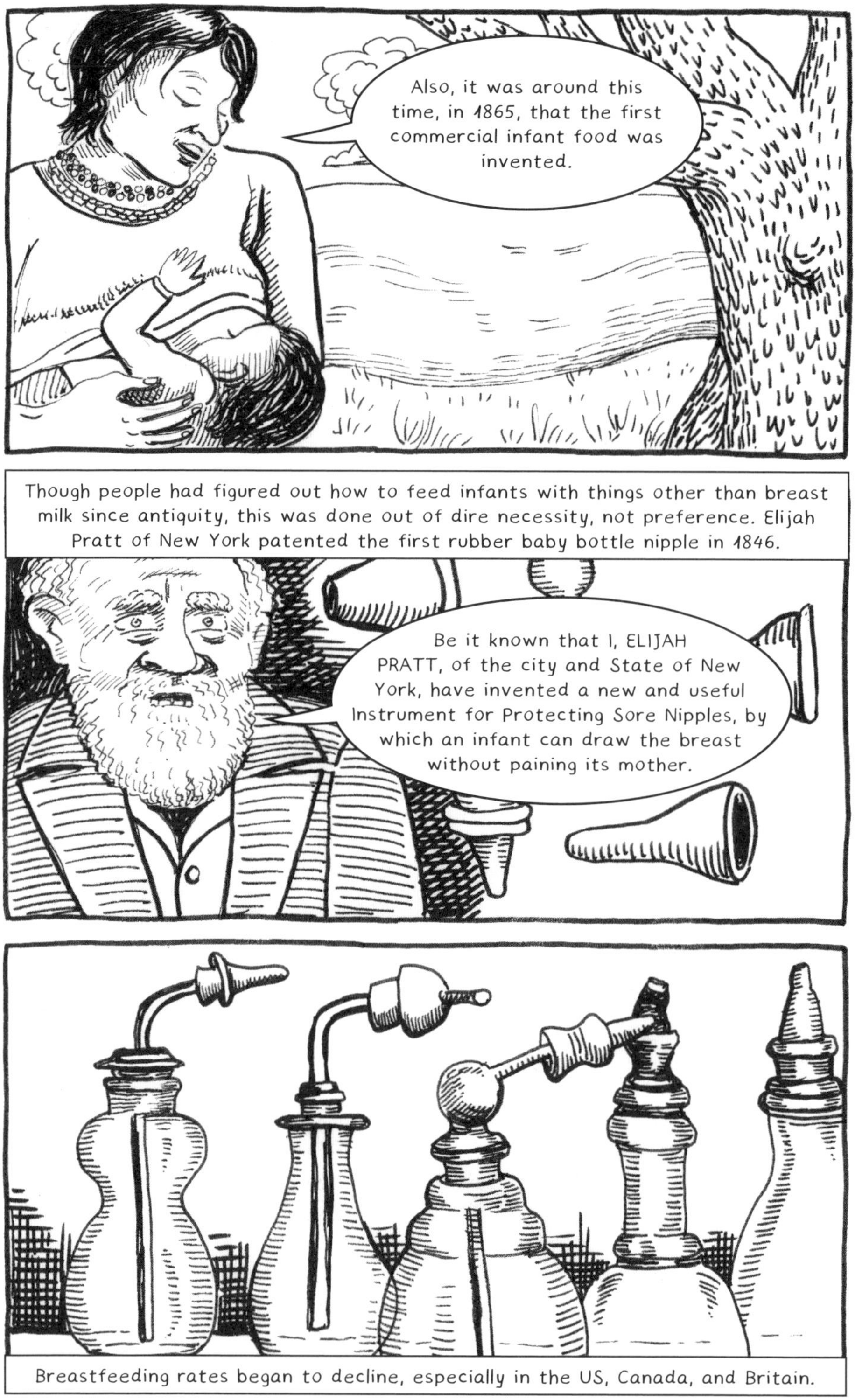
Also, it was around this time, in 1865, that the first commercial infant food was invented.
Though people had figured out how to feed infants with things other than breast milk since antiquity, this was done out of dire necessity, not preference. Elijah Pratt of New York patented the first rubber baby bottle nipple in 1846.
Be it known that I, ELIJAH PRATT, of the city and State of New York, have invented a new and useful Instrument for Protecting Sore Nipples, by which an infant can draw the breast without paining its mother.
Breastfeeding rates began to decline, especially in the US, Canada, and Britain.

Queen Victoria, after whom the Victorian Era is named, was quite an influencer, and she didn't think much of breastfeeding.

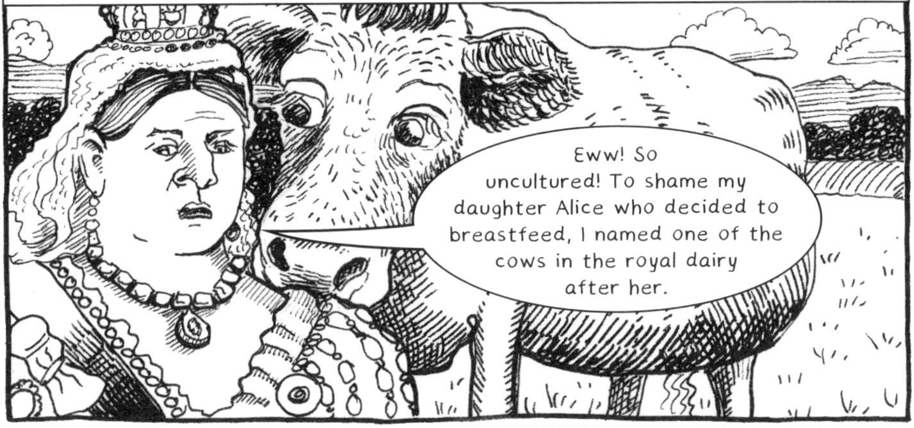

Eww! So uncultured! To shame my daughter Alice who decided to breastfeed, I named one of the cows in the royal dairy after her.

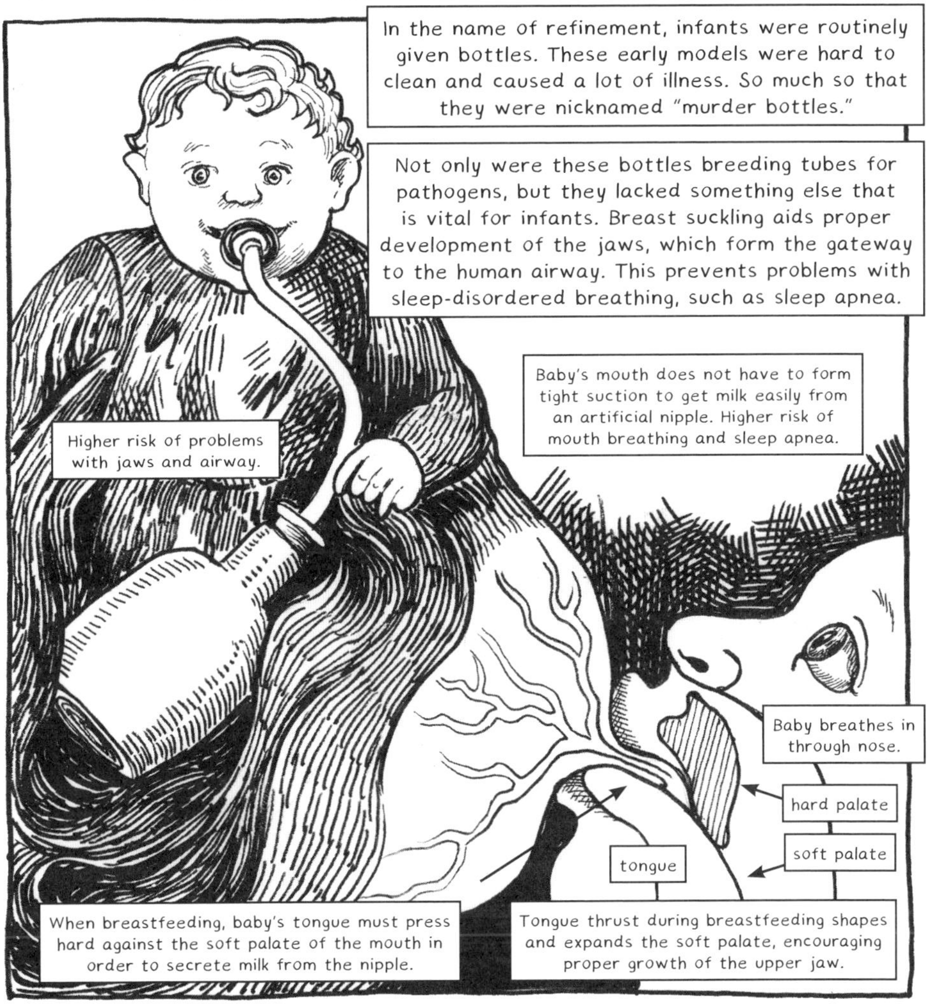

In the name of refinement, infants were routinely given bottles. These early models were hard to clean and caused a lot of illness. So much so that they were nicknamed "murder bottles."
Not only were these bottles breeding tubes for pathogens, but they lacked something else that is vital for infants. Breast suckling aids proper development of the jaws, which form the gateway to the human airway. This prevents problems with sleep-disordered breathing, such as sleep apnea.
Baby's mouth does not have to form tight suction to get milk easily from an artificial nipple. Higher risk of mouth breathing and sleep apnea.
Higher risk of problems with jaws and airway.
Baby breathes in through nose.
hard palate
soft palate
tongue
When breastfeeding, baby's tongue must press hard against the soft palate of the mouth in order to secrete milk from the nipple.
Tongue thrust during breastfeeding shapes and expands the soft palate, encouraging proper growth of the upper jaw.

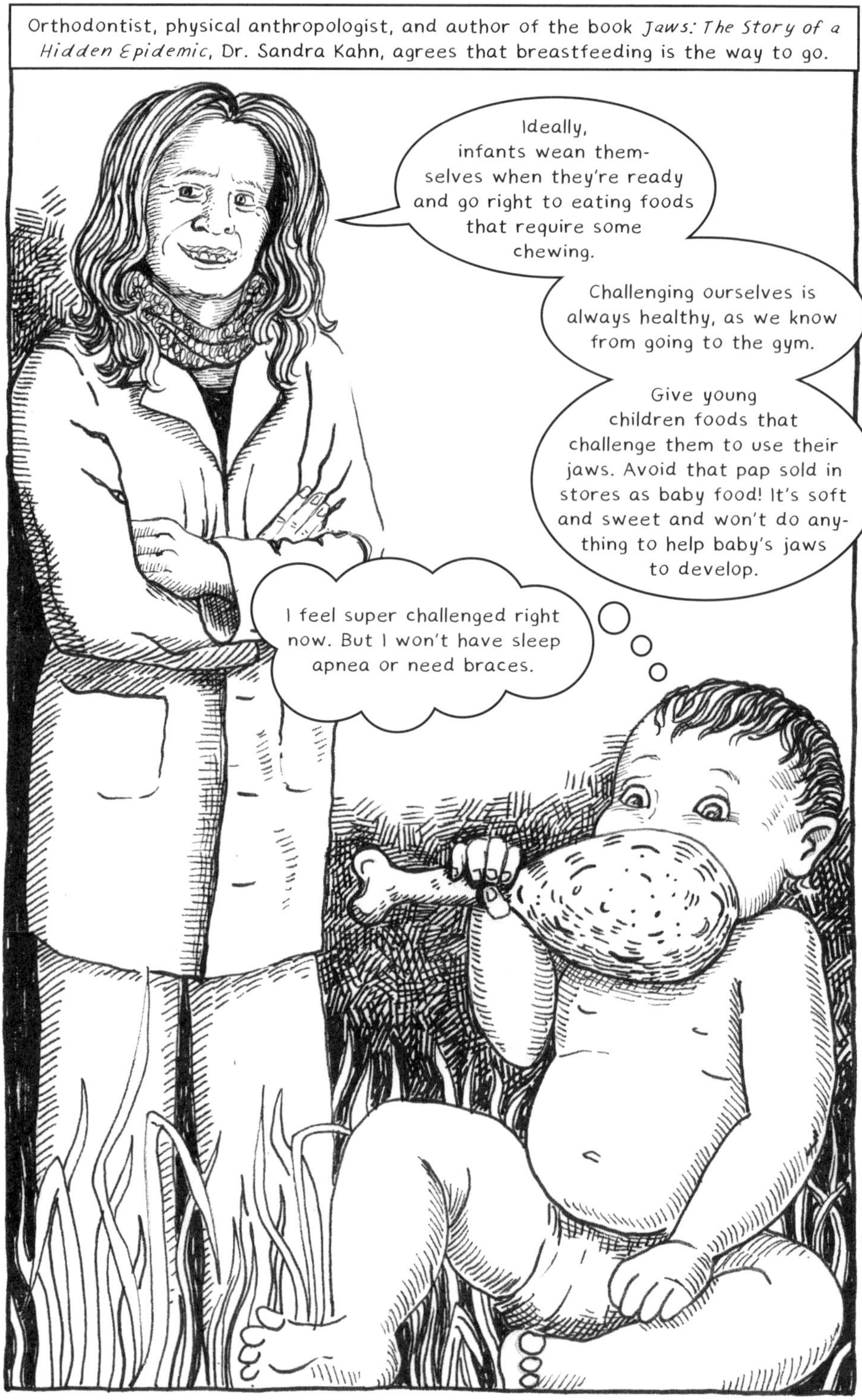
Orthodontist, physical anthropologist, and author of the book *Jaws: The Story of a Hidden Epidemic*, Dr. Sandra Kahn, agrees that breastfeeding is the way to go.
Ideally, infants wean themselves when they're ready and go right to eating foods that require some chewing.
Challenging ourselves is always healthy, as we know from going to the gym.
Give young children foods that challenge them to use their jaws. Avoid that pap sold in stores as baby food! It's soft and sweet and won't do anything to help baby's jaws to develop.
I feel super challenged right now. But I won't have sleep apnea or need braces.

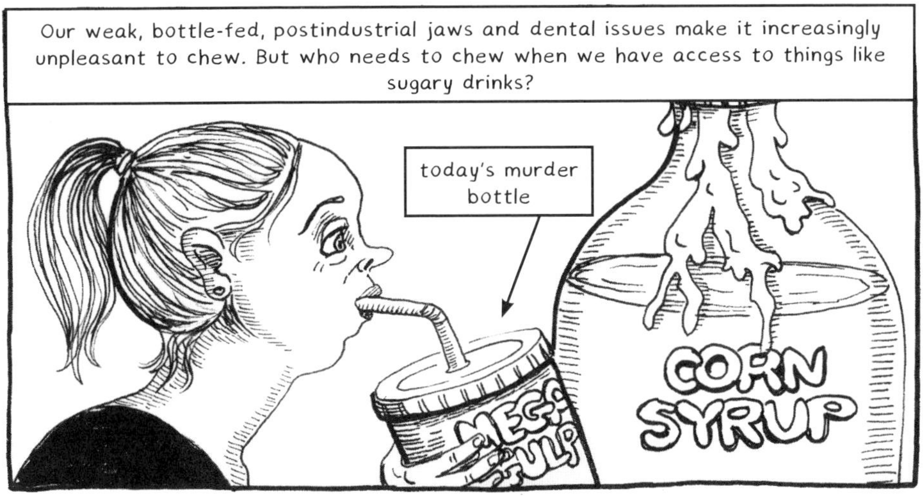
Our weak, bottle-fed, postindustrial jaws and dental issues make it increasingly unpleasant to chew. But who needs to chew when we have access to things like sugary drinks?
today's murder bottle
CORN SYRUP

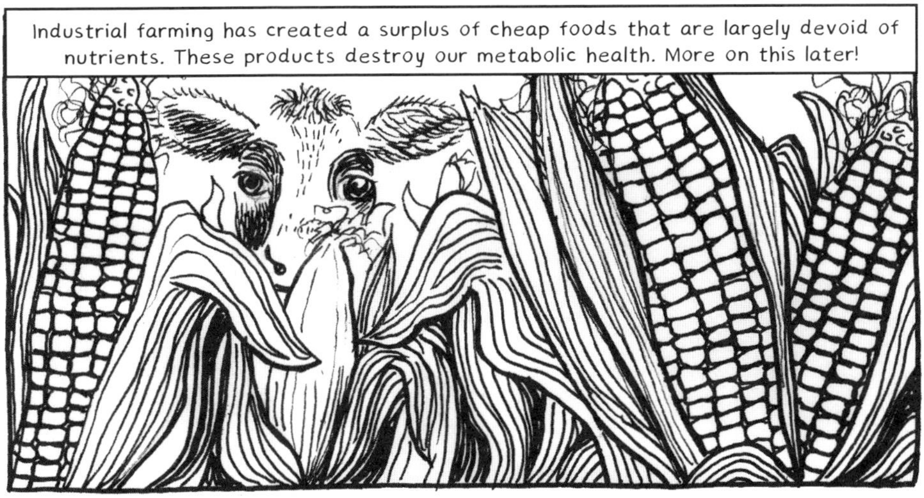
Industrial farming has created a surplus of cheap foods that are largely devoid of nutrients. These products destroy our metabolic health. More on this later!

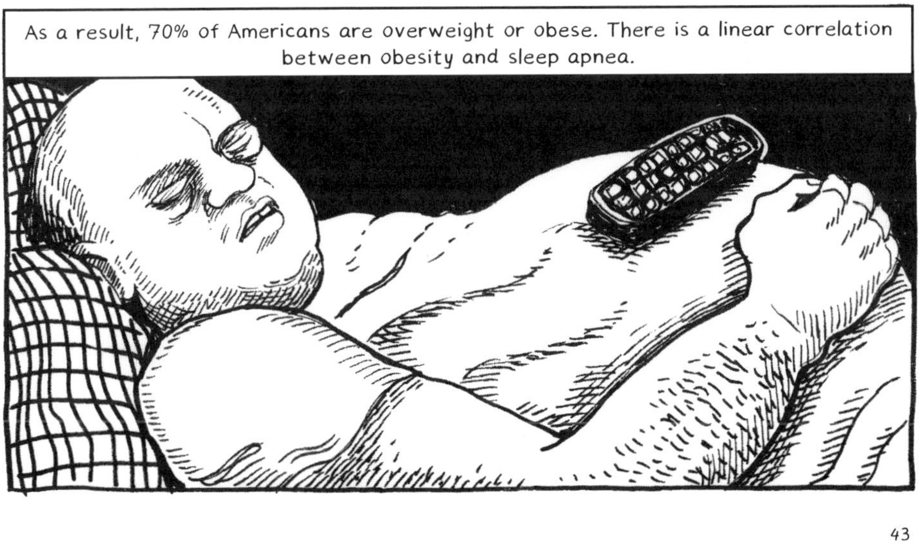
As a result, 70% of Americans are overweight or obese. There is a linear correlation between obesity and sleep apnea.

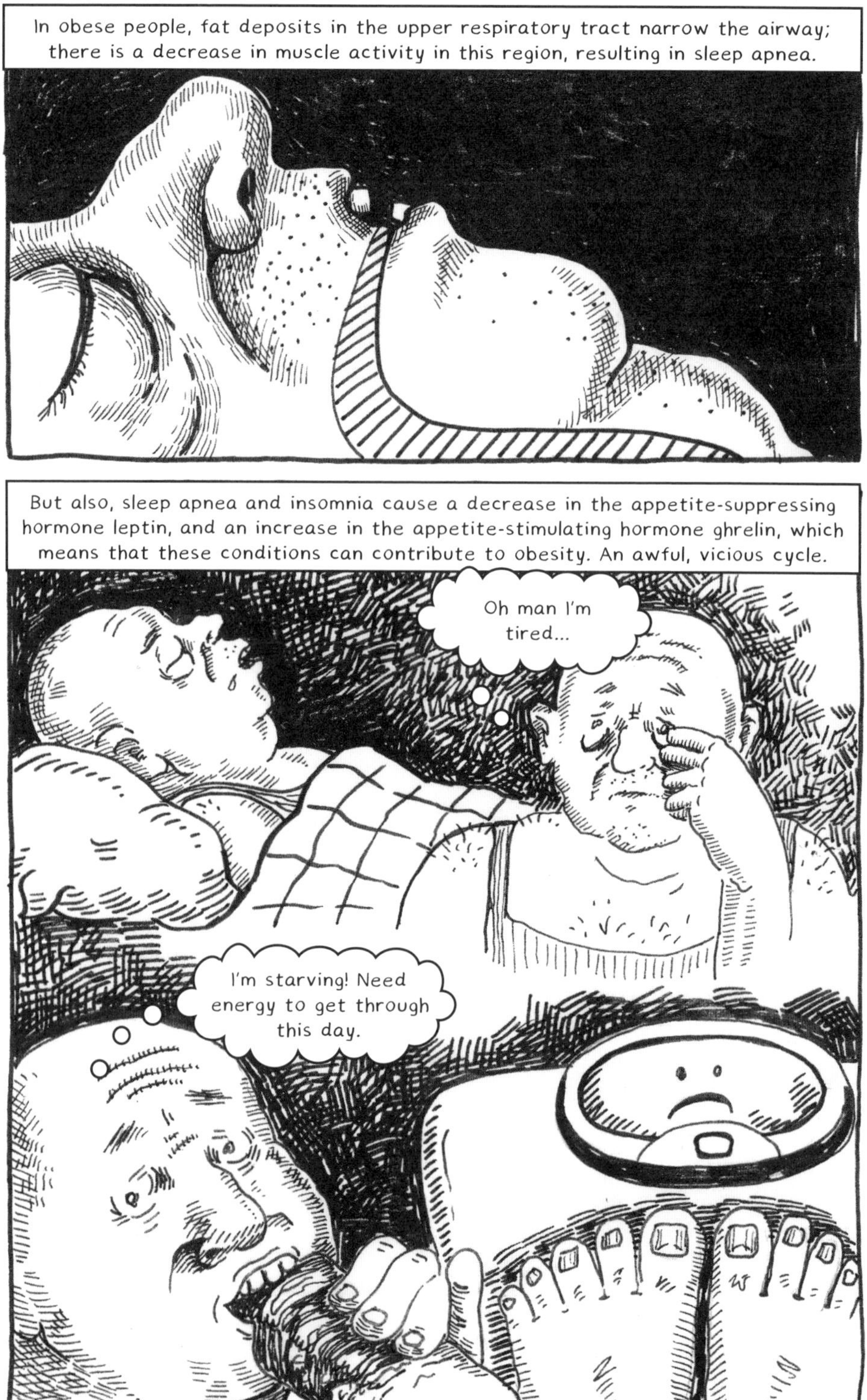
In obese people, fat deposits in the upper respiratory tract narrow the airway; there is a decrease in muscle activity in this region, resulting in sleep apnea.
But also, sleep apnea and insomnia cause a decrease in the appetite-suppressing hormone leptin, and an increase in the appetite-stimulating hormone ghrelin, which means that these conditions can contribute to obesity. An awful, vicious cycle.
Oh man I'm tired...
I'm starving! Need energy to get through this day.

In my case, I have never been obese. I never had braces, and my jaw looks pretty normal. I was bottle-fed, though. In 1970 in Germany when I was born, breastfeeding frequency was at a low point. Had this affected me physiologically somehow?

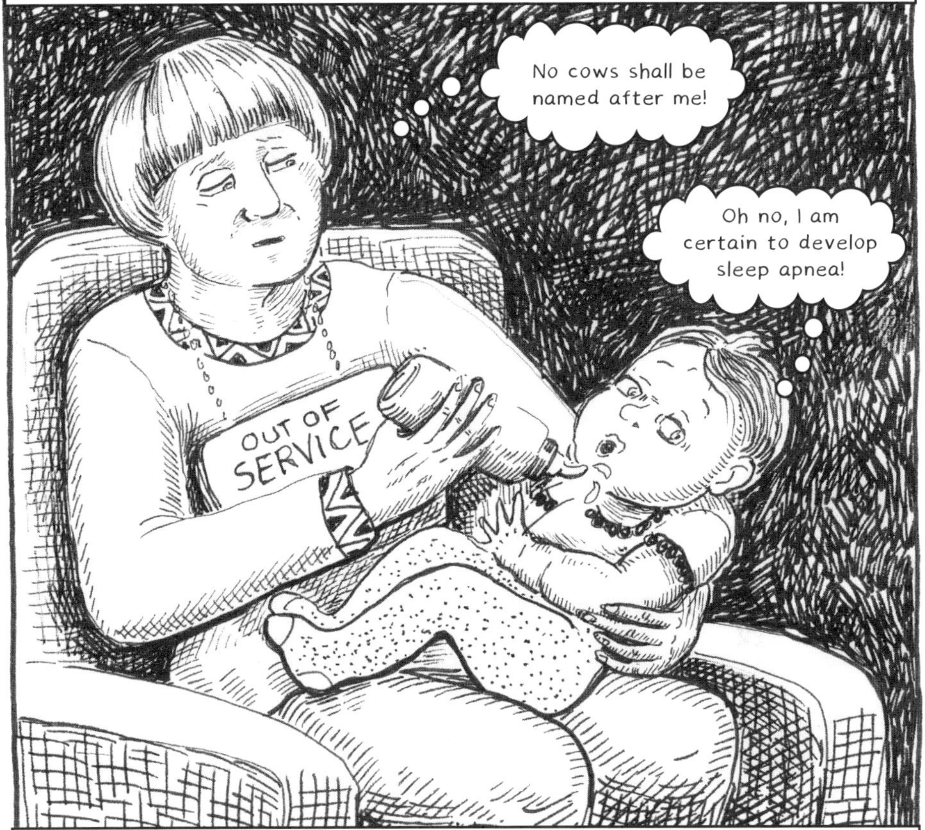
No cows shall be named after me!
OUT OF SERVICE
Oh no, I am certain to develop sleep apnea!

Is my sleep apnea related to the fact that I was bottle-fed? I'll never know for sure. All I can do today is learn how to manage my condition, for better sleep.

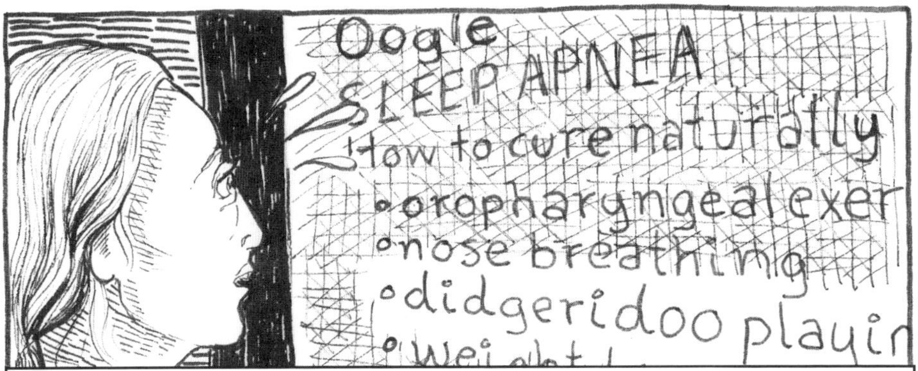
Oogle
SLEEP APNEA
How to cure naturally
oropharyngeal exer
nose breathing
didgeridoo playin

I've come to the realization that human health problems, at their root, are connected to the health and habitats of all other species on this planet, and that healing is only possible when we fully understand these interconnections. Take the didgeridoo, for example, which I came across in my research for treatments...

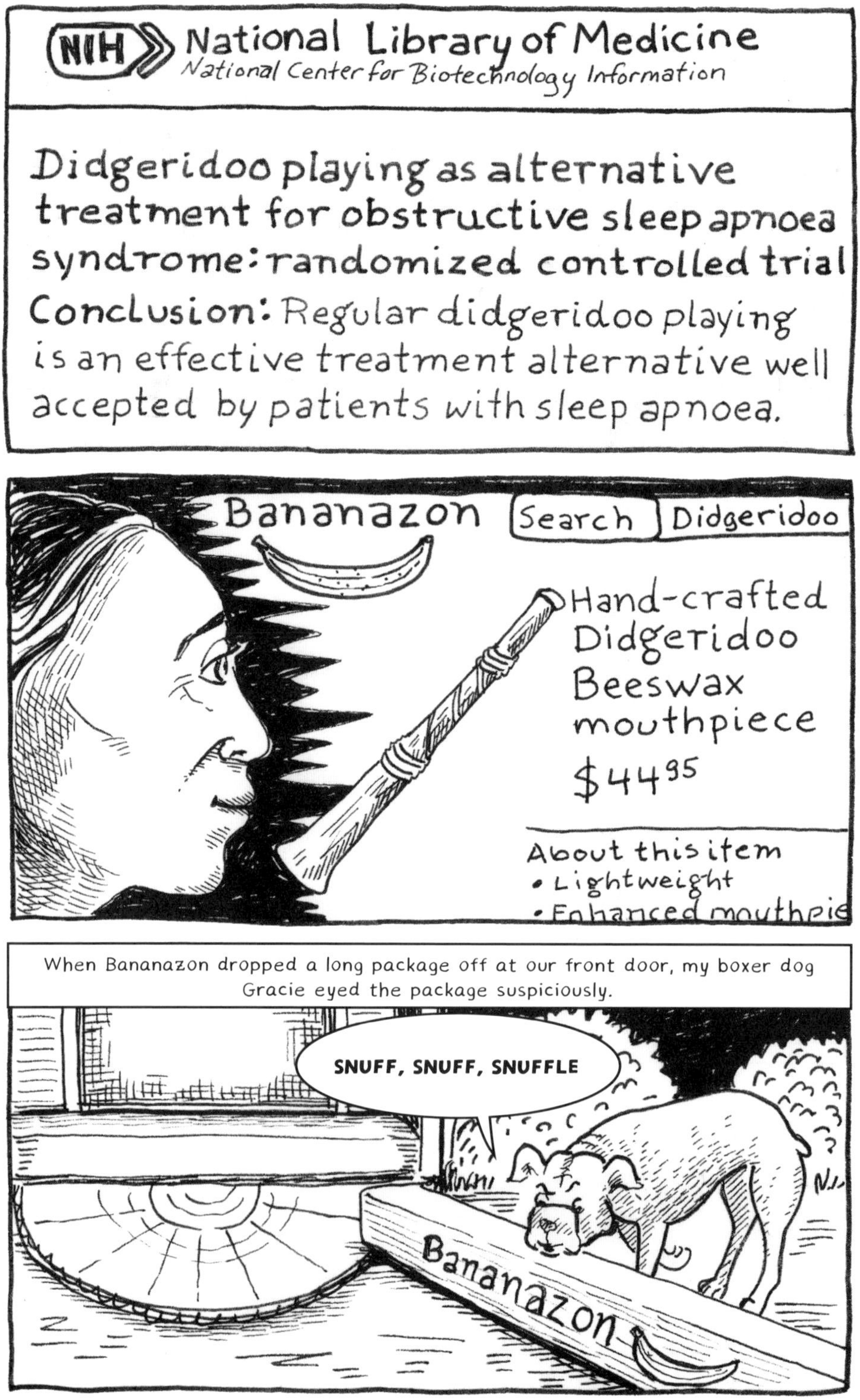
NIH National Library of Medicine
National Center for Biotechnology Information
Didgeridoo playing as alternative treatment for obstructive sleep apnoea syndrome: randomized controlled trial
Conclusion: Regular didgeridoo playing is an effective treatment alternative well accepted by patients with sleep apnoea.
Bananazon
Search
Didgeridoo
Hand-crafted Didgeridoo Beeswax mouthpiece
$44.95
About this item
• Lightweight
• Enhanced mouthpie
When Bananazon dropped a long package off at our front door, my boxer dog Gracie eyed the package suspiciously.
SNUFF, SNUFF, SNUFFLE
Bananazon

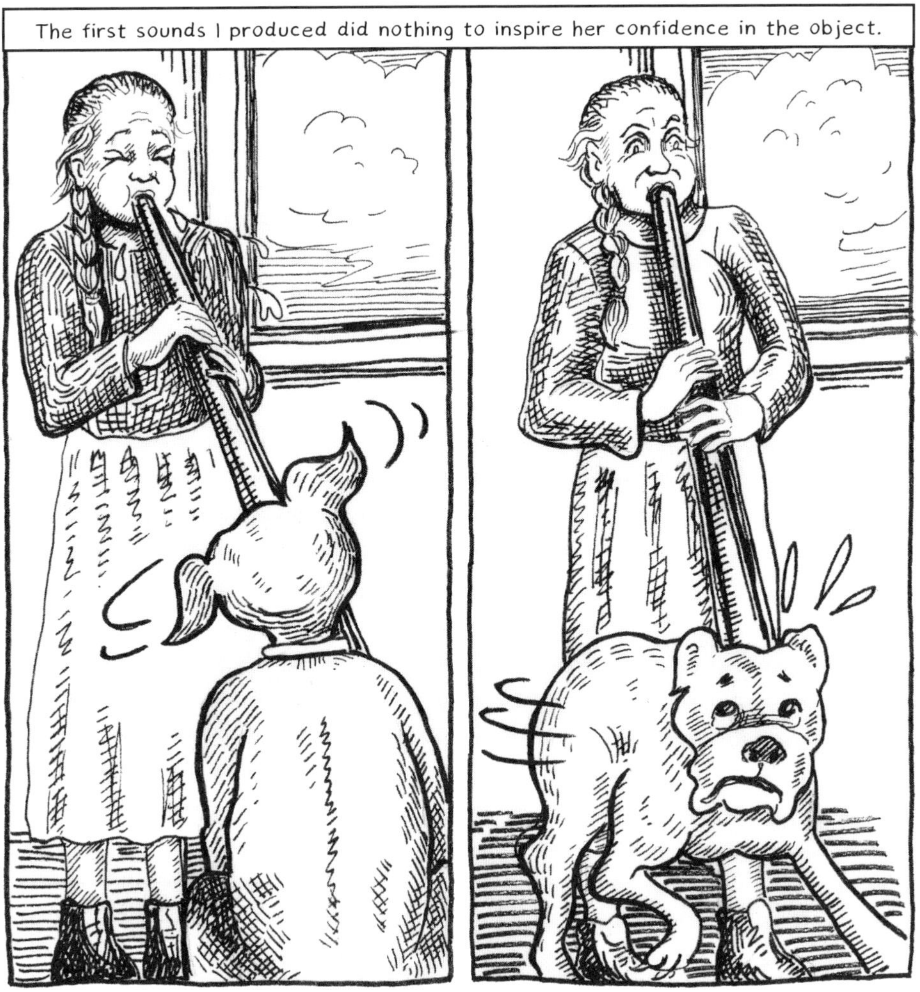
The first sounds I produced did nothing to inspire her confidence in the object.

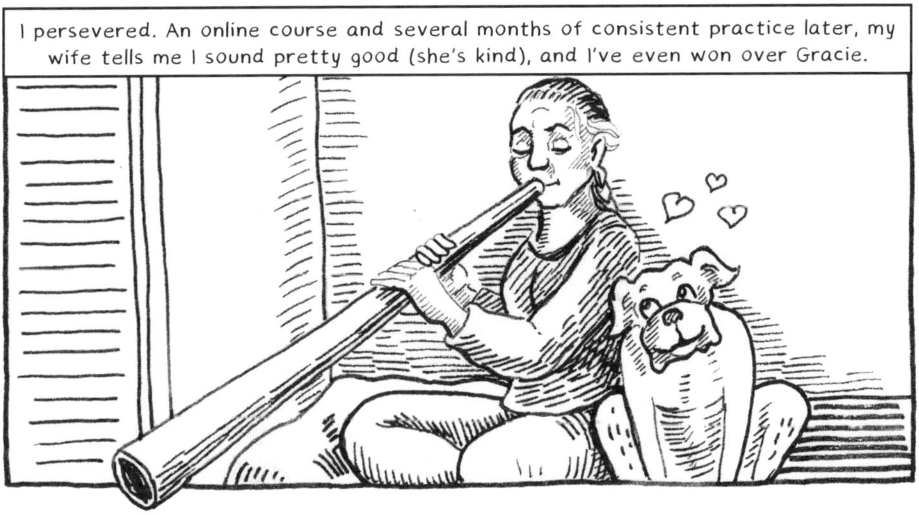
I persevered. An online course and several months of consistent practice later, my wife tells me I sound pretty good (she's kind), and I've even won over Gracie.

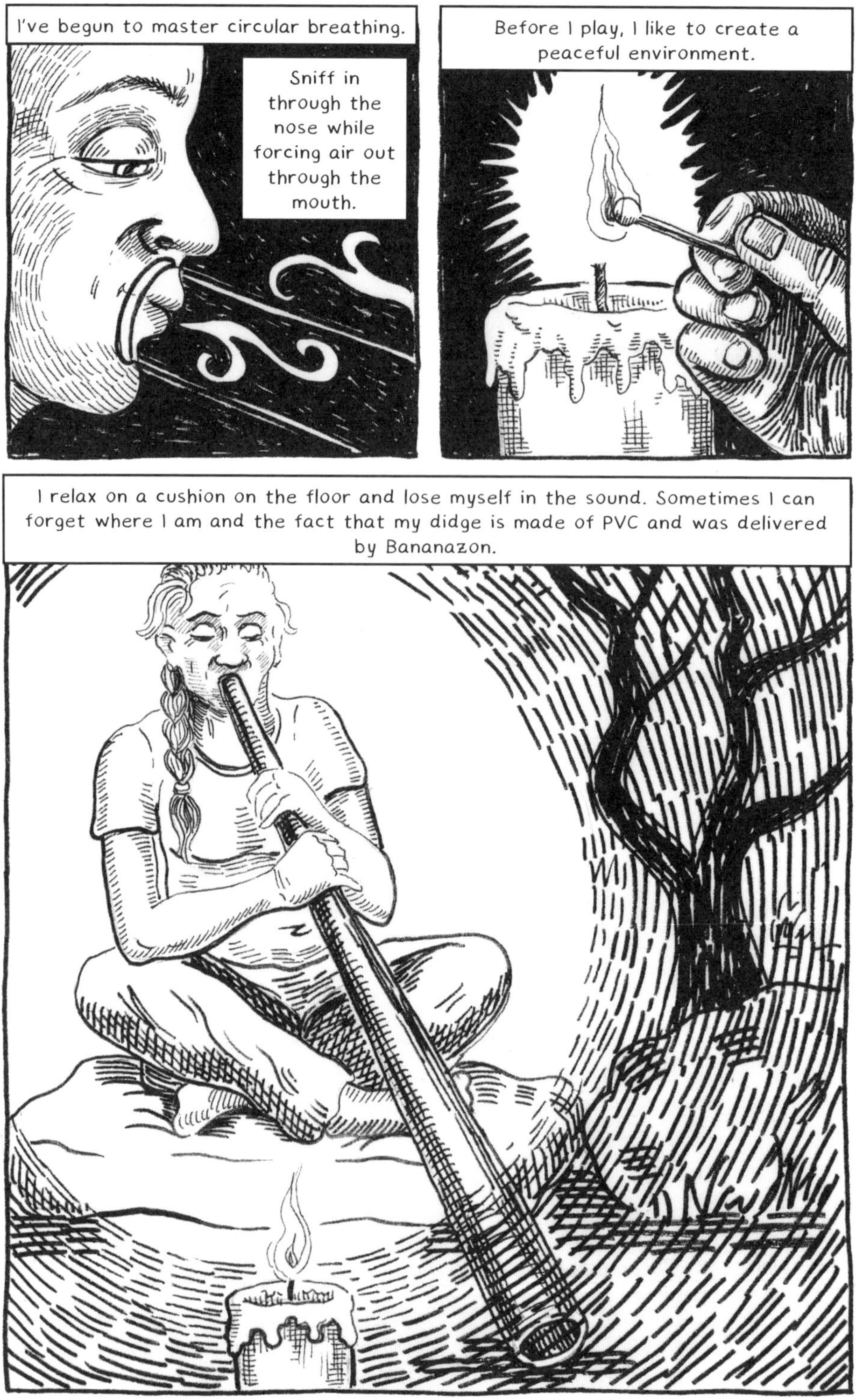
I've begun to master circular breathing.
Sniff in through the nose while forcing air out through the mouth.
Before I play, I like to create a peaceful environment.
I relax on a cushion on the floor and lose myself in the sound. Sometimes I can forget where I am and the fact that my didge is made of PVC and was delivered by Bananazon.

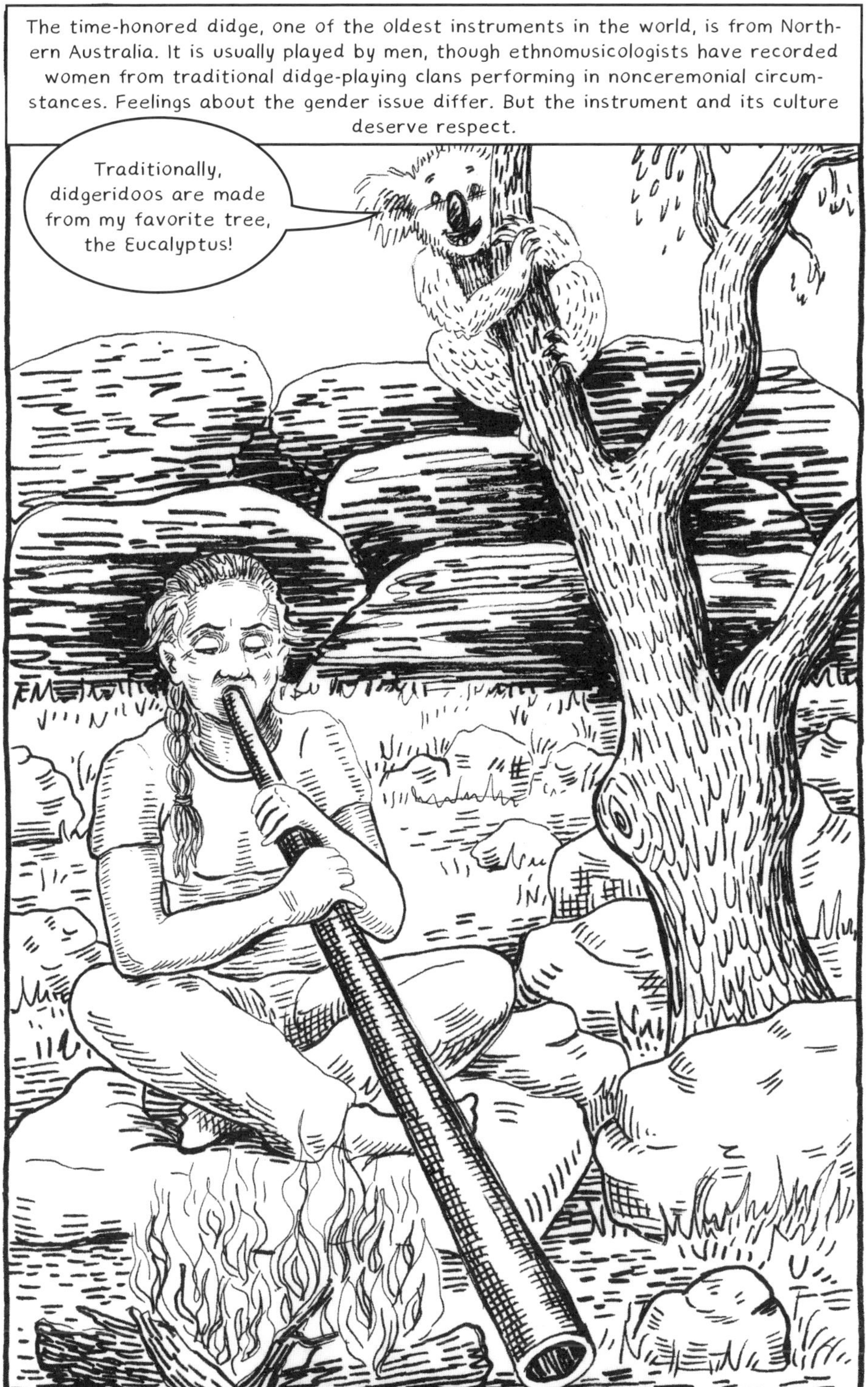
The time-honored didge, one of the oldest instruments in the world, is from Northern Australia. It is usually played by men, though ethnomusicologists have recorded women from traditional didge-playing clans performing in nonceremonial circumstances. Feelings about the gender issue differ. But the instrument and its culture deserve respect.
Traditionally, didgeridoos are made from my favorite tree, the Eucalyptus!

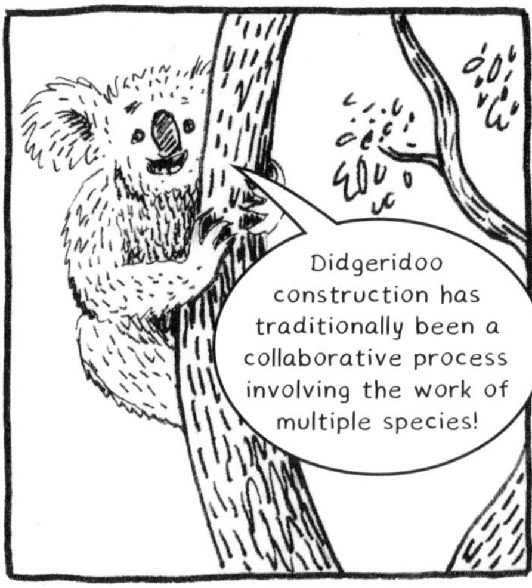
Didgeridoo construction has traditionally been a collaborative process involving the work of multiple species!

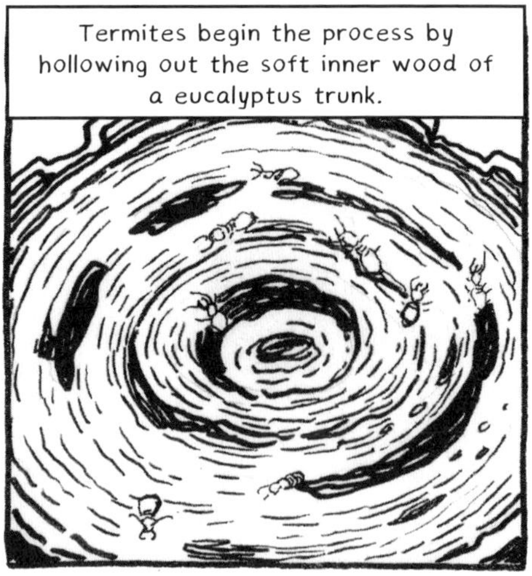
Termites begin the process by hollowing out the soft inner wood of a eucalyptus trunk.

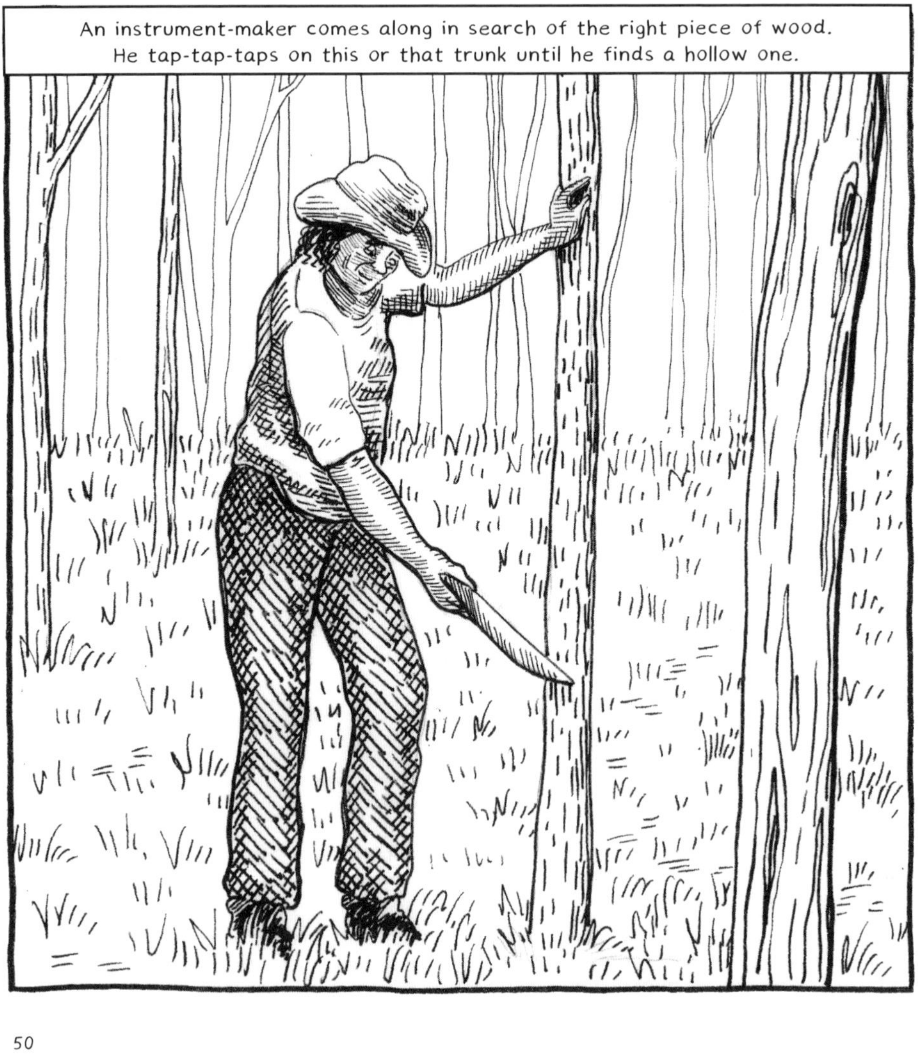
An instrument-maker comes along in search of the right piece of wood. He tap-tap-taps on this or that trunk until he finds a hollow one.

Once he's made his selection, he fells the tree...

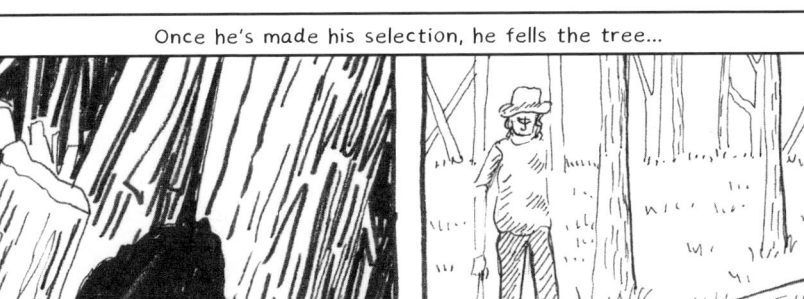

...and strips the bark and cleans out the termites' leftover grit.

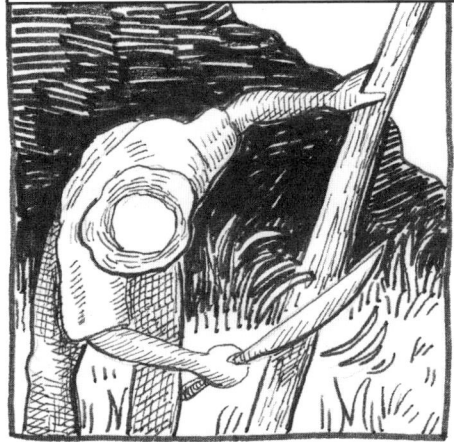
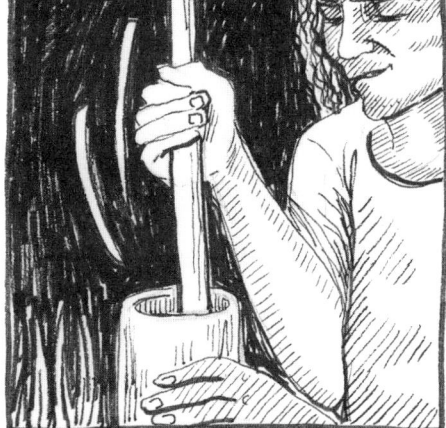

Then he gathers wax from the hive of the little sugar bee, a stingless species native to Australia. The sugar bees' wax is used for making the mouthpiece of the didgeridoo and for plugging any holes in the wood.

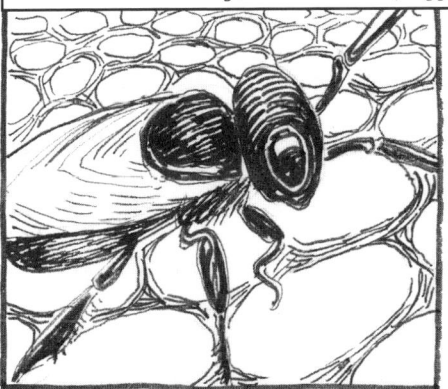
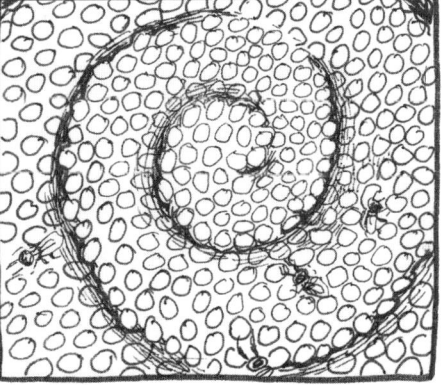

Wax works well for the mouthpiece because it creates an opening that's just the right size for the musician. And when the wax warms up while the instrument is being played, the musician can get a good tight seal for his lips.

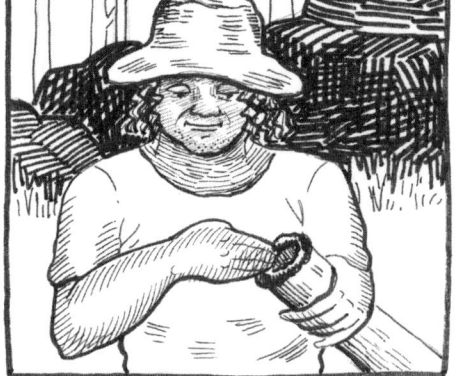 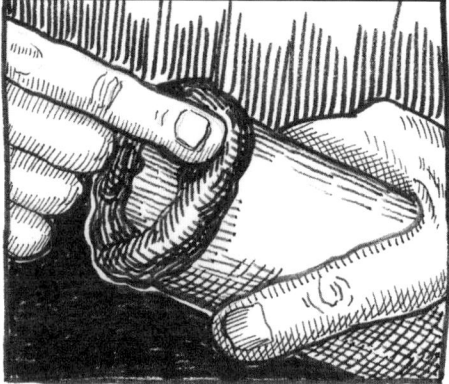

After assembly, the didgeridoo is customarily painted using natural pigments...

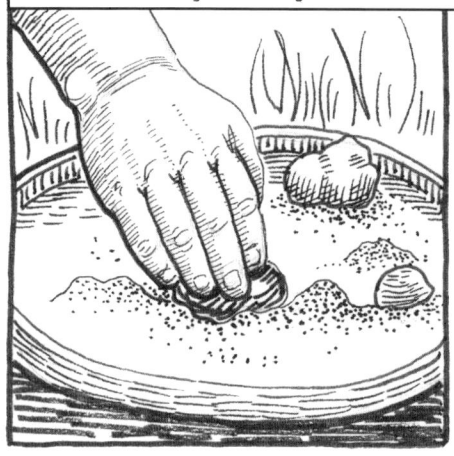 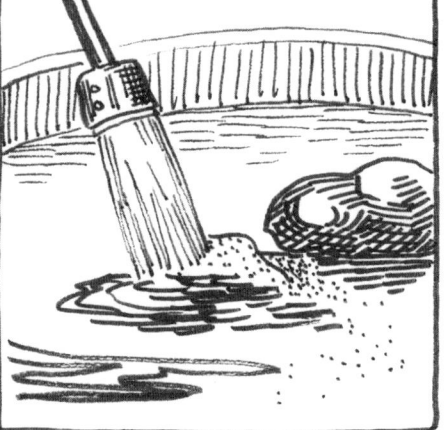

...and is decorated with designs passed down from earlier generations.

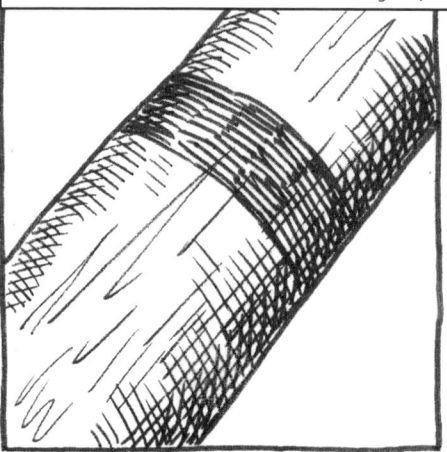 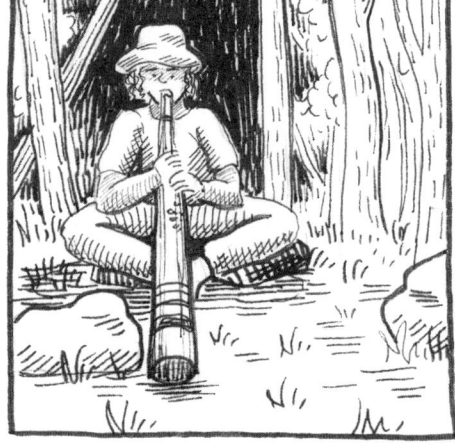

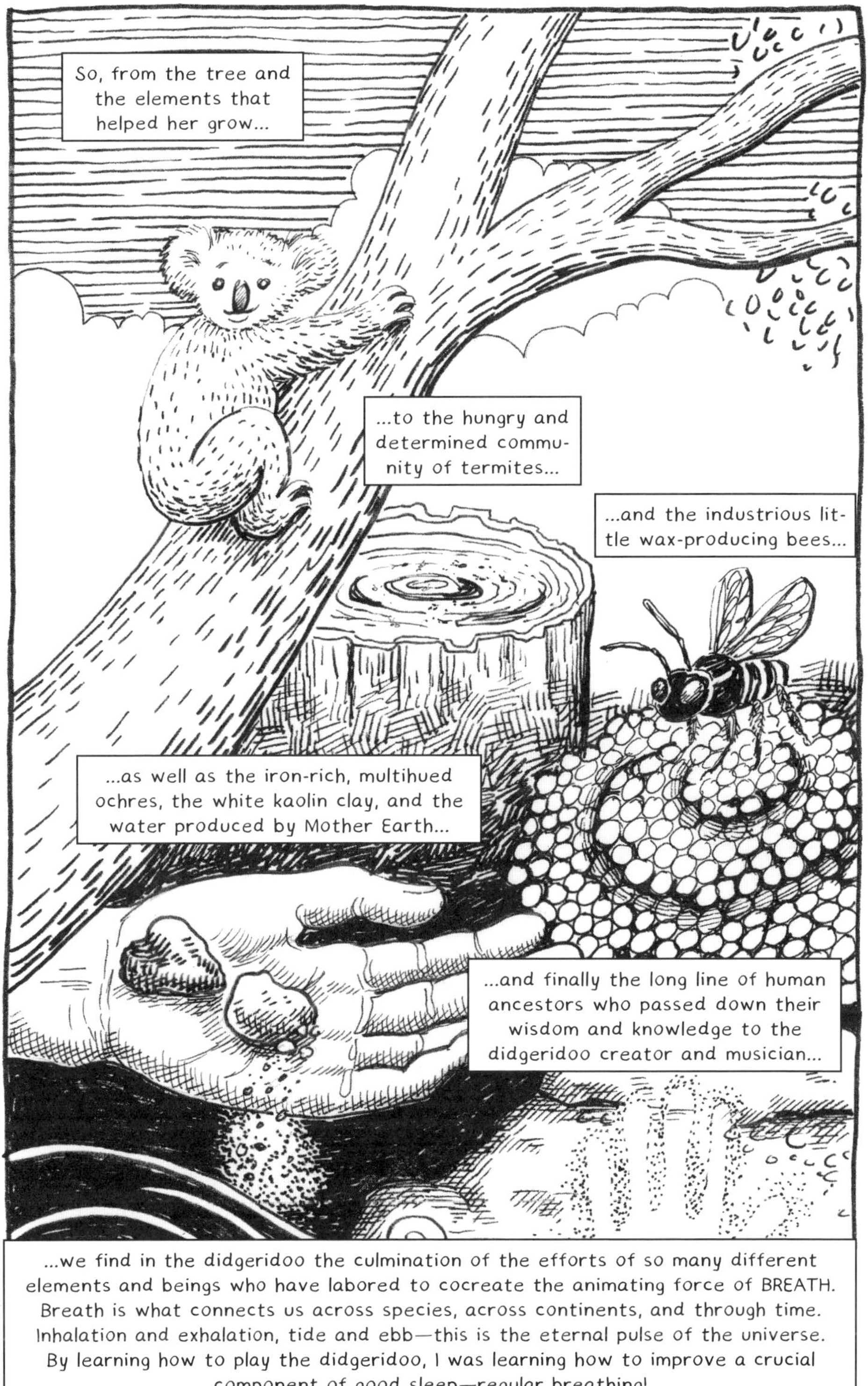
So, from the tree and the elements that helped her grow...
...to the hungry and determined community of termites...
...and the industrious little wax-producing bees...
...as well as the iron-rich, multihued ochres, the white kaolin clay, and the water produced by Mother Earth...
...and finally the long line of human ancestors who passed down their wisdom and knowledge to the didgeridoo creator and musician...
...we find in the didgeridoo the culmination of the efforts of so many different elements and beings who have labored to cocreate the animating force of BREATH. Breath is what connects us across species, across continents, and through time. Inhalation and exhalation, tide and ebb—this is the eternal pulse of the universe. By learning how to play the didgeridoo, I was learning how to improve a crucial component of good sleep—regular breathing!

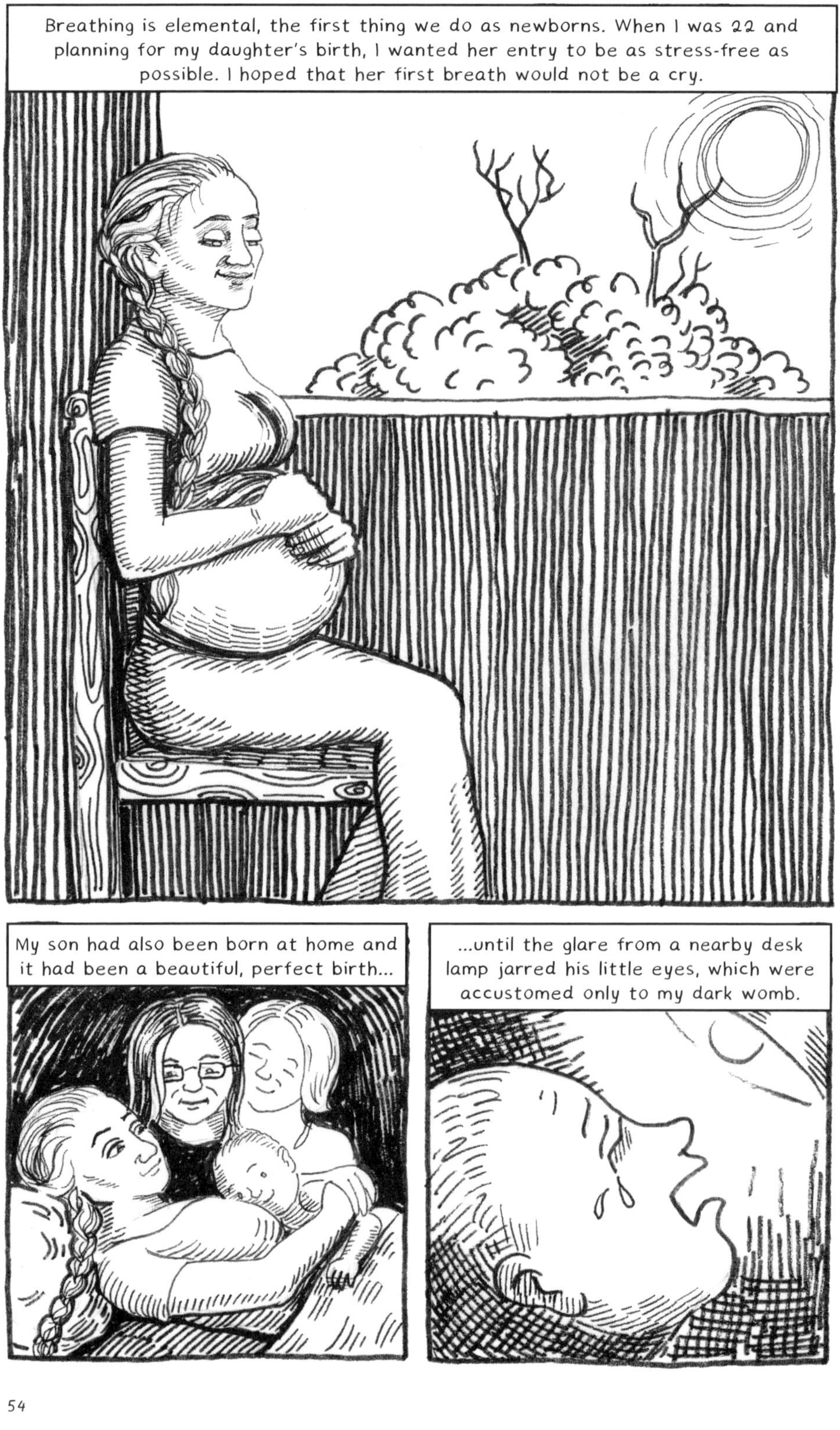
Breathing is elemental, the first thing we do as newborns. When I was 22 and planning for my daughter's birth, I wanted her entry to be as stress-free as possible. I hoped that her first breath would not be a cry.
My son had also been born at home and it had been a beautiful, perfect birth...
...until the glare from a nearby desk lamp jarred his little eyes, which were accustomed only to my dark womb.

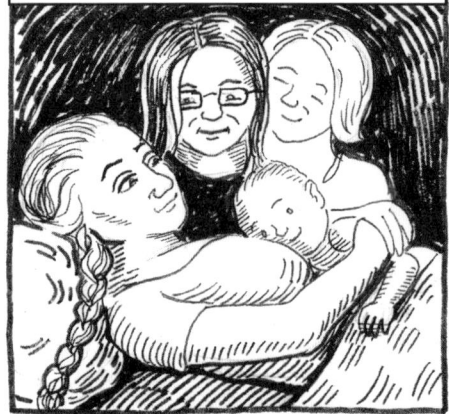

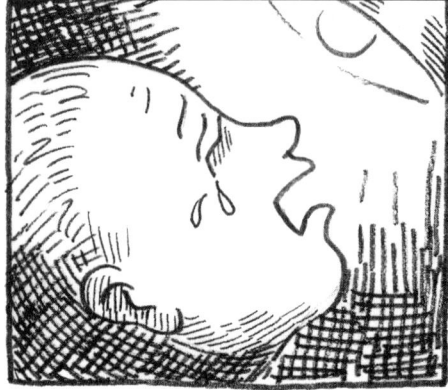

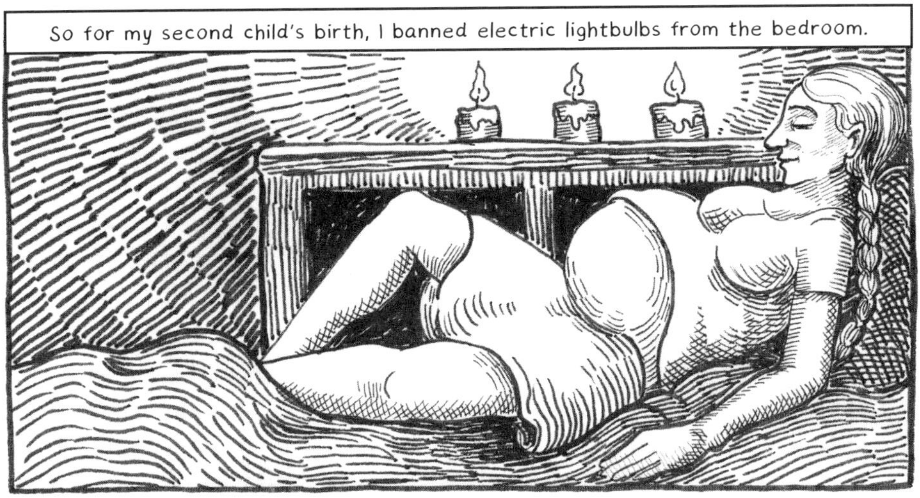
So for my second child's birth, I banned electric lightbulbs from the bedroom.

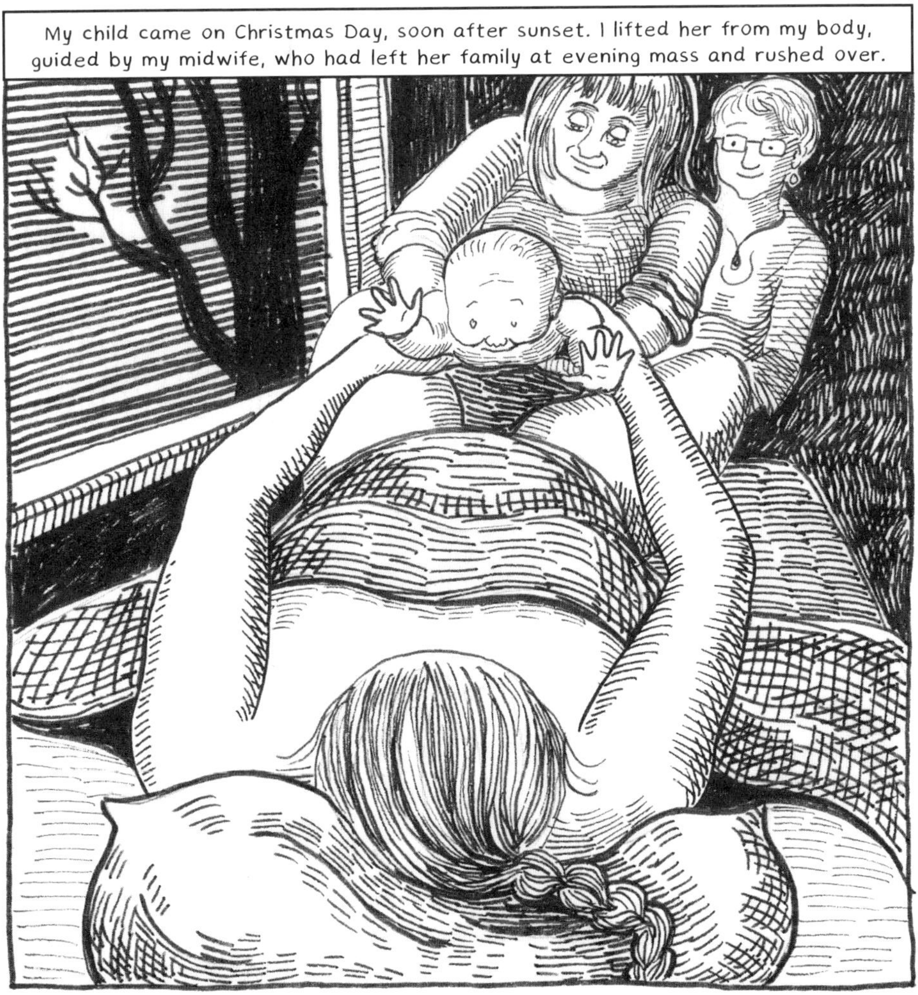
My child came on Christmas Day, soon after sunset. I lifted her from my body, guided by my midwife, who had left her family at evening mass and rushed over.

My little one's arms shot out toward me, her lungs filled with air for the very first time, and her first sound rang out calm and clear.

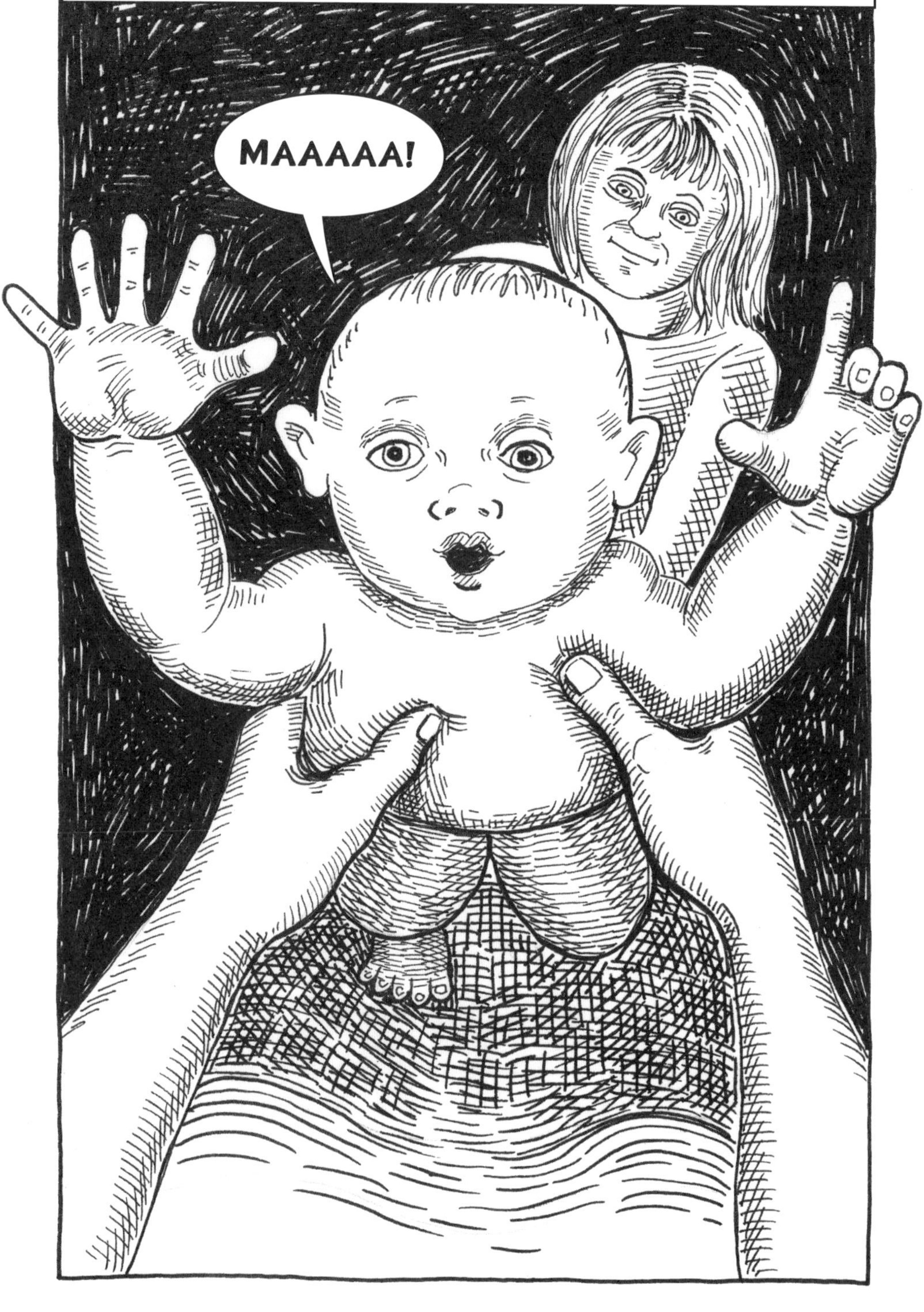
MAAAAA!

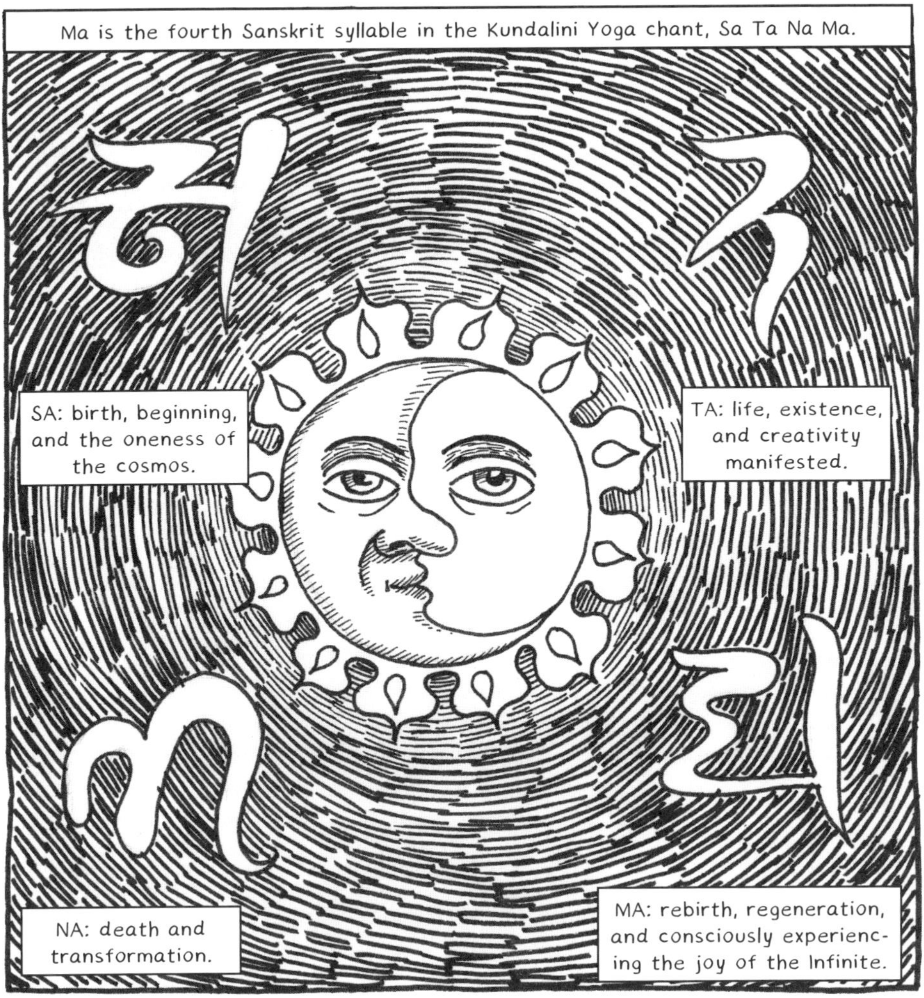
Ma is the fourth Sanskrit syllable in the Kundalini Yoga chant, Sa Ta Na Ma.
SA: birth, beginning, and the oneness of the cosmos.
TA: life, existence, and creativity manifested.
NA: death and transformation.
MA: rebirth, regeneration, and consciously experiencing the joy of the Infinite.

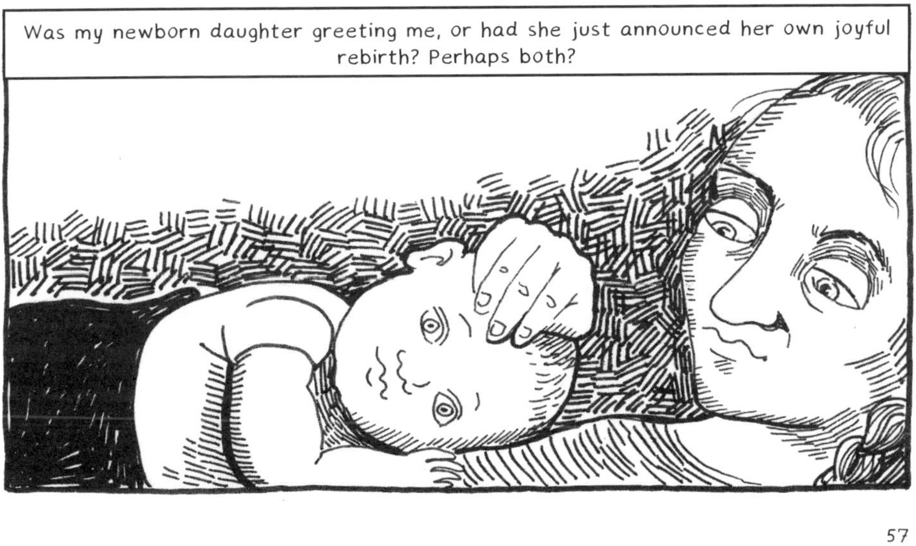
Was my newborn daughter greeting me, or had she just announced her own joyful rebirth? Perhaps both?

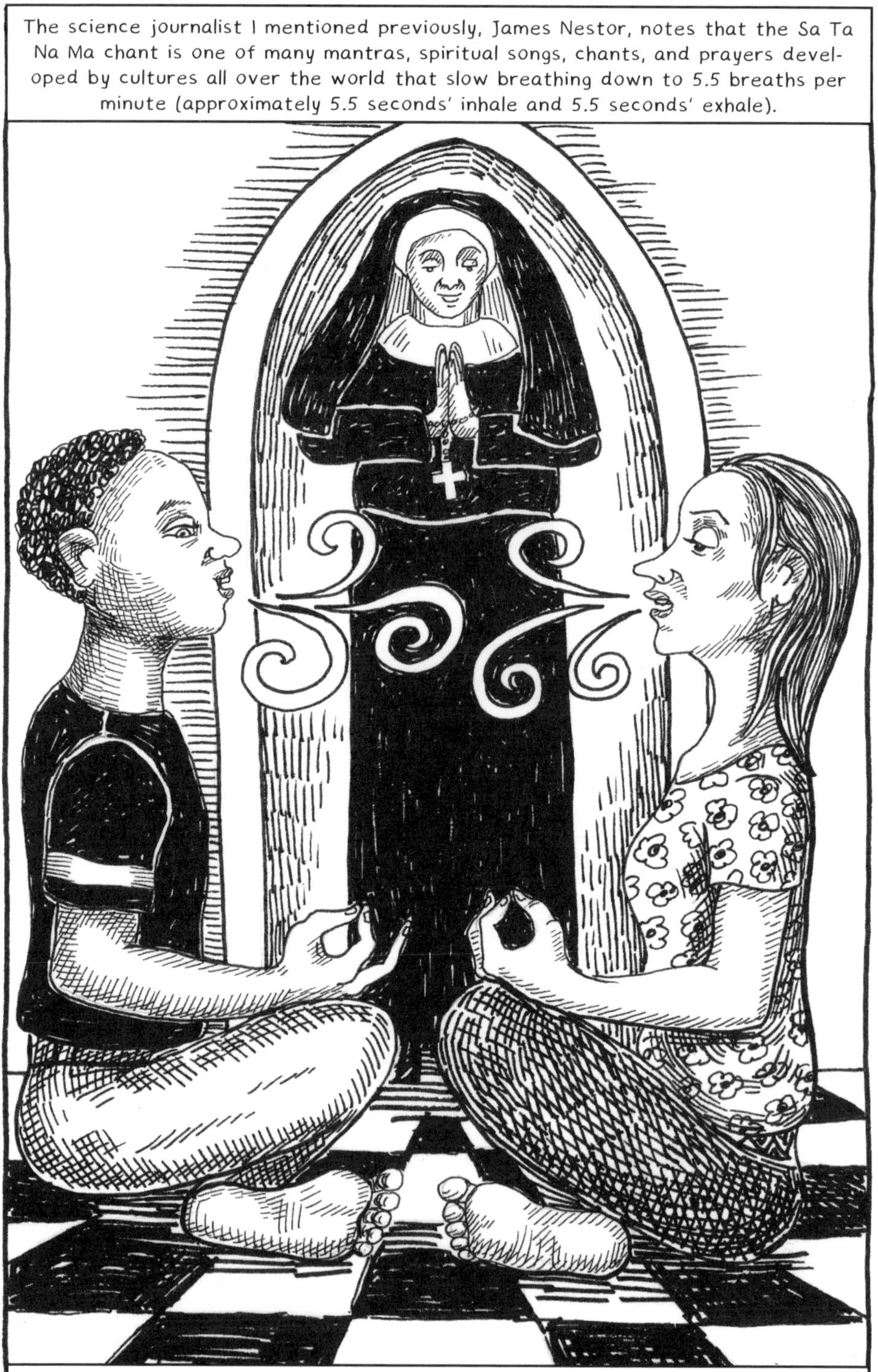
The science journalist I mentioned previously, James Nestor, notes that the Sa Ta Na Ma chant is one of many mantras, spiritual songs, chants, and prayers developed by cultures all over the world that slow breathing down to 5.5 breaths per minute (approximately 5.5 seconds' inhale and 5.5 seconds' exhale).
Among them are the Kirtan Kriya chant (Sa Ta Na Ma), Om Mane Padme Hum, OM, Ave Maria, and the original Latin version of the rosary.

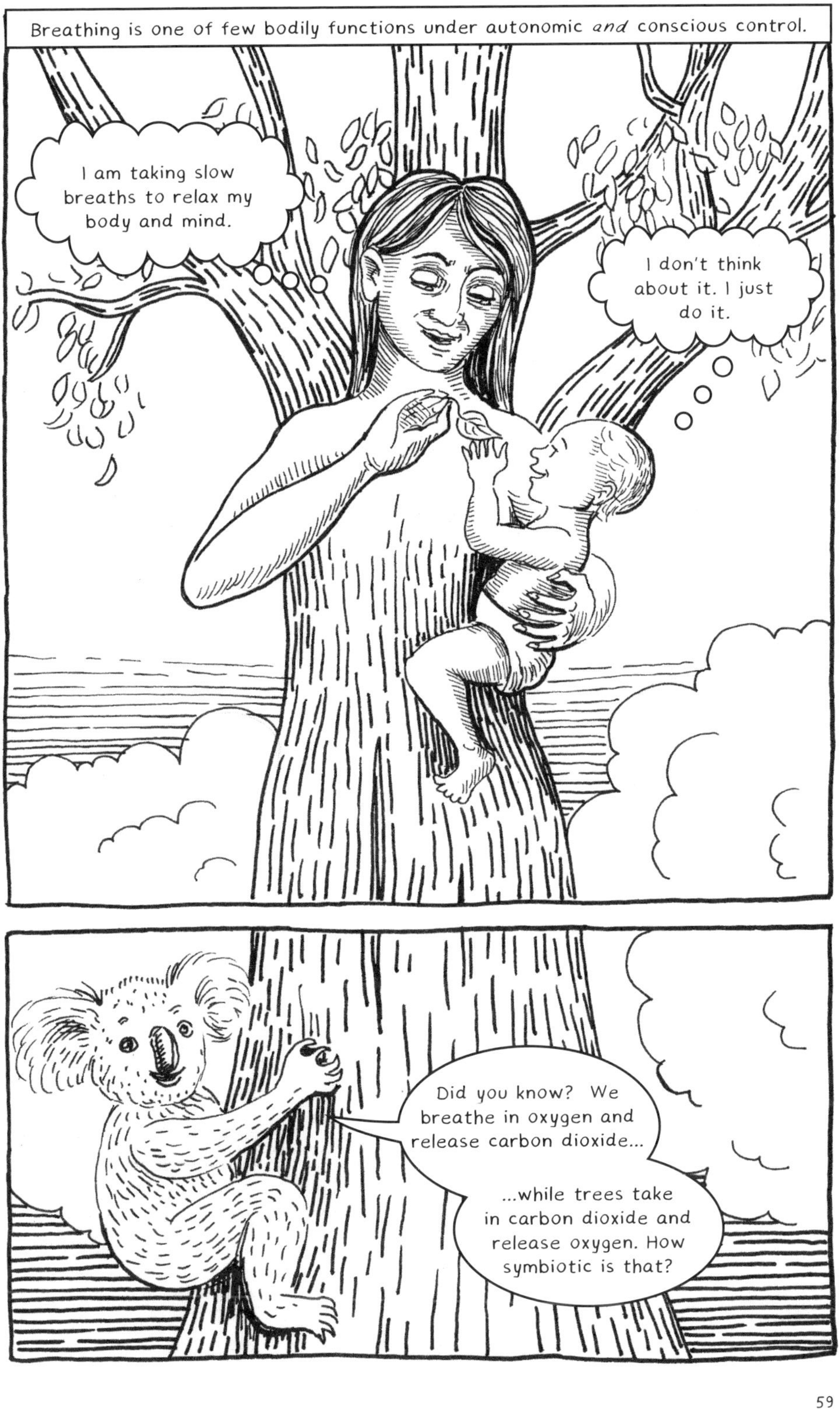

Breathing is one of few bodily functions under autonomic *and* conscious control.
I am taking slow breaths to relax my body and mind.
I don't think about it. I just do it.
Did you know? We breathe in oxygen and release carbon dioxide...
...while trees take in carbon dioxide and release oxygen. How symbiotic is that?

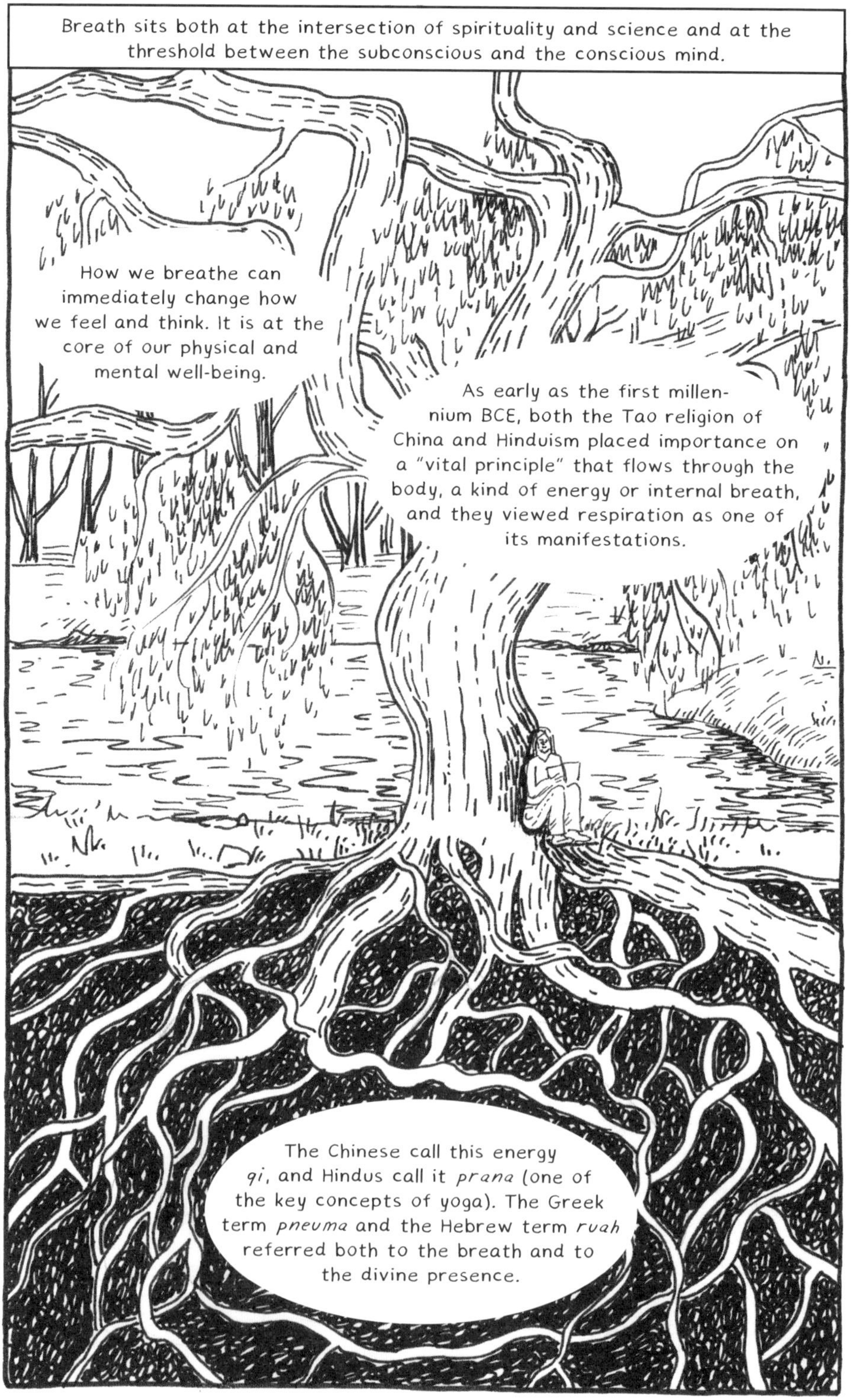
Breath sits both at the intersection of spirituality and science and at the threshold between the subconscious and the conscious mind.
How we breathe can immediately change how we feel and think. It is at the core of our physical and mental well-being.
As early as the first millennium BCE, both the Tao religion of China and Hinduism placed importance on a "vital principle" that flows through the body, a kind of energy or internal breath, and they viewed respiration as one of its manifestations.
The Chinese call this energy *qi*, and Hindus call it *prana* (one of the key concepts of yoga). The Greek term *pneuma* and the Hebrew term *ruah* referred both to the breath and to the divine presence.

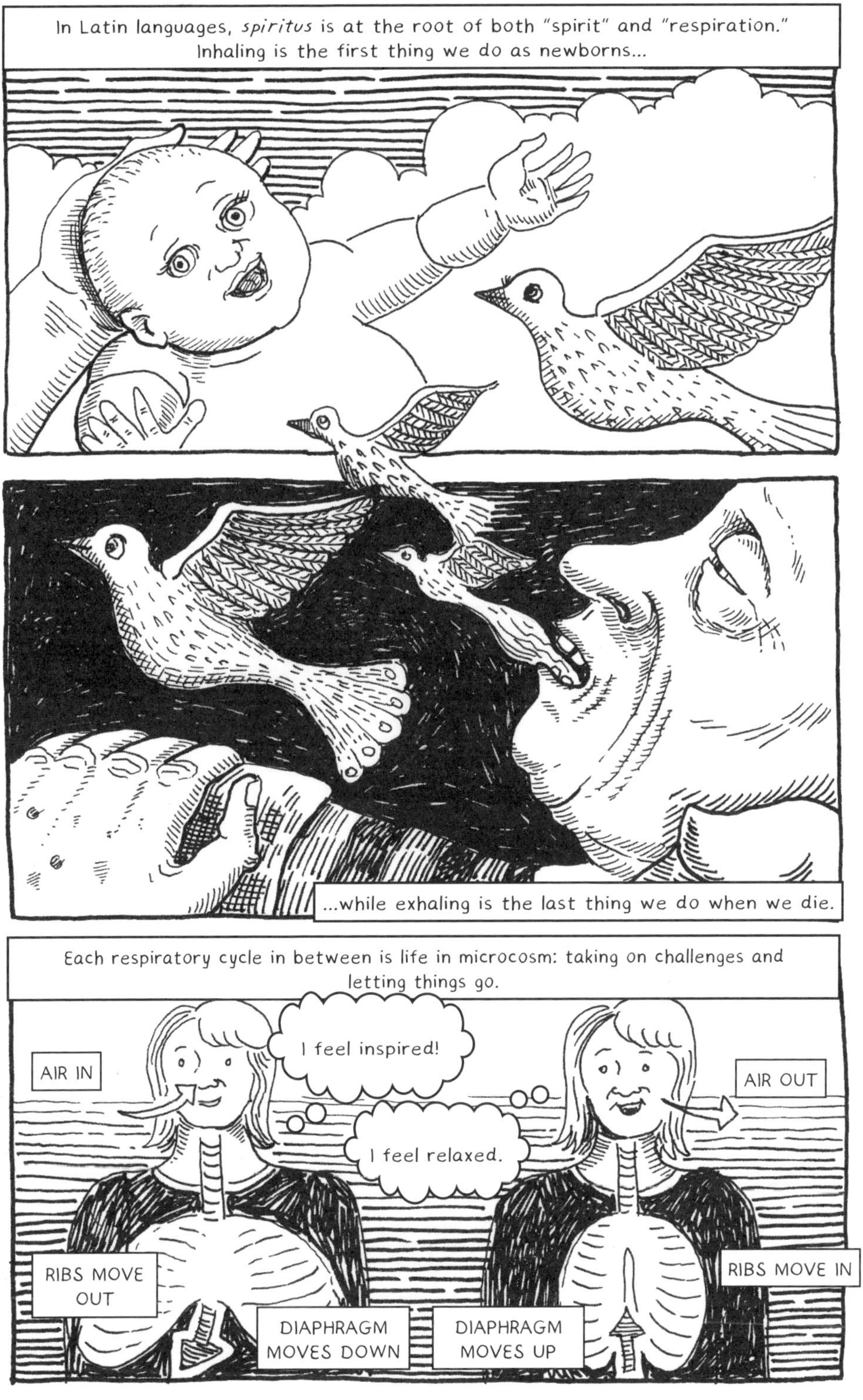

In Latin languages, *spiritus* is at the root of both "spirit" and "respiration." Inhaling is the first thing we do as newborns...
...while exhaling is the last thing we do when we die.
Each respiratory cycle in between is life in microcosm: taking on challenges and letting things go.
AIR IN
I feel inspired!
I feel relaxed.
AIR OUT
RIBS MOVE OUT
DIAPHRAGM MOVES DOWN
DIAPHRAGM MOVES UP
RIBS MOVE IN

Inhaling activates oxygenation and the sympathetic nervous system (SNS), which actually isn't very sympathetic at all. When it is activated, the SNS stimulates the body's fight, flight, or freeze response. The SNS corresponds with the YANG principle in Chinese medicine.

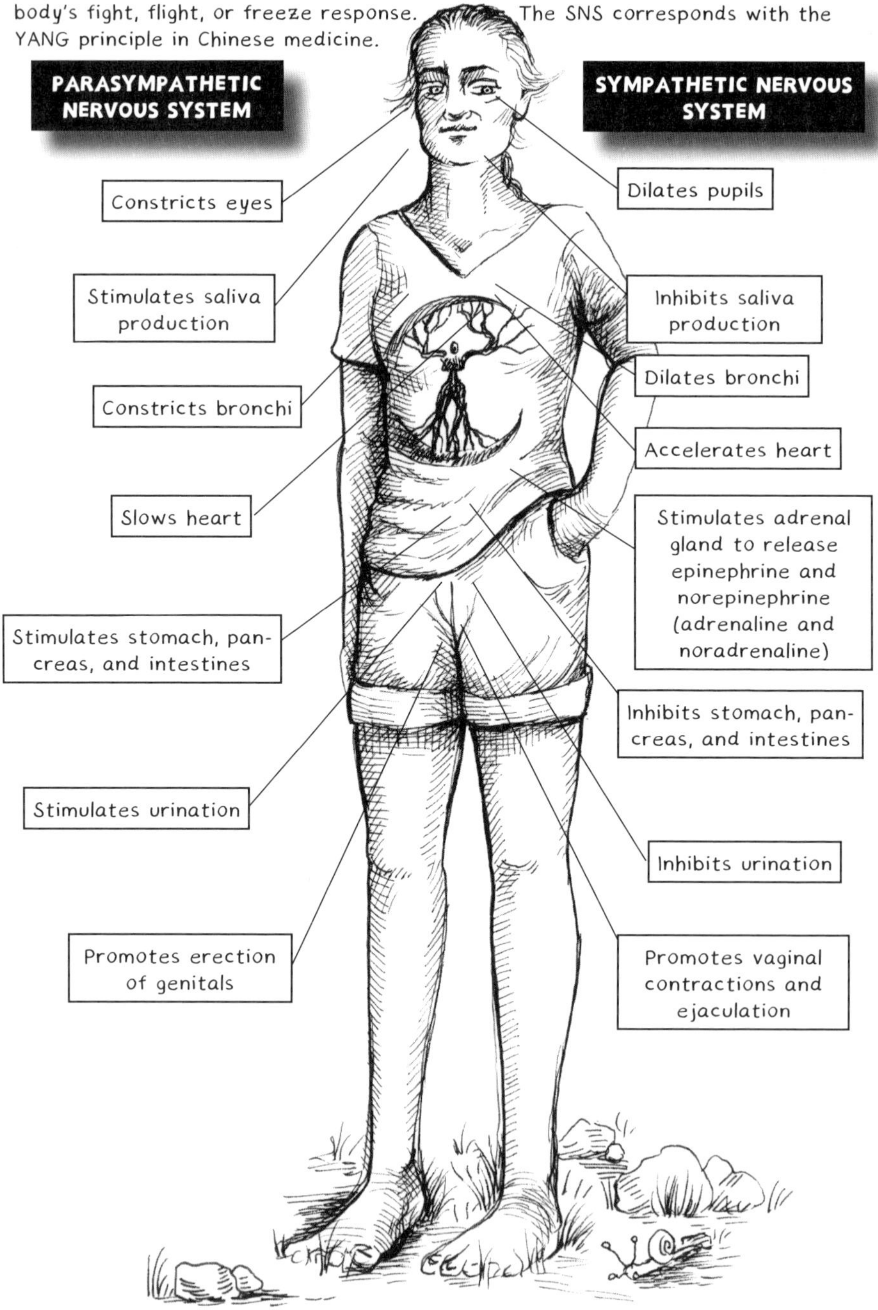

PARASYMPATHETIC NERVOUS SYSTEM
Constricts eyes
Stimulates saliva production
Constricts bronchi
Slows heart
Stimulates stomach, pancreas, and intestines
Stimulates urination
Promotes erection of genitals
SYMPATHETIC NERVOUS SYSTEM
Dilates pupils
Inhibits saliva production
Dilates bronchi
Accelerates heart
Stimulates adrenal gland to release epinephrine and norepinephrine (adrenaline and noradrenaline)
Inhibits stomach, pancreas, and intestines
Inhibits urination
Promotes vaginal contractions and ejaculation

Exhaling expels carbon dioxide and stimulates the parasympathetic nervous system (PNS), the network of nerves that relaxes the body after stress or danger. The PNS also helps run life-sustaining processes, like digestion, during times when we feel safe and relaxed. The PNS corresponds with the YIN principle in Chinese medicine.

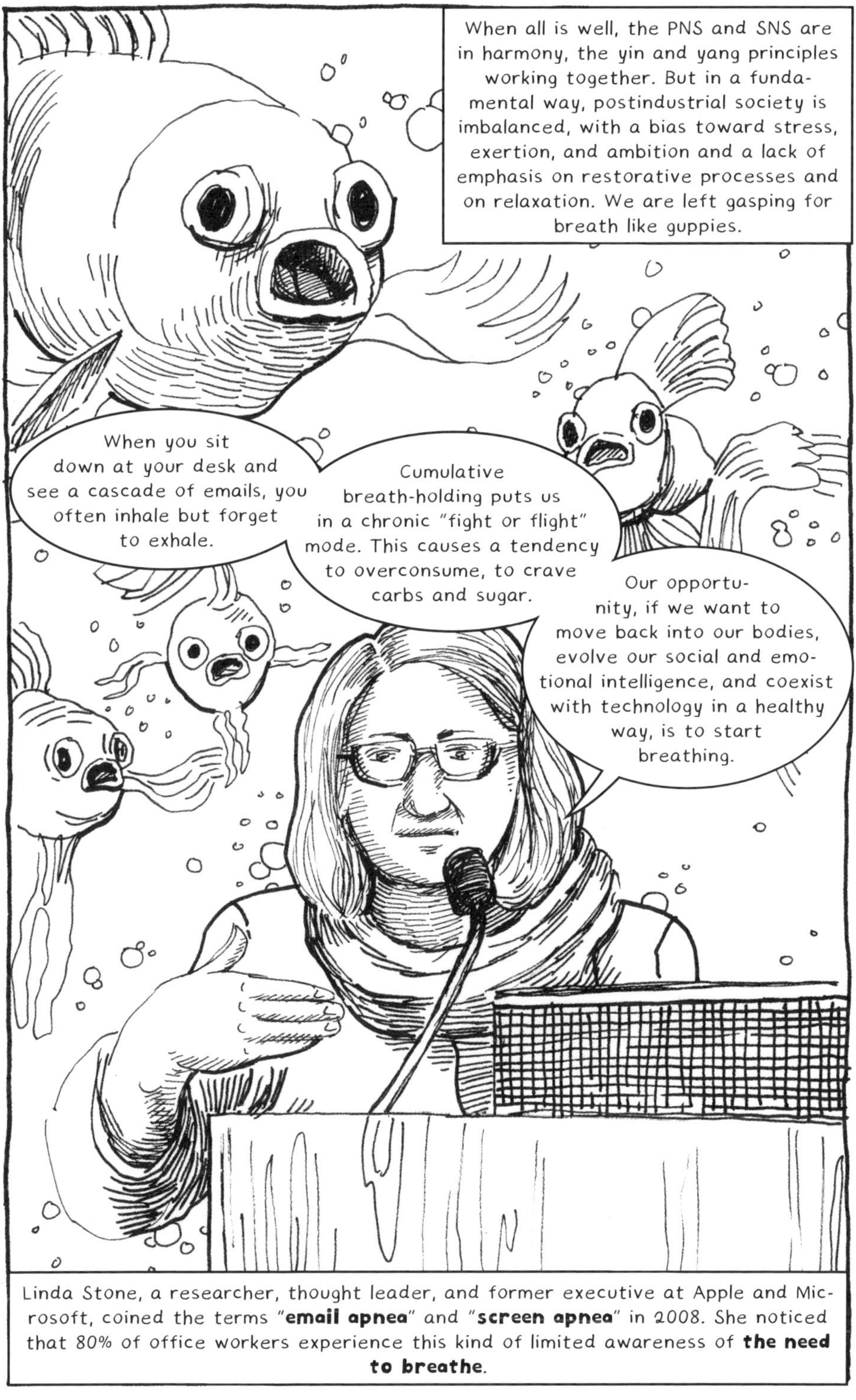
When all is well, the PNS and SNS are in harmony, the yin and yang principles working together. But in a fundamental way, postindustrial society is imbalanced, with a bias toward stress, exertion, and ambition and a lack of emphasis on restorative processes and on relaxation. We are left gasping for breath like guppies.
When you sit down at your desk and see a cascade of emails, you often inhale but forget to exhale.
Cumulative breath-holding puts us in a chronic "fight or flight" mode. This causes a tendency to overconsume, to crave carbs and sugar.
Our opportunity, if we want to move back into our bodies, evolve our social and emotional intelligence, and coexist with technology in a healthy way, is to start breathing.
Linda Stone, a researcher, thought leader, and former executive at Apple and Microsoft, coined the terms "**email apnea**" and "**screen apnea**" in 2008. She noticed that 80% of office workers experience this kind of limited awareness of **the need to breathe**.

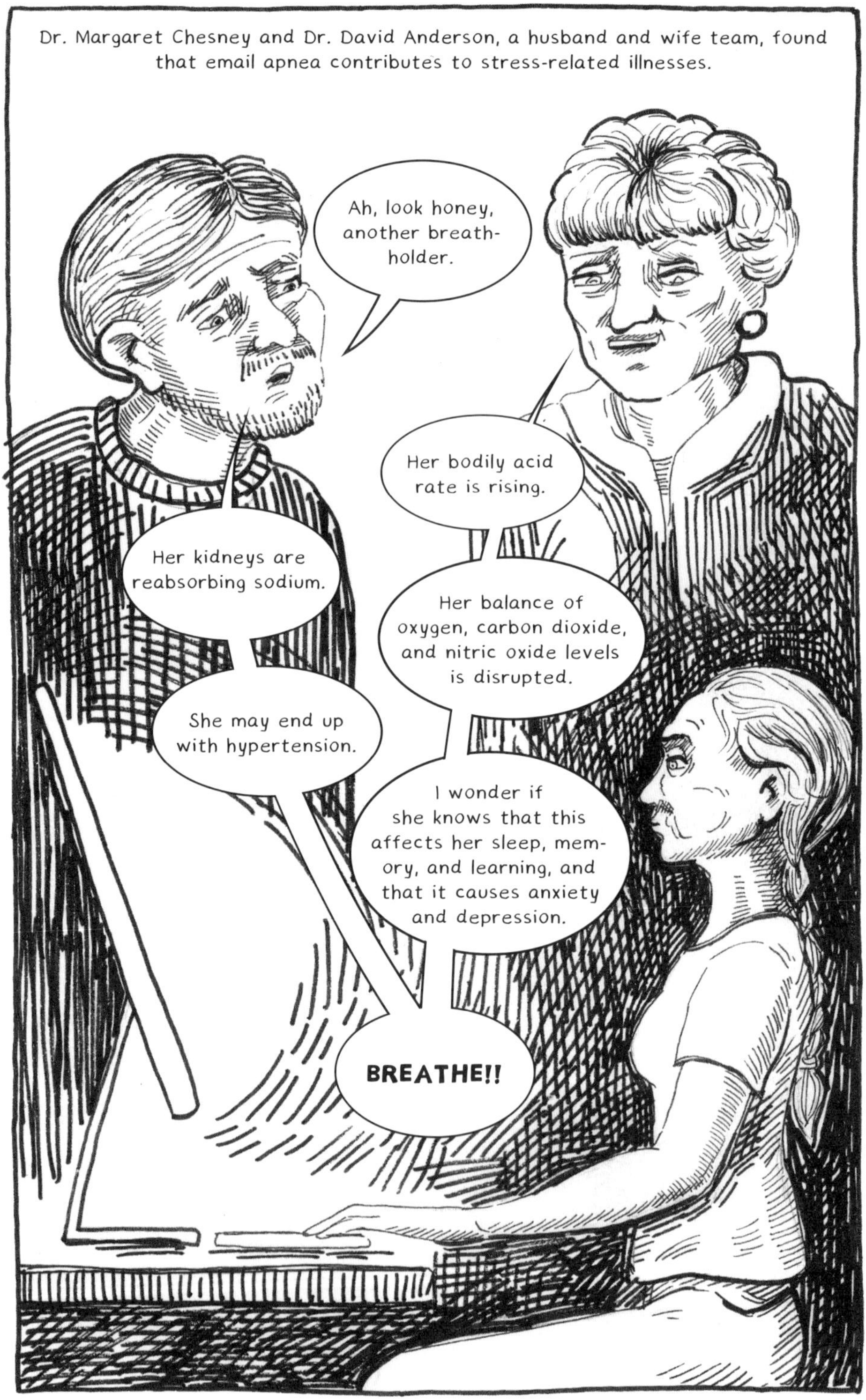
Dr. Margaret Chesney and Dr. David Anderson, a husband and wife team, found that email apnea contributes to stress-related illnesses.
Ah, look honey, another breath-holder.
Her bodily acid rate is rising.
Her kidneys are reabsorbing sodium.
Her balance of oxygen, carbon dioxide, and nitric oxide levels is disrupted.
She may end up with hypertension.
I wonder if she knows that this affects her sleep, memory, and learning, and that it causes anxiety and depression.
BREATHE!!

As the pace of productivity accelerates, and as social and environmental threats pile up, we're becoming an increasingly anxious species. It's a vicious cycle: Anxiety affects our ability to breathe and to sleep calmly, and our persistent lack of calm and sleep exacerbates all of the problems that lead to our anxiety in the first place!

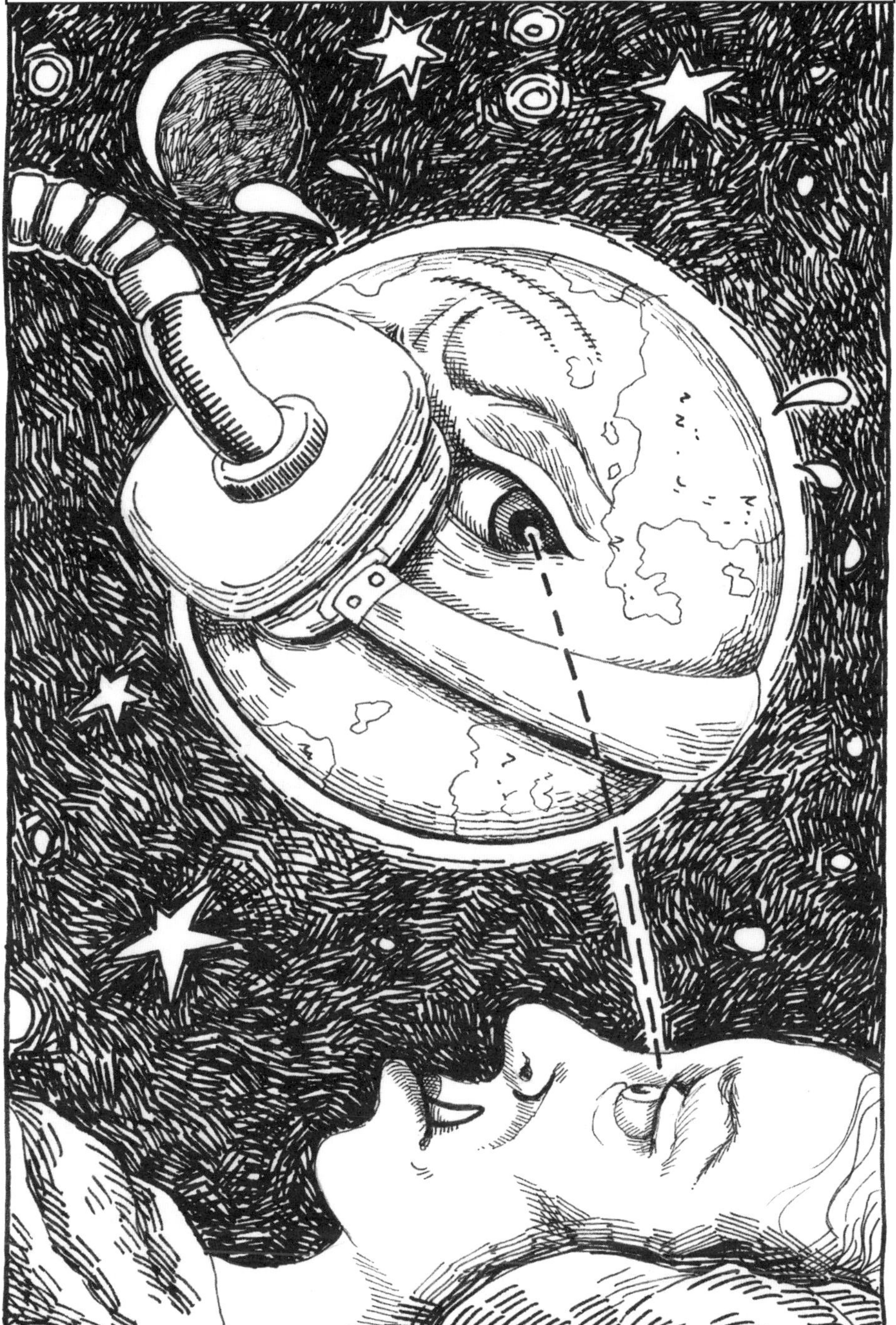

There is an opportunity here to stop, pause, and relearn how to breathe. Many of us today did not grow up doing the things that require conscious breathing, such as chanting, singing, playing the didgeridoo, or meditating. It can be helpful to do one or more of these things daily, especially before bed each evening.

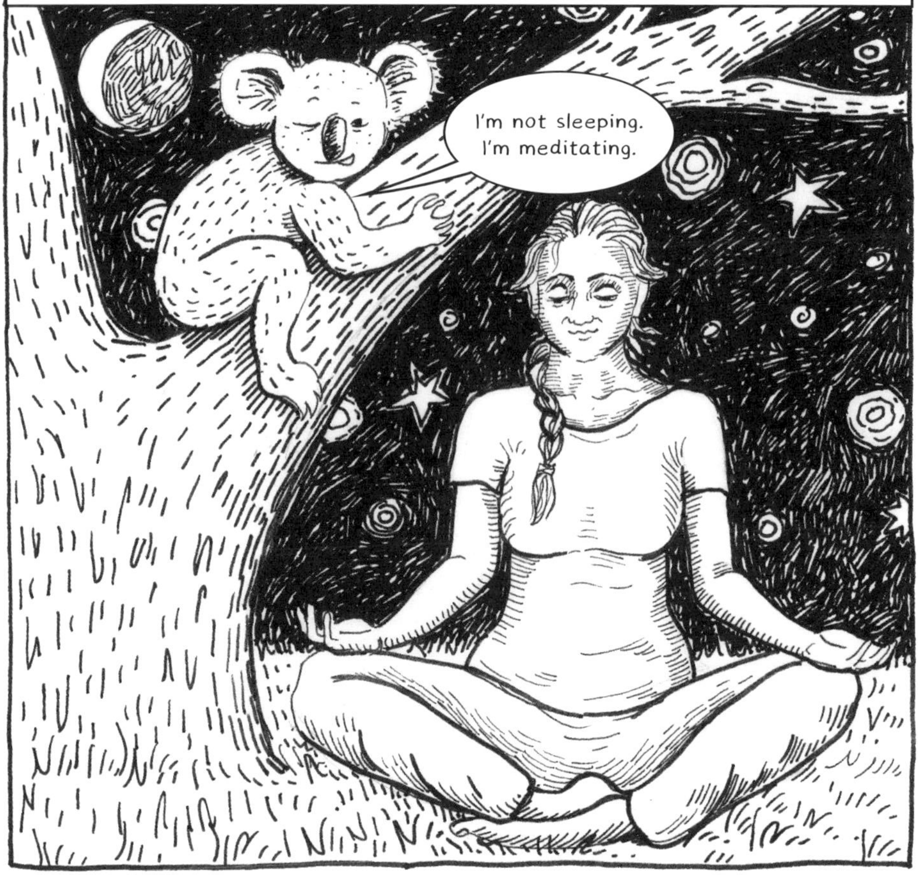
I'm not sleeping. I'm meditating.

Dr. Matt Walker, aka the Sleep Diplomat, would agree.

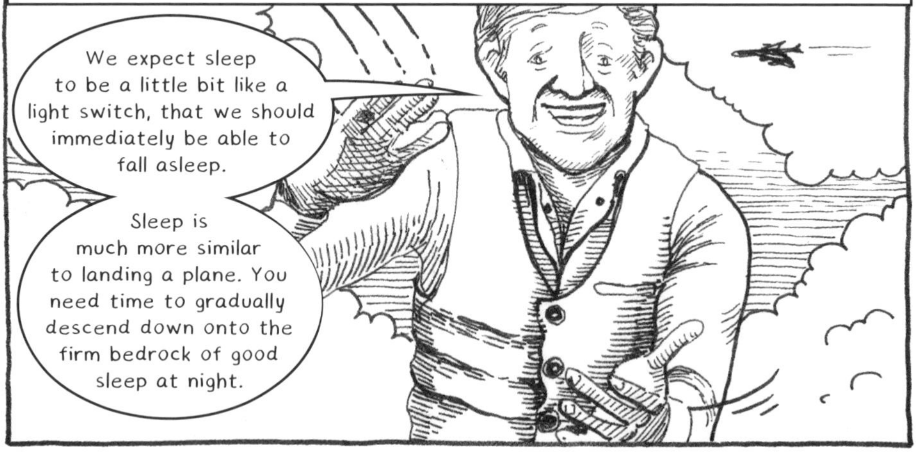
We expect sleep to be a little bit like a light switch, that we should immediately be able to fall asleep.
Sleep is much more similar to landing a plane. You need time to gradually descend down onto the firm bedrock of good sleep at night.

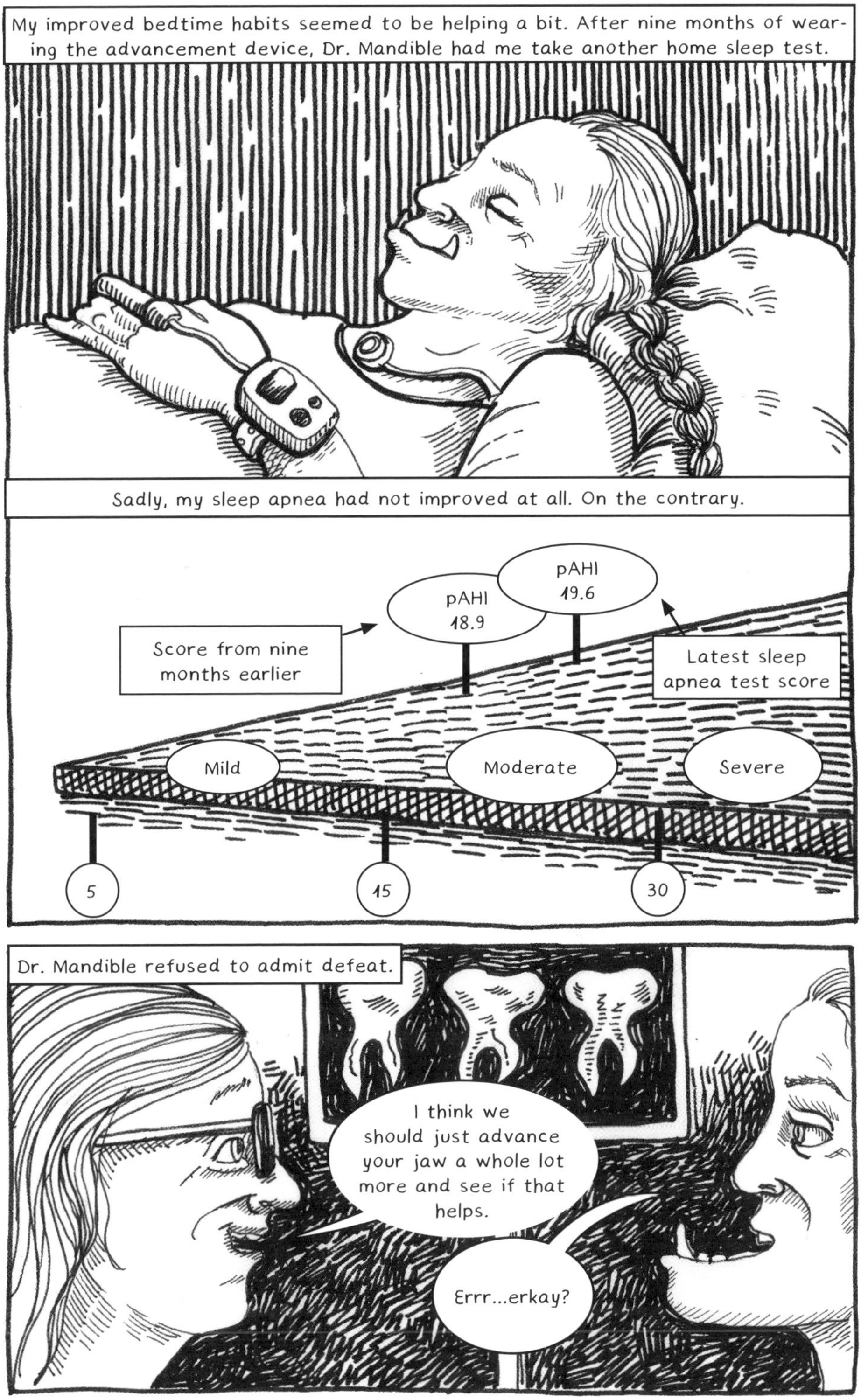
My improved bedtime habits seemed to be helping a bit. After nine months of wearing the advancement device, Dr. Mandible had me take another home sleep test.
Sadly, my sleep apnea had not improved at all. On the contrary.
Score from nine months earlier
pAHI 18.9
pAHI 19.6
Latest sleep apnea test score
Mild
Moderate
Severe
5
15
30
Dr. Mandible refused to admit defeat.
I think we should just advance your jaw a whole lot more and see if that helps.
Errr...erkay?

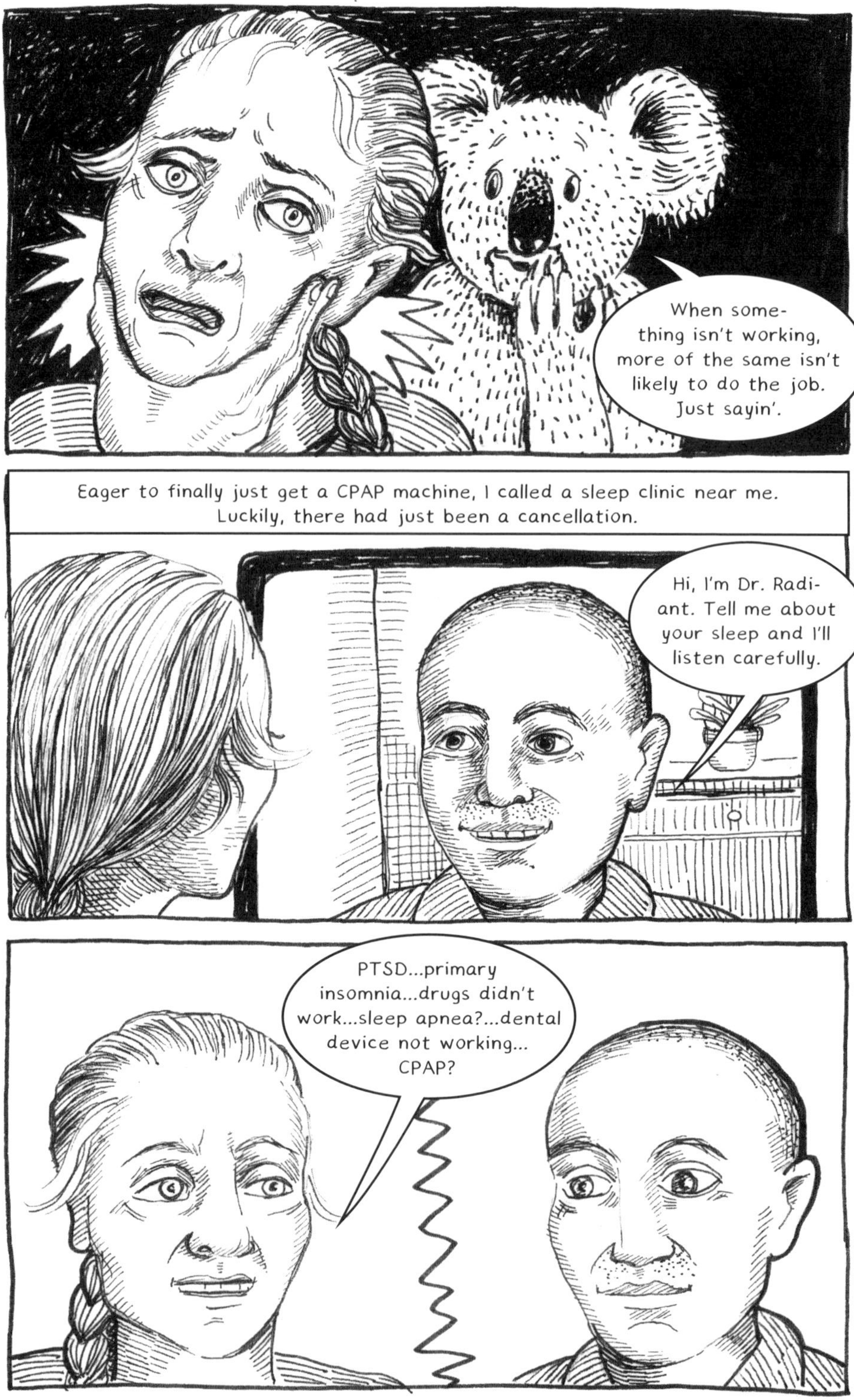
When some-thing isn't working, more of the same isn't likely to do the job. Just sayin'.
Eager to finally just get a CPAP machine, I called a sleep clinic near me. Luckily, there had just been a cancellation.
Hi, I'm Dr. Radi-ant. Tell me about your sleep and I'll listen carefully.
PTSD...primary insomnia...drugs didn't work...sleep apnea?...dental device not working... CPAP?

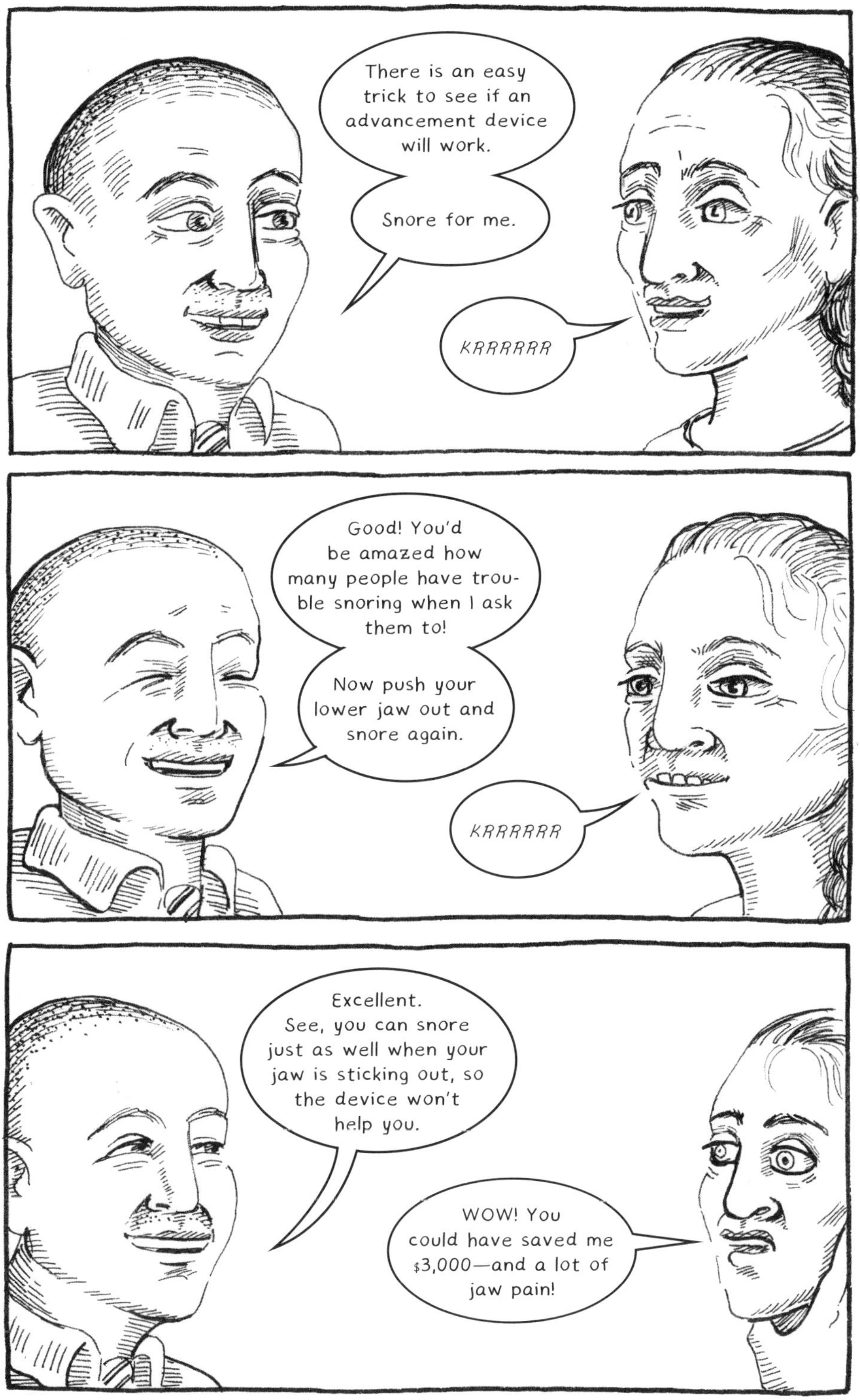
There is an easy trick to see if an advancement device will work.
Snore for me.
KRRRRRR
Good! You'd be amazed how many people have trouble snoring when I ask them to!
Now push your lower jaw out and snore again.
KRRRRRR
Excellent. See, you can snore just as well when your jaw is sticking out, so the device won't help you.
WOW! You could have saved me $3,000—and a lot of jaw pain!

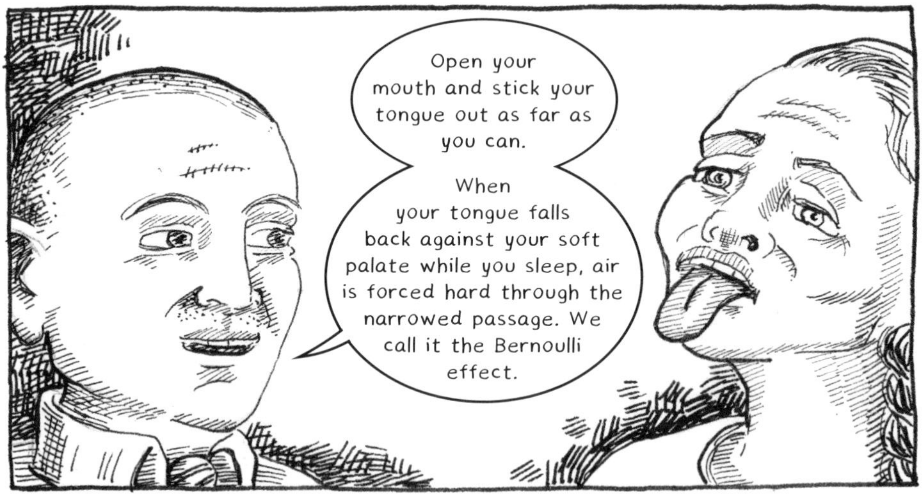
Open your mouth and stick your tongue out as far as you can.
When your tongue falls back against your soft palate while you sleep, air is forced hard through the narrowed passage. We call it the Bernoulli effect.

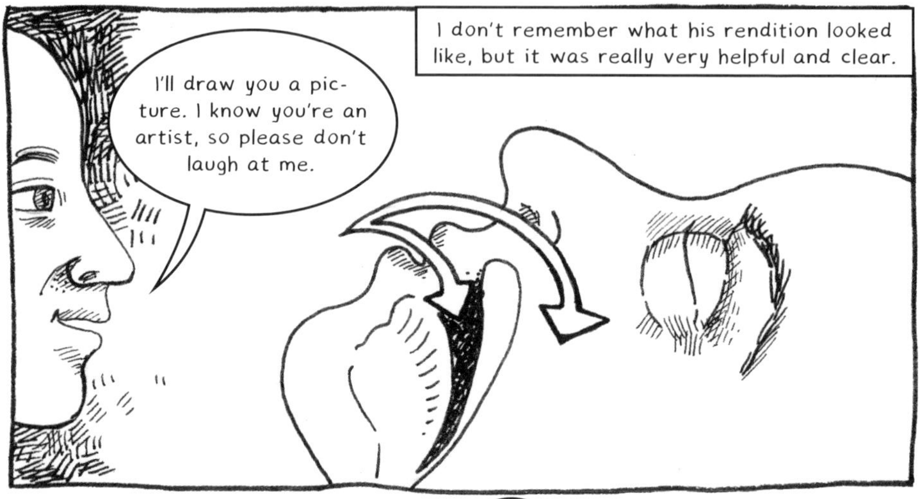
I don't remember what his rendition looked like, but it was really very helpful and clear.
I'll draw you a picture. I know you're an artist, so please don't laugh at me.

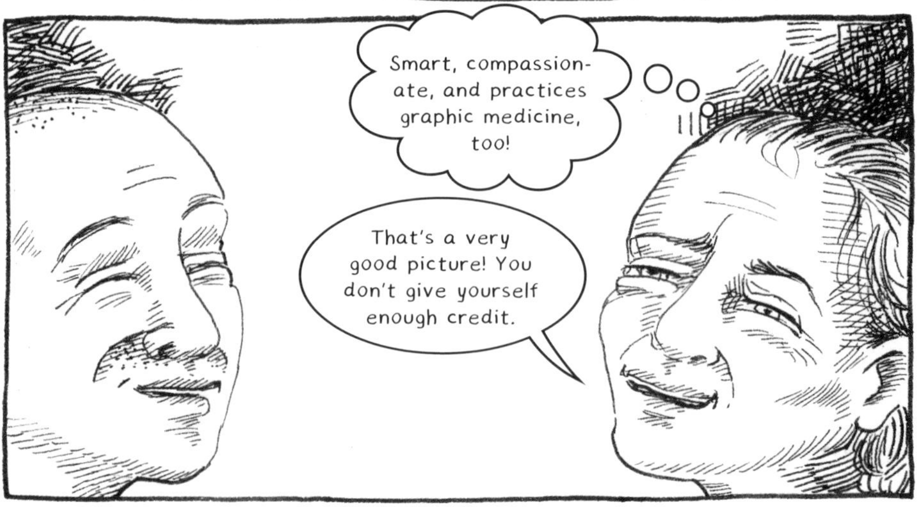
Smart, compassionate, and practices graphic medicine, too!
That's a very good picture! You don't give yourself enough credit.

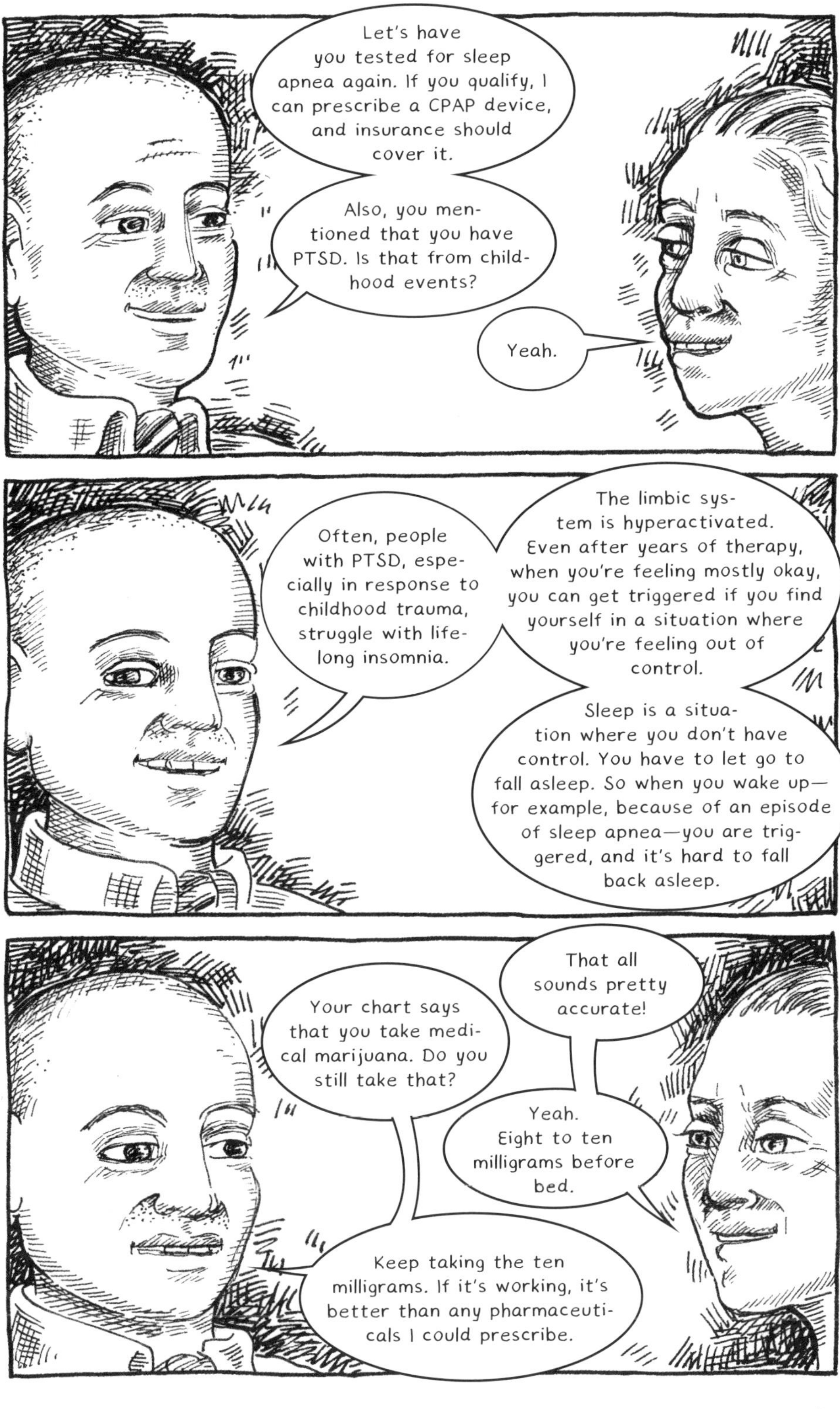
Let's have you tested for sleep apnea again. If you qualify, I can prescribe a CPAP device, and insurance should cover it.
Also, you mentioned that you have PTSD. Is that from childhood events?
Yeah.
Often, people with PTSD, especially in response to childhood trauma, struggle with lifelong insomnia.
The limbic system is hyperactivated. Even after years of therapy, when you're feeling mostly okay, you can get triggered if you find yourself in a situation where you're feeling out of control.
Sleep is a situation where you don't have control. You have to let go to fall asleep. So when you wake up—for example, because of an episode of sleep apnea—you are triggered, and it's hard to fall back asleep.
Your chart says that you take medical marijuana. Do you still take that?
That all sounds pretty accurate!
Yeah. Eight to ten milligrams before bed.
Keep taking the ten milligrams. If it's working, it's better than any pharmaceuticals I could prescribe.

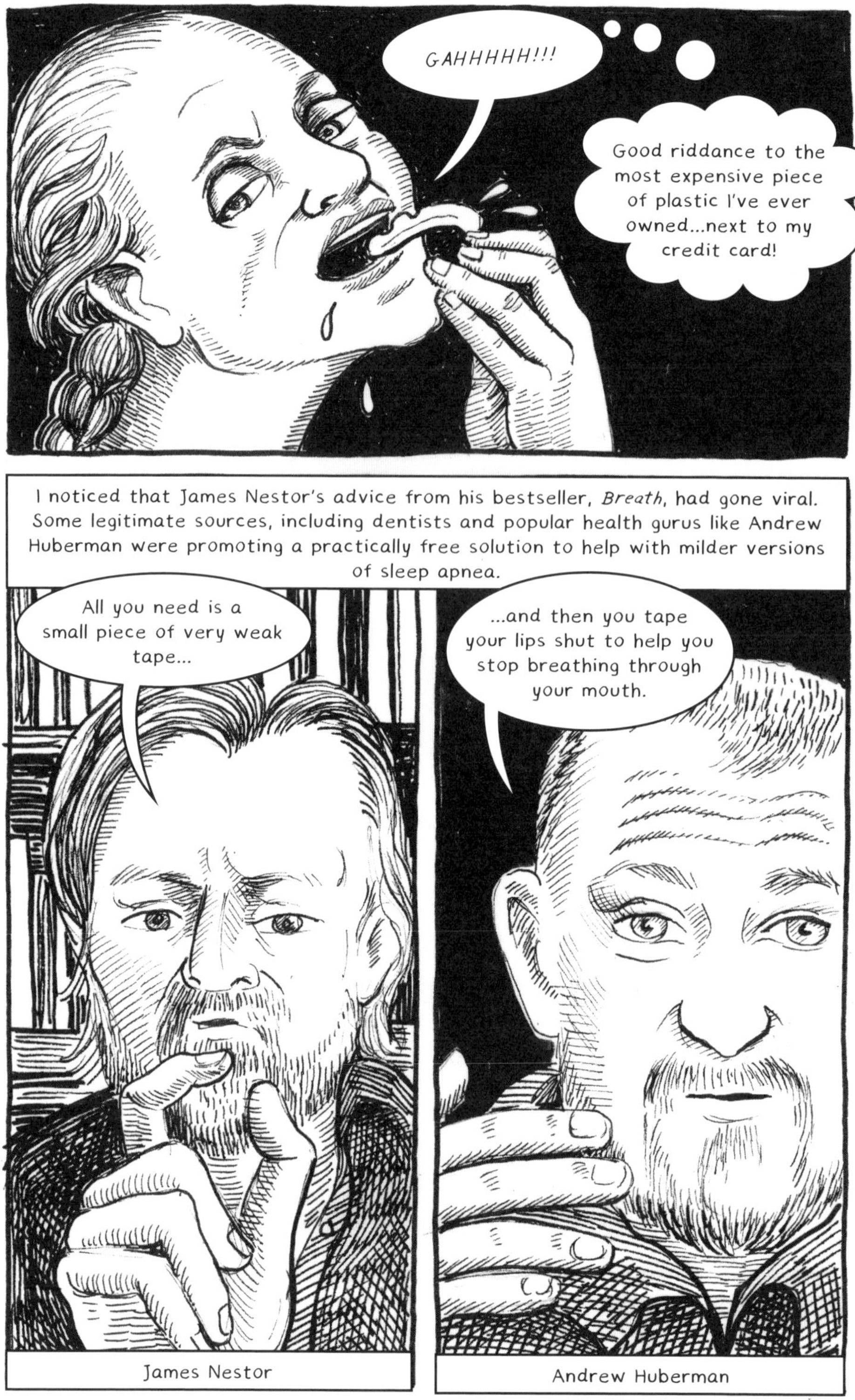
GAHHHHH!!!
Good riddance to the most expensive piece of plastic I've ever owned...next to my credit card!
I noticed that James Nestor's advice from his bestseller, *Breath*, had gone viral. Some legitimate sources, including dentists and popular health gurus like Andrew Huberman were promoting a practically free solution to help with milder versions of sleep apnea.
All you need is a small piece of very weak tape...
...and then you tape your lips shut to help you stop breathing through your mouth.
James Nestor
Andrew Huberman

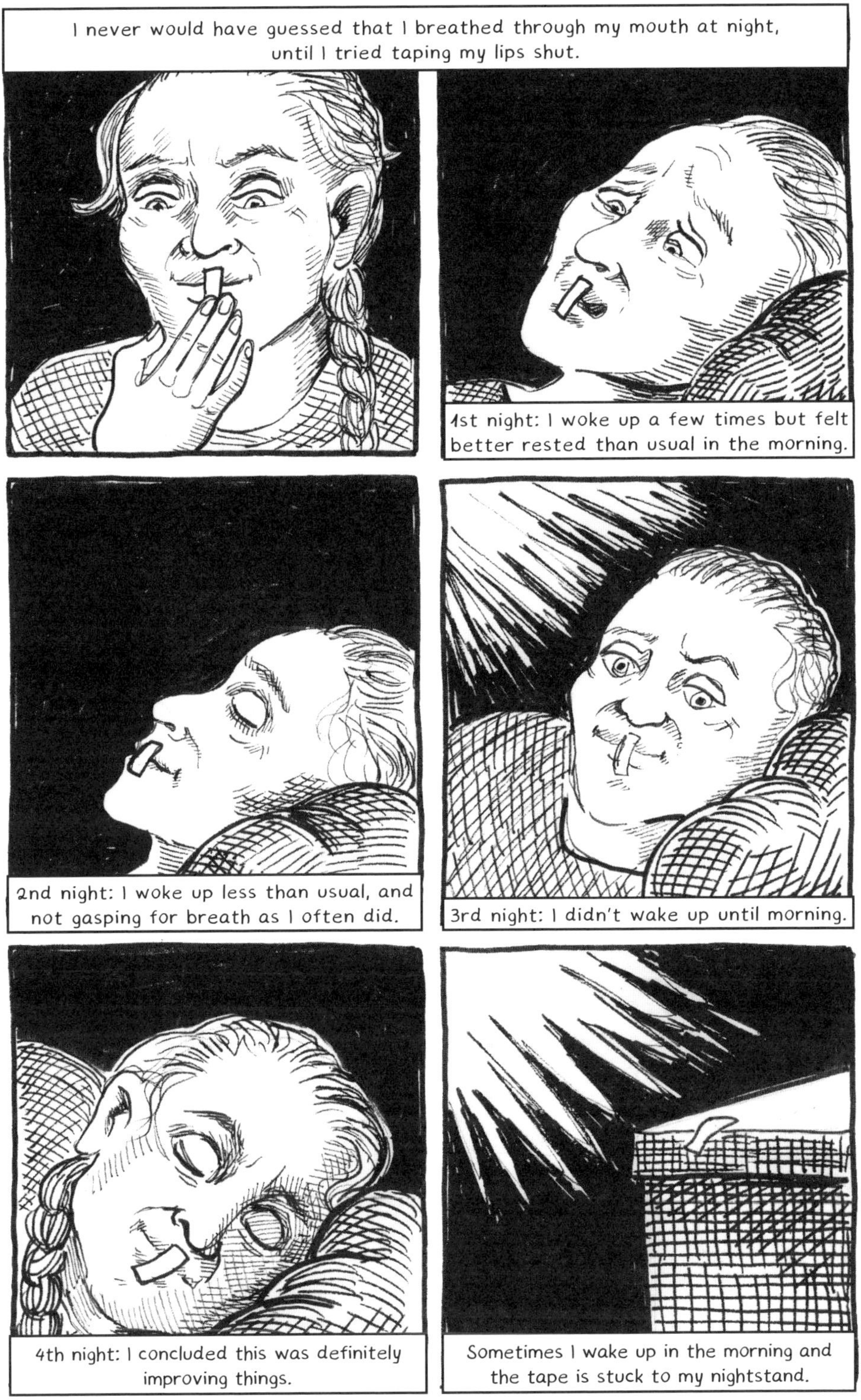
I never would have guessed that I breathed through my mouth at night, until I tried taping my lips shut.
1st night: I woke up a few times but felt better rested than usual in the morning.
2nd night: I woke up less than usual, and not gasping for breath as I often did.
3rd night: I didn't wake up until morning.
4th night: I concluded this was definitely improving things.
Sometimes I wake up in the morning and the tape is stuck to my nightstand.

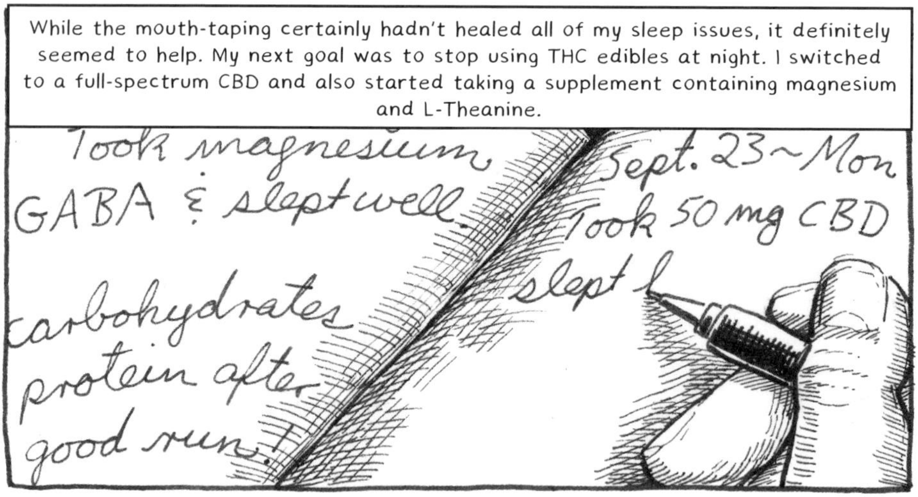
While the mouth-taping certainly hadn't healed all of my sleep issues, it definitely seemed to help. My next goal was to stop using THC edibles at night. I switched to a full-spectrum CBD and also started taking a supplement containing magnesium and L-Theanine.
Took magnesium GABA & slept well.
carbohydrates protein after good run!
Sept. 23~Mon
Took 50 mg CBD
slept l

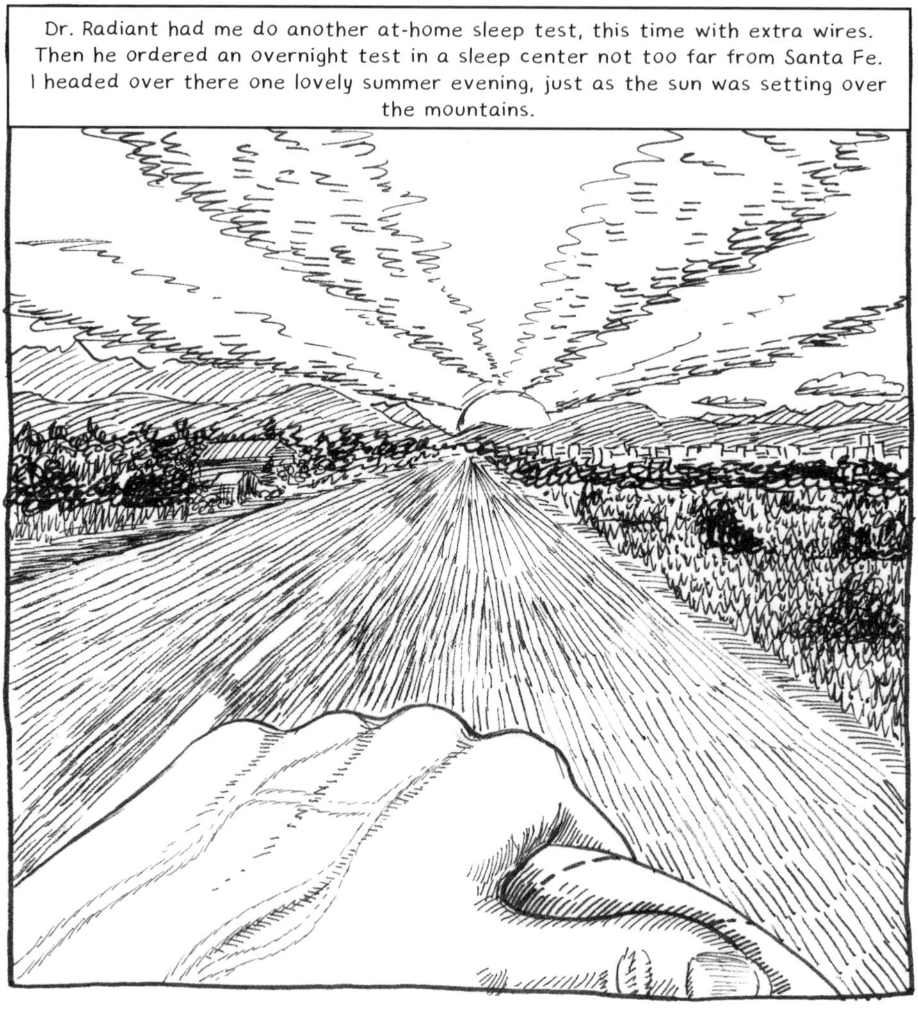
Dr. Radiant had me do another at-home sleep test, this time with extra wires. Then he ordered an overnight test in a sleep center not too far from Santa Fe. I headed over there one lovely summer evening, just as the sun was setting over the mountains.

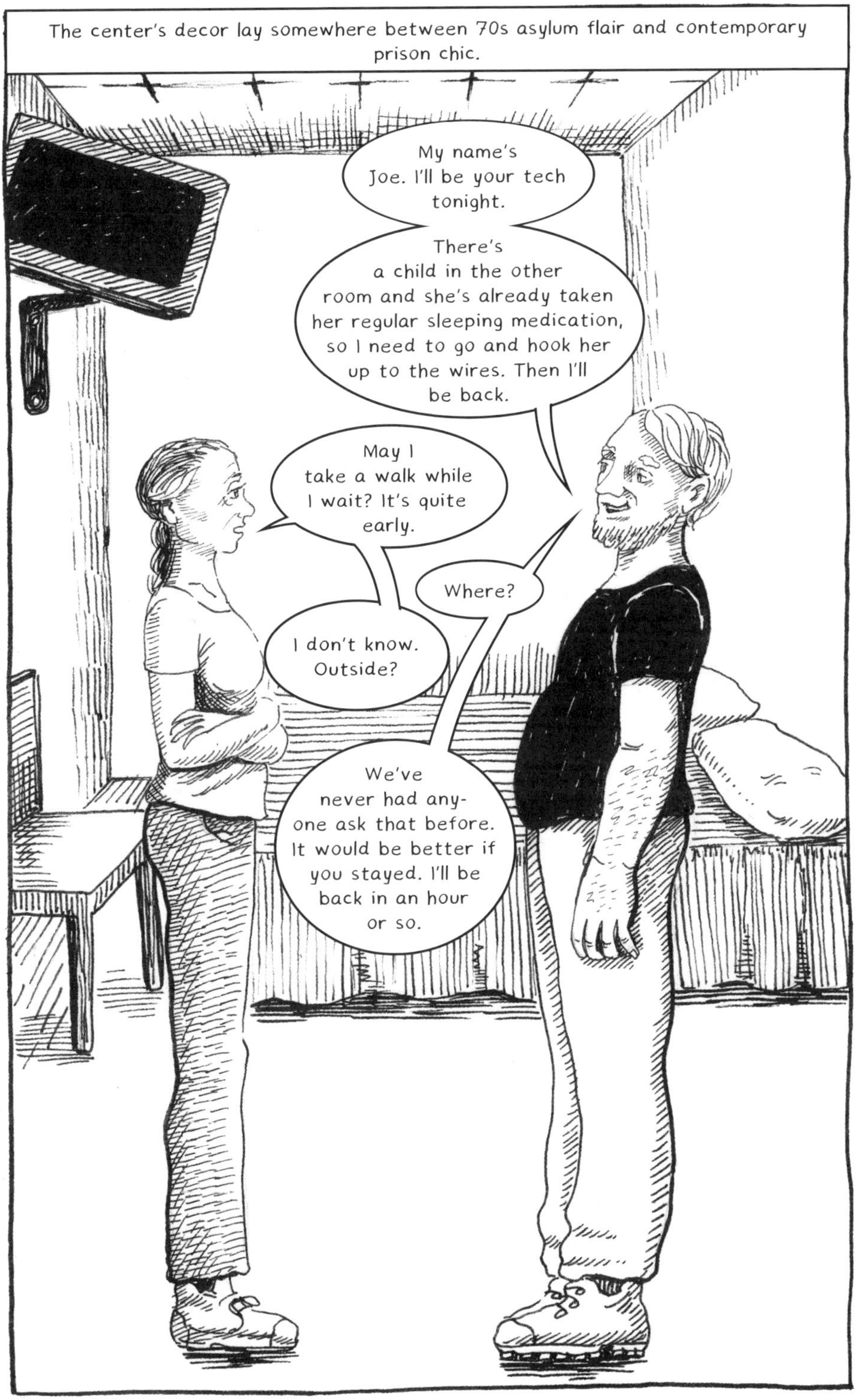
The center's decor lay somewhere between 70s asylum flair and contemporary prison chic.
My name's Joe. I'll be your tech tonight.
There's a child in the other room and she's already taken her regular sleeping medication, so I need to go and hook her up to the wires. Then I'll be back.
May I take a walk while I wait? It's quite early.
Where?
I don't know. Outside?
We've never had any-one ask that before. It would be better if you stayed. I'll be back in an hour or so.

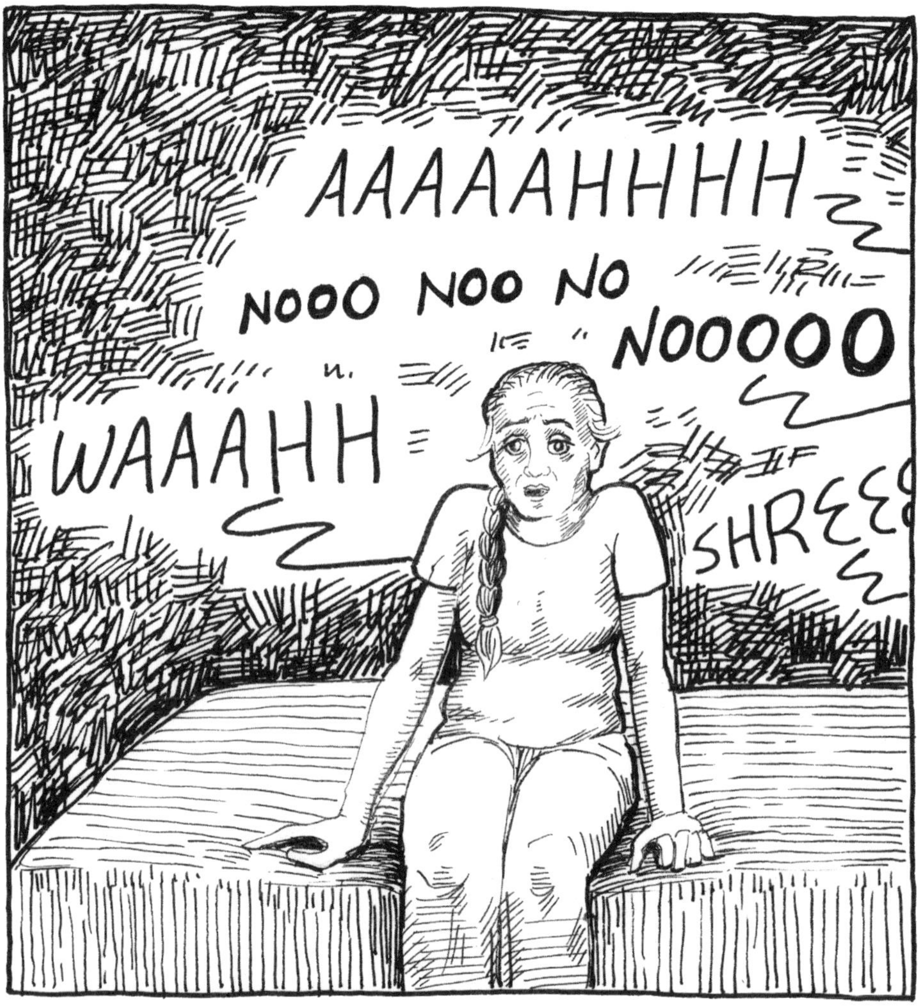
AAAAAHHHH
NOOO NOO NO
NOOOOO
WAAAHH
SHREE

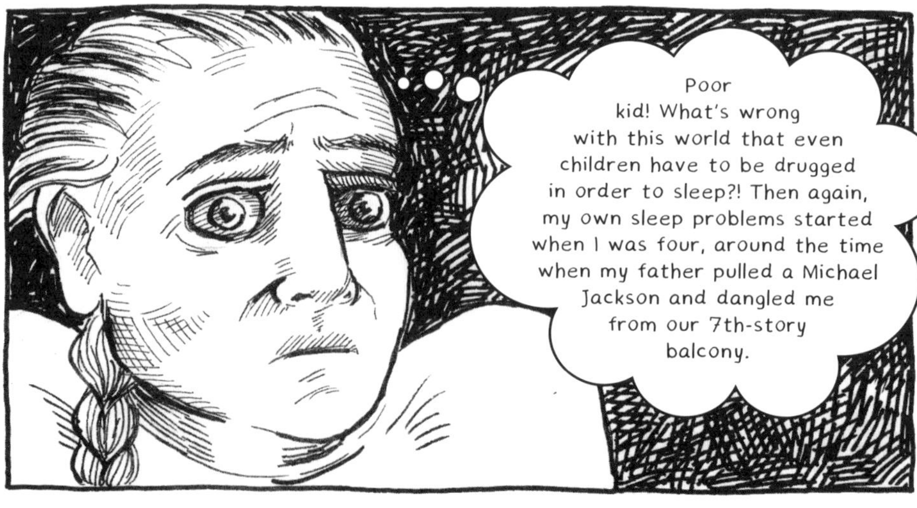
Poor kid! What's wrong with this world that even children have to be drugged in order to sleep?! Then again, my own sleep problems started when I was four, around the time when my father pulled a Michael Jackson and dangled me from our 7th-story balcony.

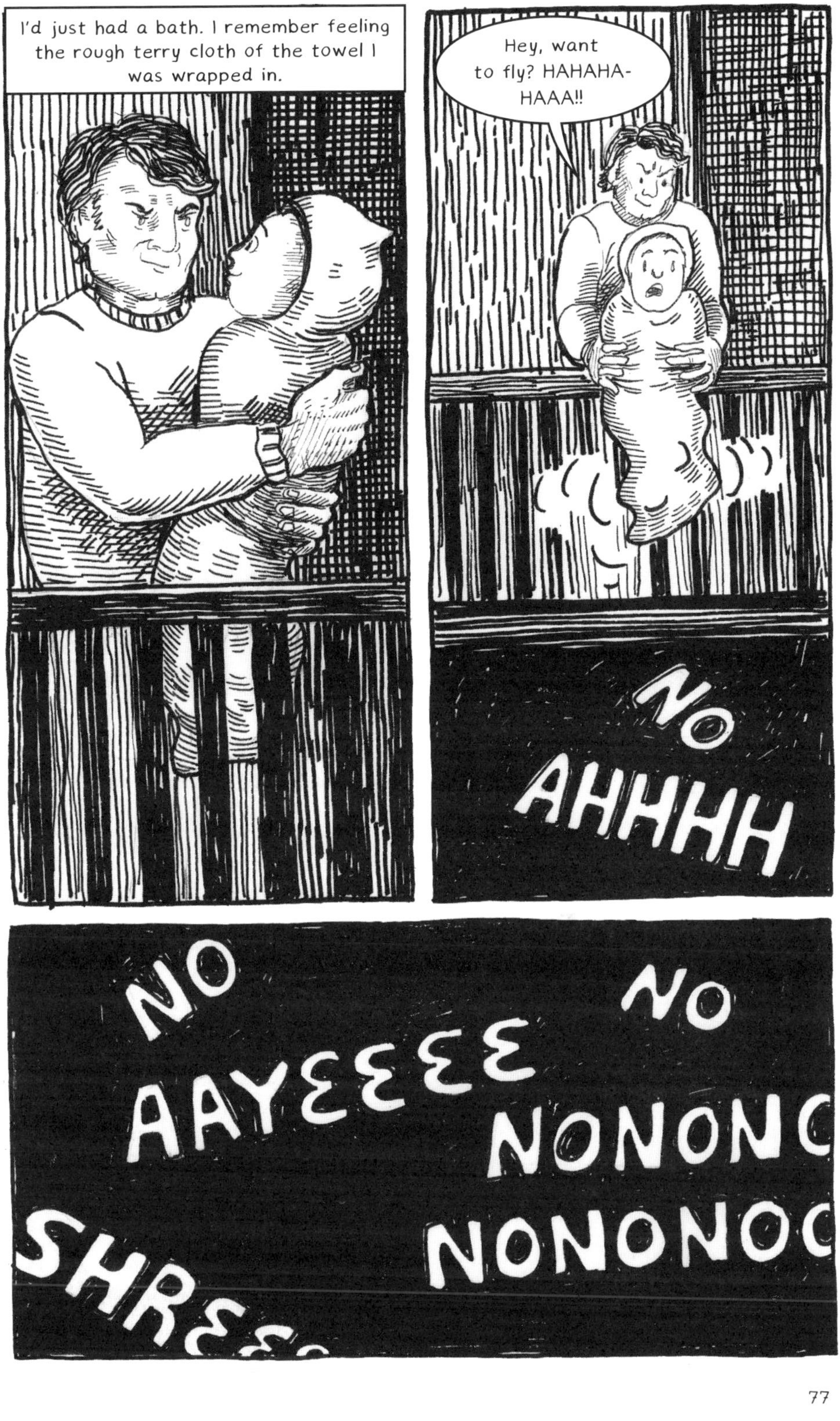

I'd just had a bath. I remember feeling the rough terry cloth of the towel I was wrapped in.
Hey, want to fly? HAHAHA-HAAA!!
NO
AHHHH
NO
NO
AAYEEEE
NONONO
NONONO
SHREE

NO
NOO
An hour and an eternity later, the screaming in the next room stopped.
Sorry about that. She really hated having the wires put on.
Let's get you hooked up now.
Just a few more...

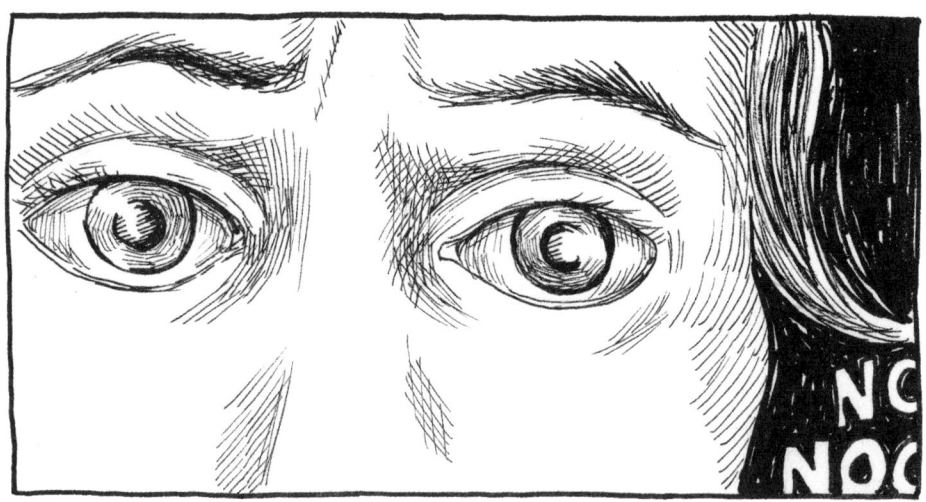

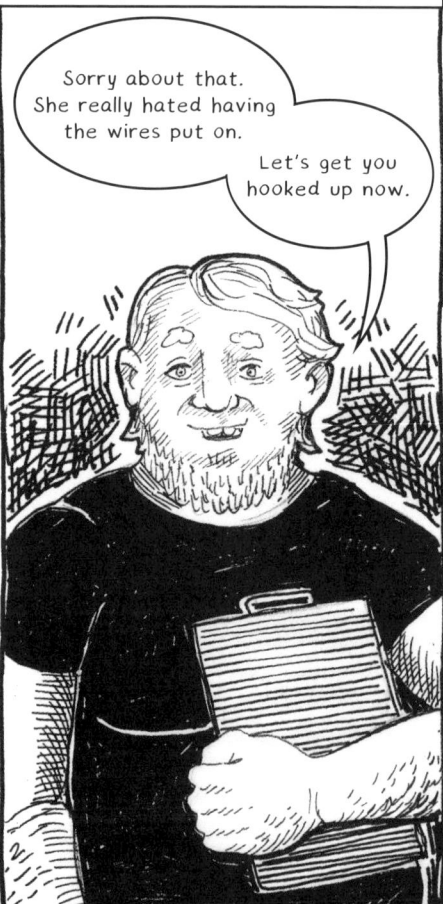

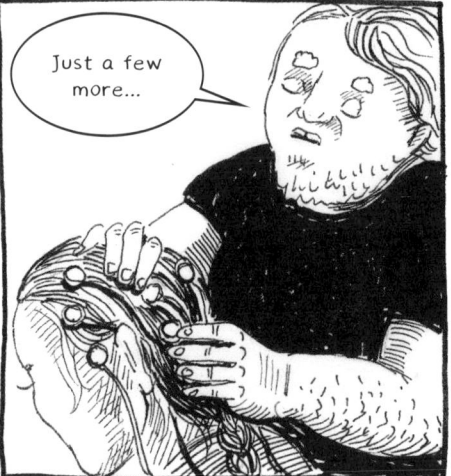

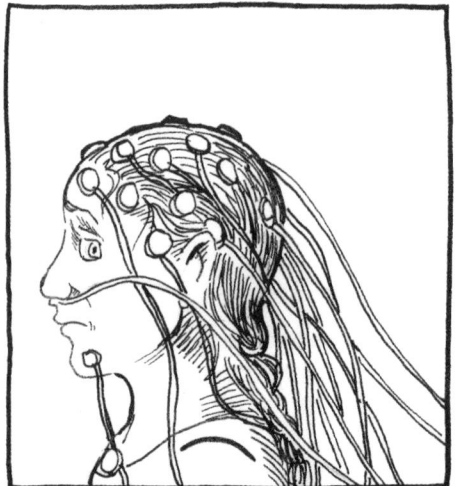

Sleep well!

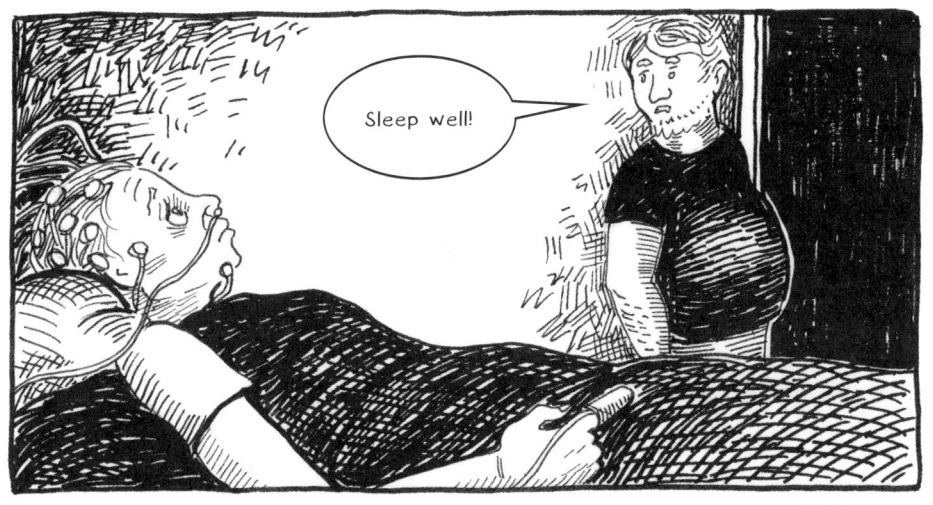

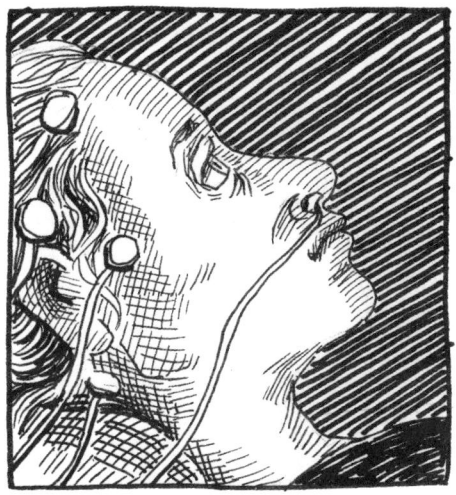

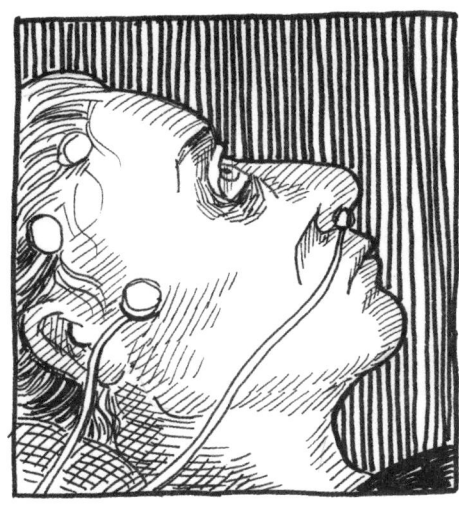

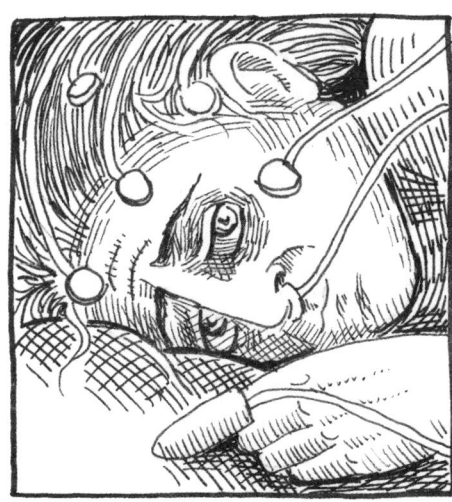

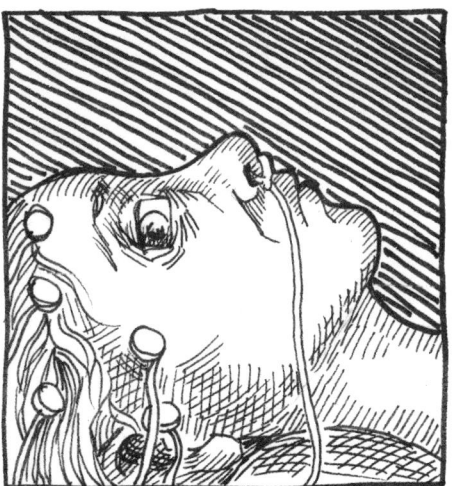

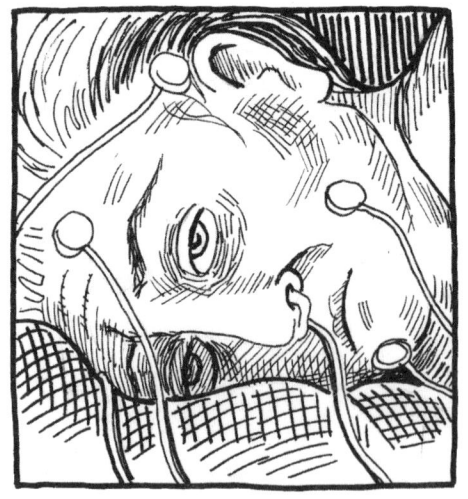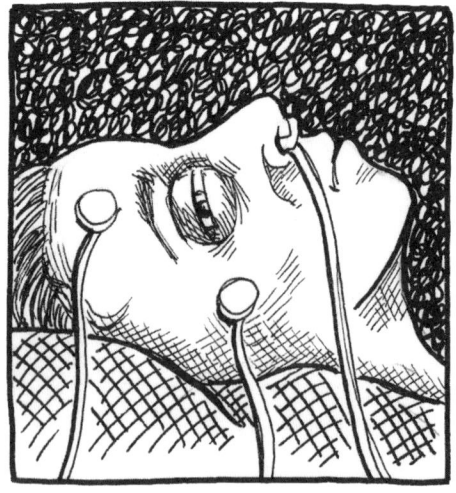

About two hours later...

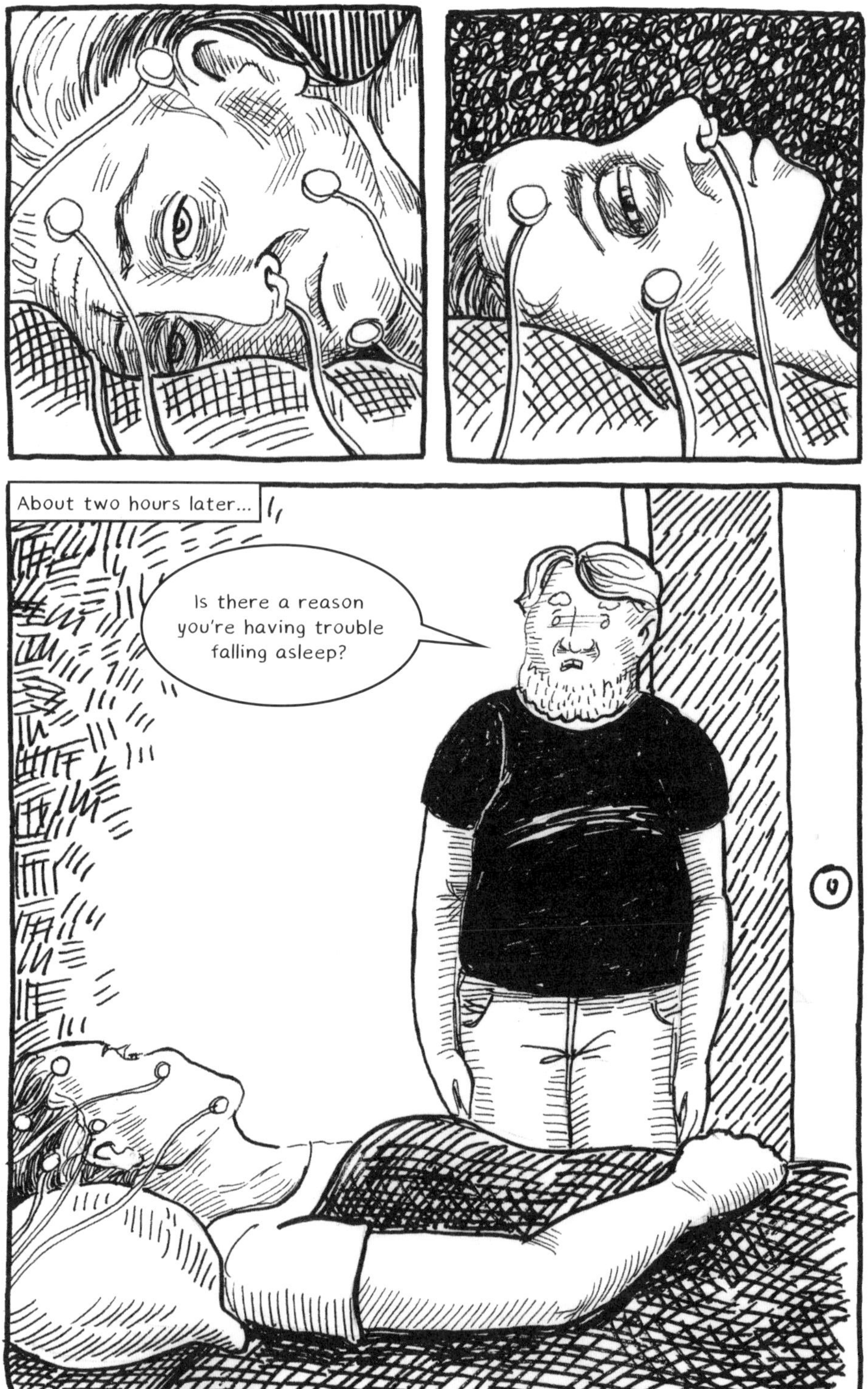

Is there a reason you're having trouble falling asleep?

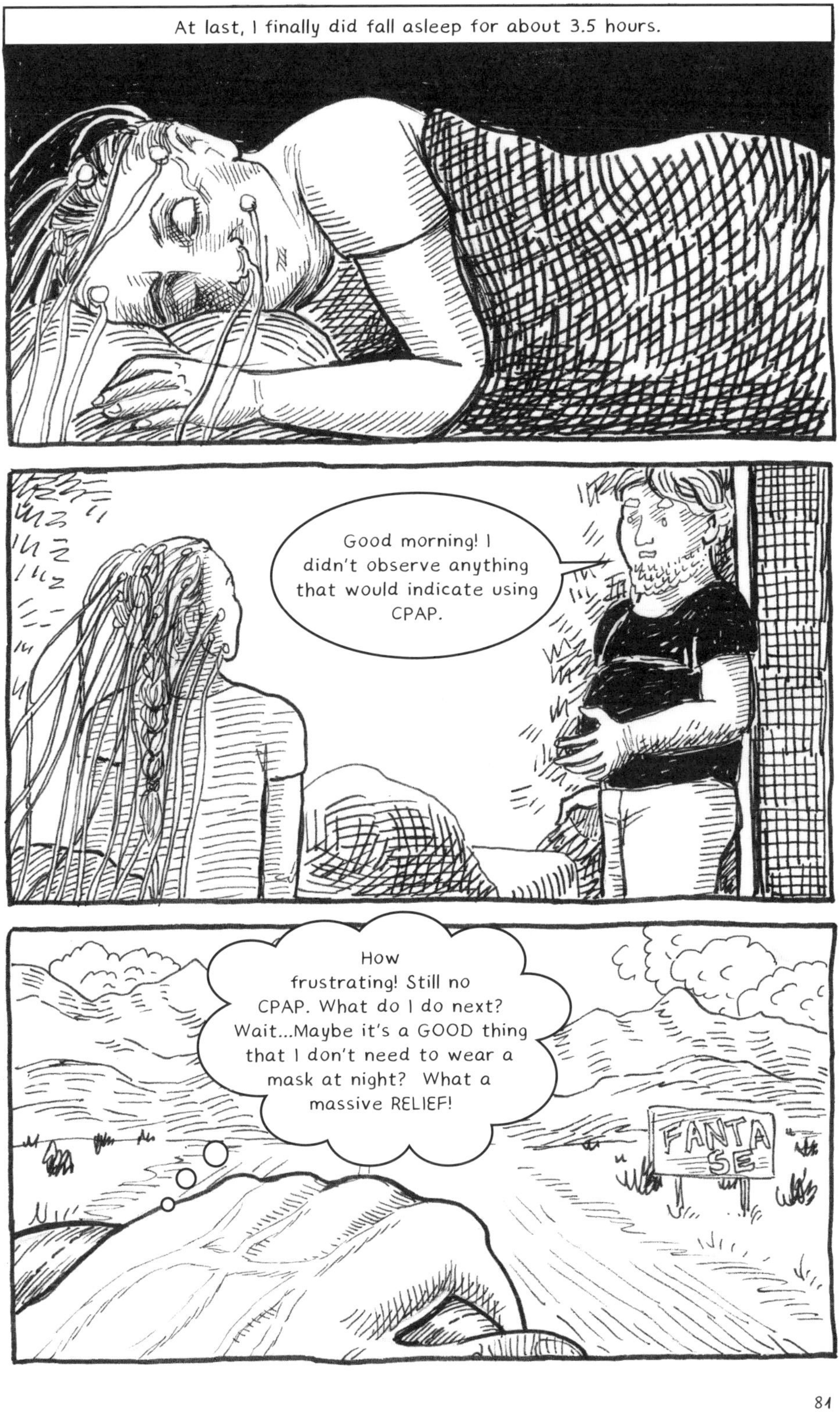
At last, I finally did fall asleep for about 3.5 hours.
Good morning! I didn't observe anything that would indicate using CPAP.
How frustrating! Still no CPAP. What do I do next? Wait...Maybe it's a GOOD thing that I don't need to wear a mask at night? What a massive RELIEF!
FANTA SE

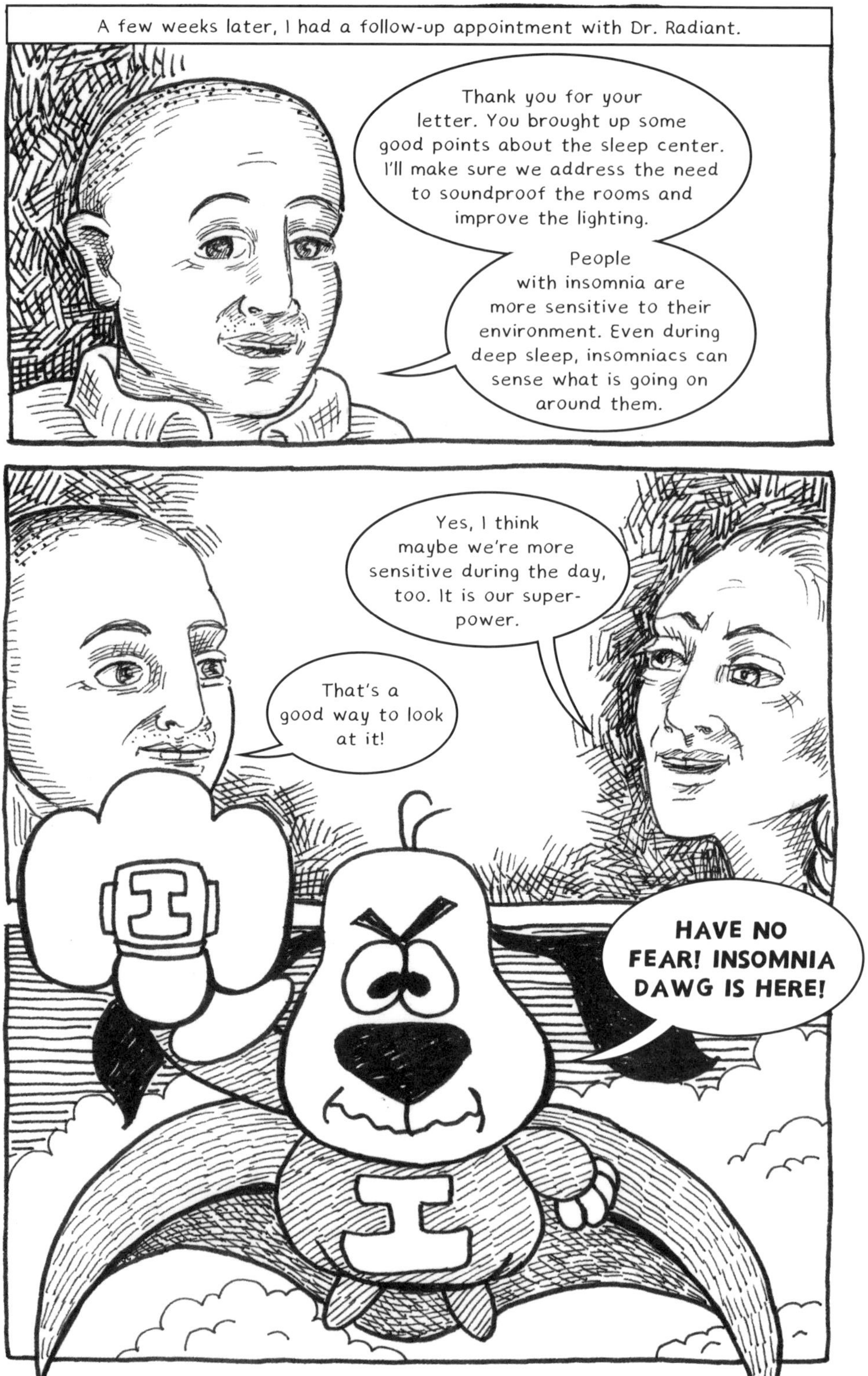
A few weeks later, I had a follow-up appointment with Dr. Radiant.
Thank you for your letter. You brought up some good points about the sleep center. I'll make sure we address the need to soundproof the rooms and improve the lighting.
People with insomnia are more sensitive to their environment. Even during deep sleep, insomniacs can sense what is going on around them.
Yes, I think maybe we're more sensitive during the day, too. It is our super-power.
That's a good way to look at it!
HAVE NO FEAR! INSOMNIA DAWG IS HERE!

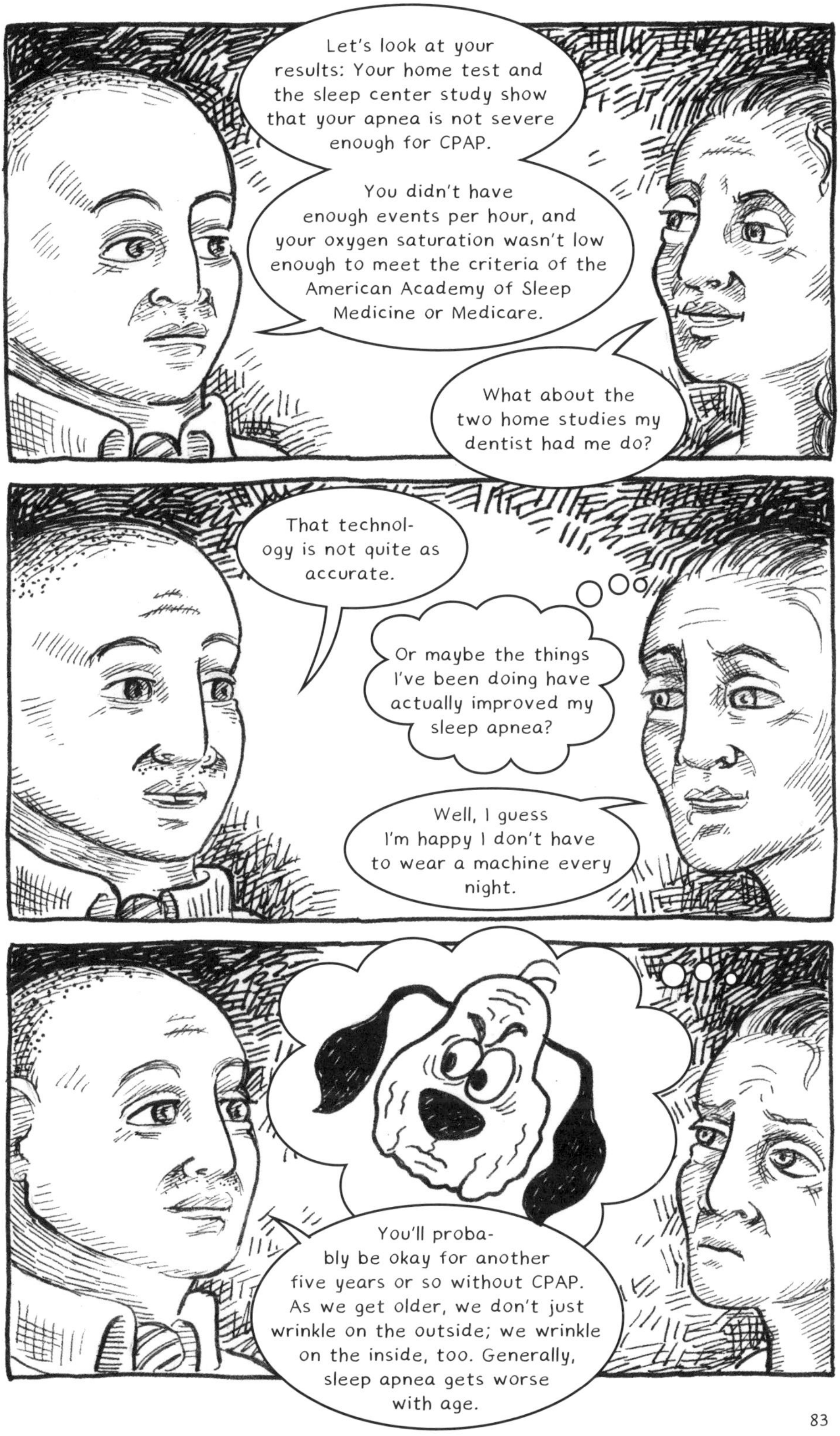

Let's look at your results: Your home test and the sleep center study show that your apnea is not severe enough for CPAP.
You didn't have enough events per hour, and your oxygen saturation wasn't low enough to meet the criteria of the American Academy of Sleep Medicine or Medicare.
What about the two home studies my dentist had me do?
That technol-ogy is not quite as accurate.
Or maybe the things I've been doing have actually improved my sleep apnea?
Well, I guess I'm happy I don't have to wear a machine every night.
You'll proba-bly be okay for another five years or so without CPAP. As we get older, we don't just wrinkle on the outside; we wrinkle on the inside, too. Generally, sleep apnea gets worse with age.

A colleague of mine told me that playing a wind instrument can help...
Yes, that was it! My colleague sent me the details of a study...
Yes! That's the one!
You mean the didgeridoo?
The Swiss one from 2006, right?
I've noticed that, in addition to strengthening oropharyngeal muscles, playing the didge requires long exhalations, thus stimulating the parasympathetic nervous system. It helps me relax.
Right!
Mouth-taping also seems to help with apnea.
Haha! I've heard of that. I'm not too convinced, though.
It seems to be helping me. I'm waking up less and grinding my teeth much less. My jaw pain is gone. And I almost never need THC anymore.
Interesting... You may find that you'll need to use the THC every now and then.

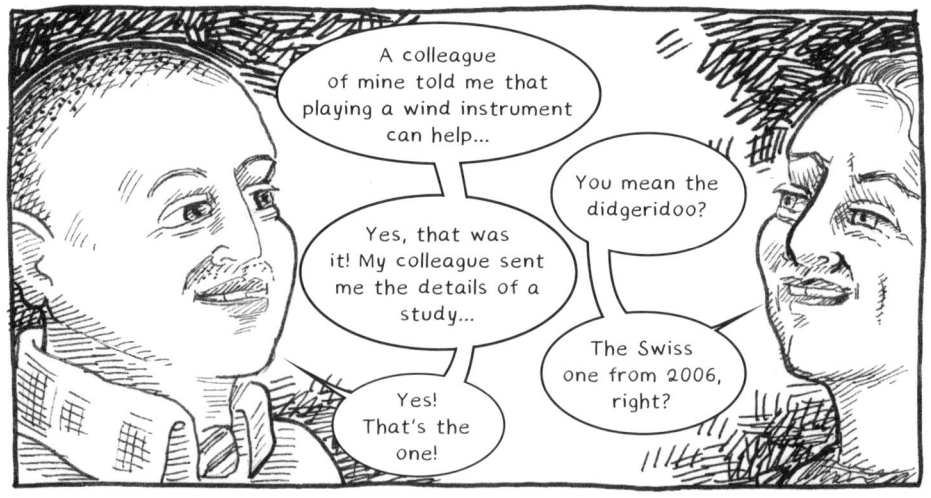

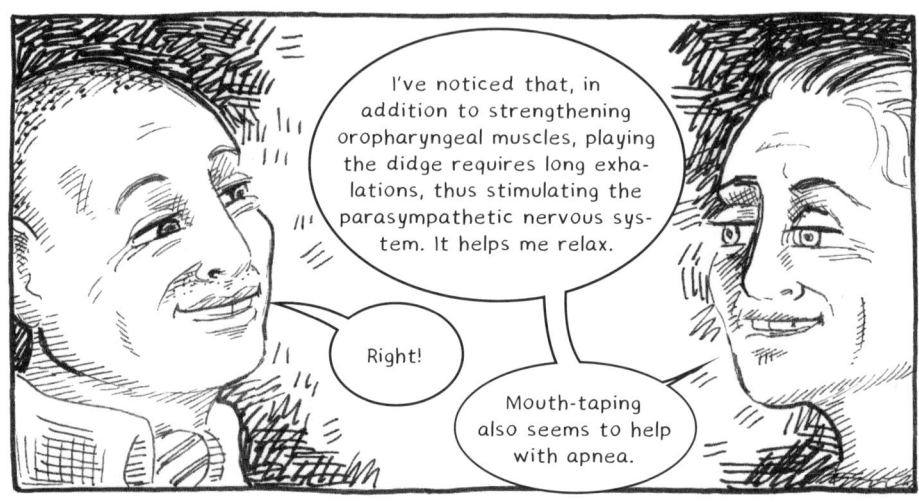

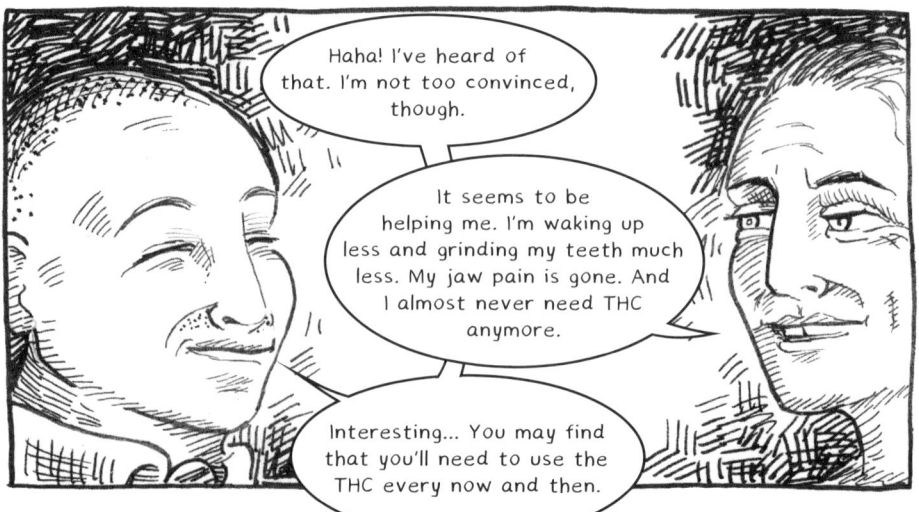

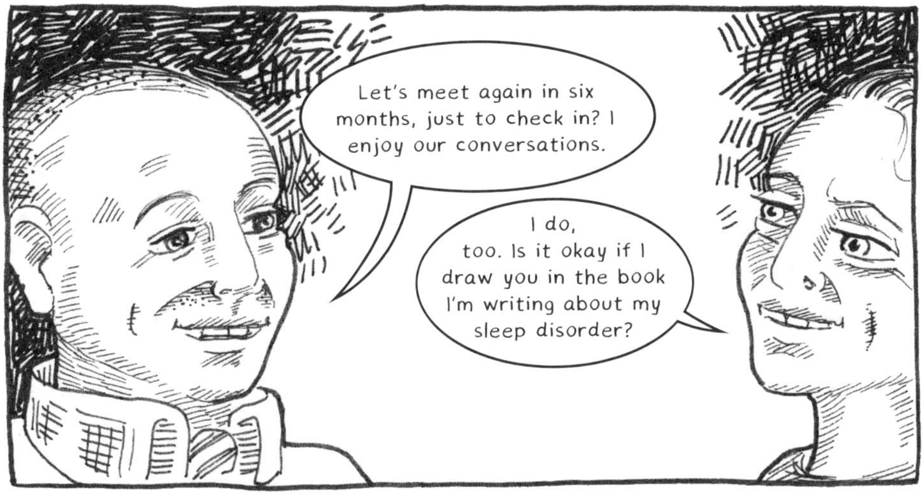
Let's meet again in six months, just to check in? I enjoy our conversations.
I do, too. Is it okay if I draw you in the book I'm writing about my sleep disorder?

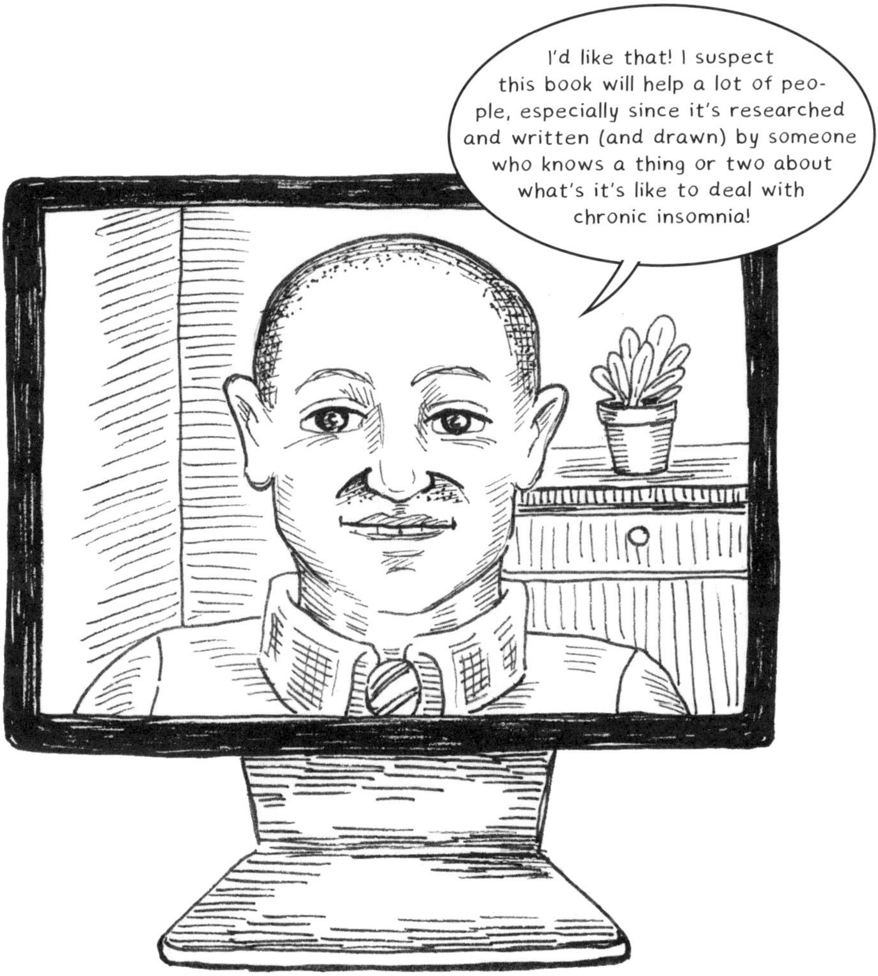
I'd like that! I suspect this book will help a lot of people, especially since it's researched and written (and drawn) by someone who knows a thing or two about what's it's like to deal with chronic insomnia!

Sleep
Hormones
Health
META-
BOLISM

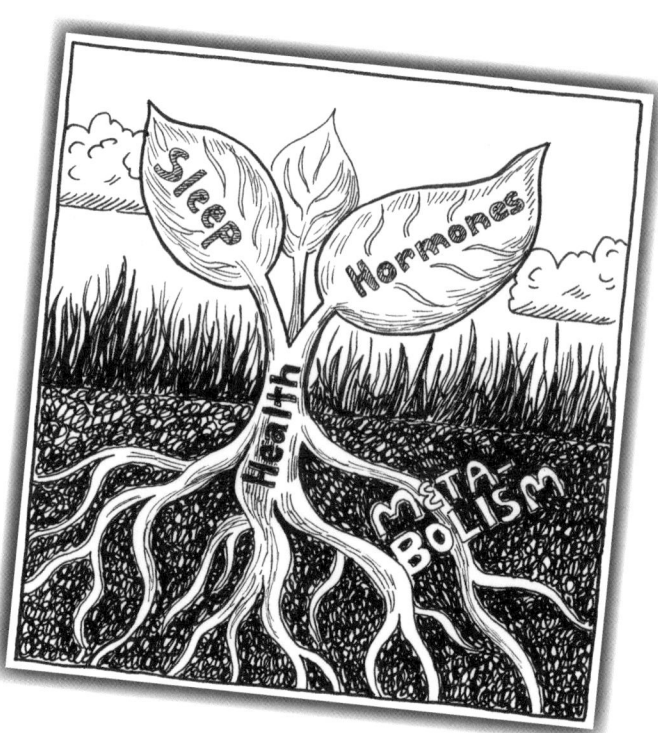

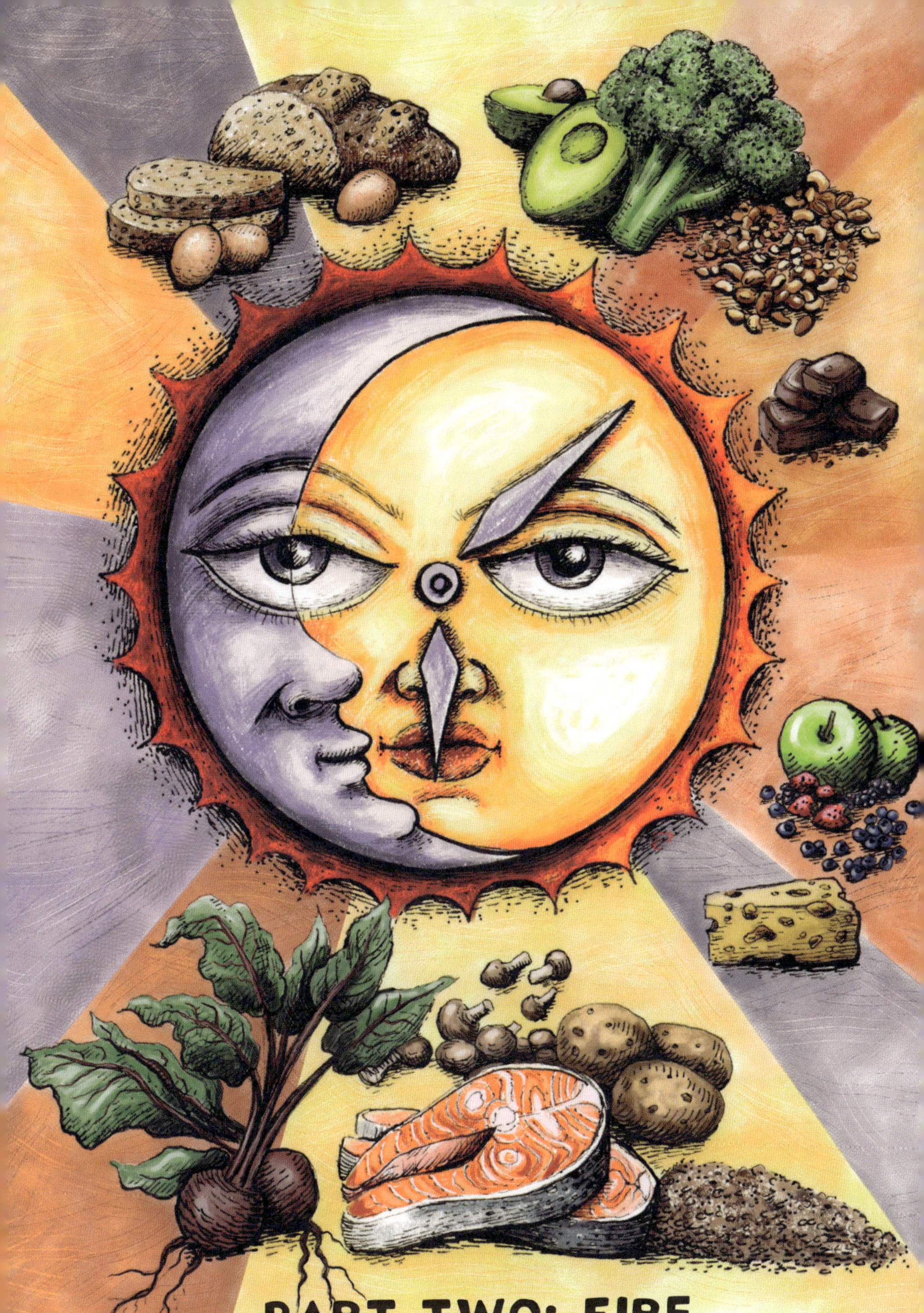

PART TWO: FIRE

The Metabolic Furnace

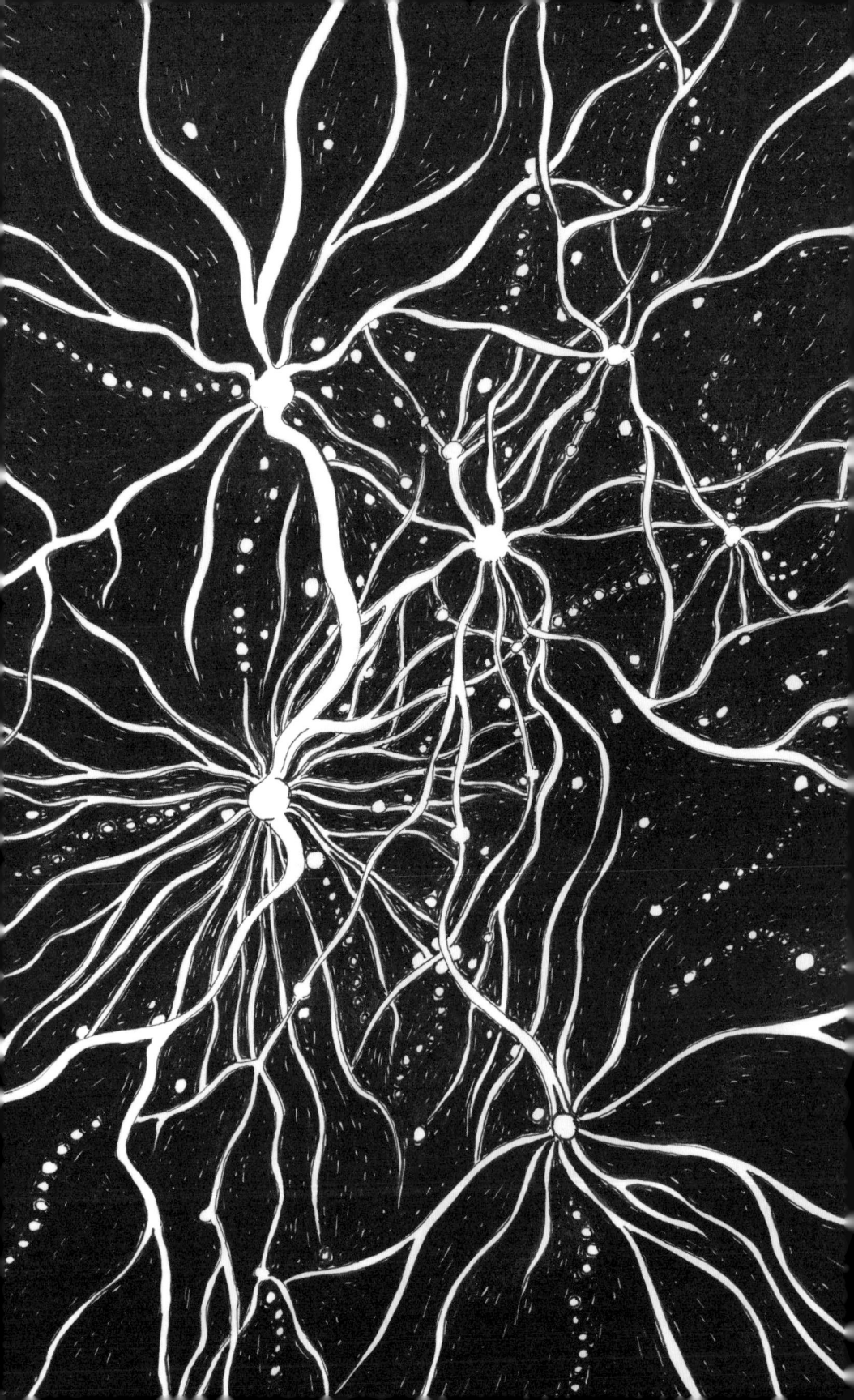

As it turns out, women are twice as likely as men to have insomnia. My own insomnia had definitely gotten worse when I was in my perimenopausal forties.
Sleep issues among peri- and postmenopausal women increase from affecting one in four women in the US to about one in two—that's half of all women! This is likely explained by hormonal shifts occurring at this stage of life, and by the generalized anxiety women feel about living in an aging woman's body in a misogynistic world.
after (post) menopause
during (peri) menopause
before (pre) menopause
JOB SEARCH
Thanks for your interest but no thanks
Sincerely, Search Team
Women in other parts of the world, like China and Japan, report fewer problems during menopause. This seems to hinge on multiple factors, including cultural attitudes.
It's harder to see my future. Prospects seem grim.
I'm so excited! I've entered my second spring!

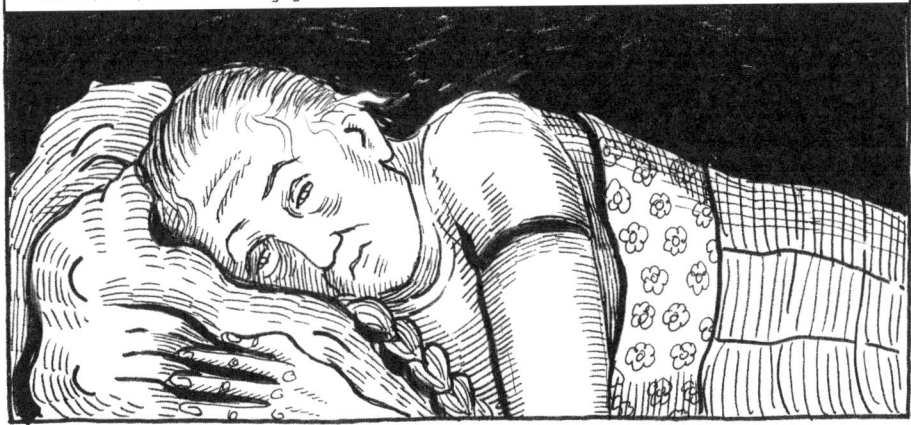

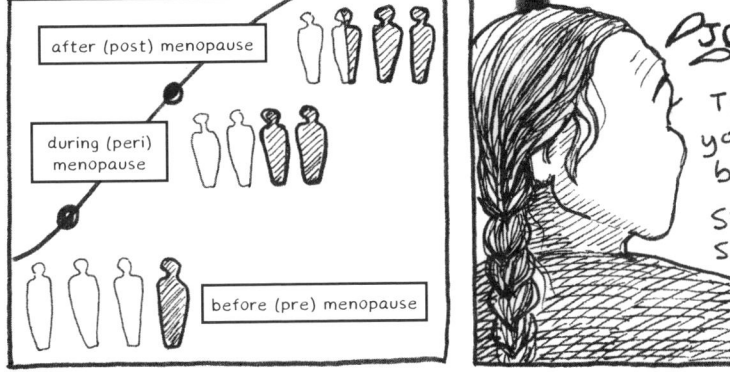

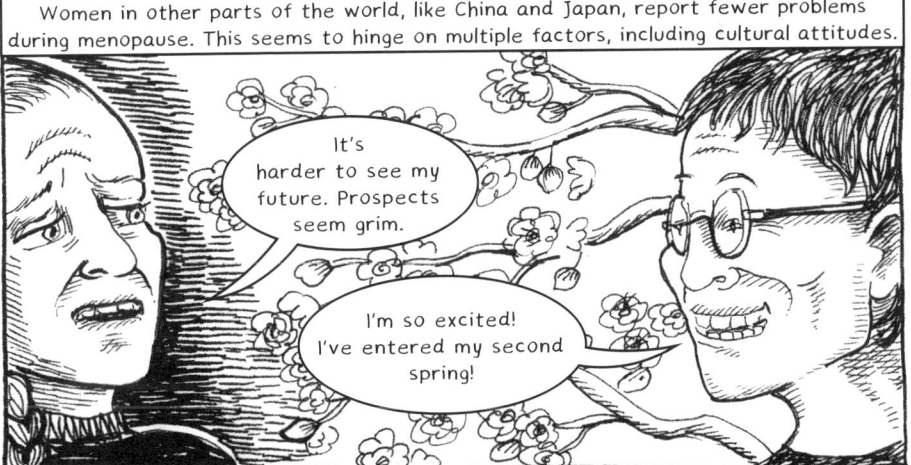

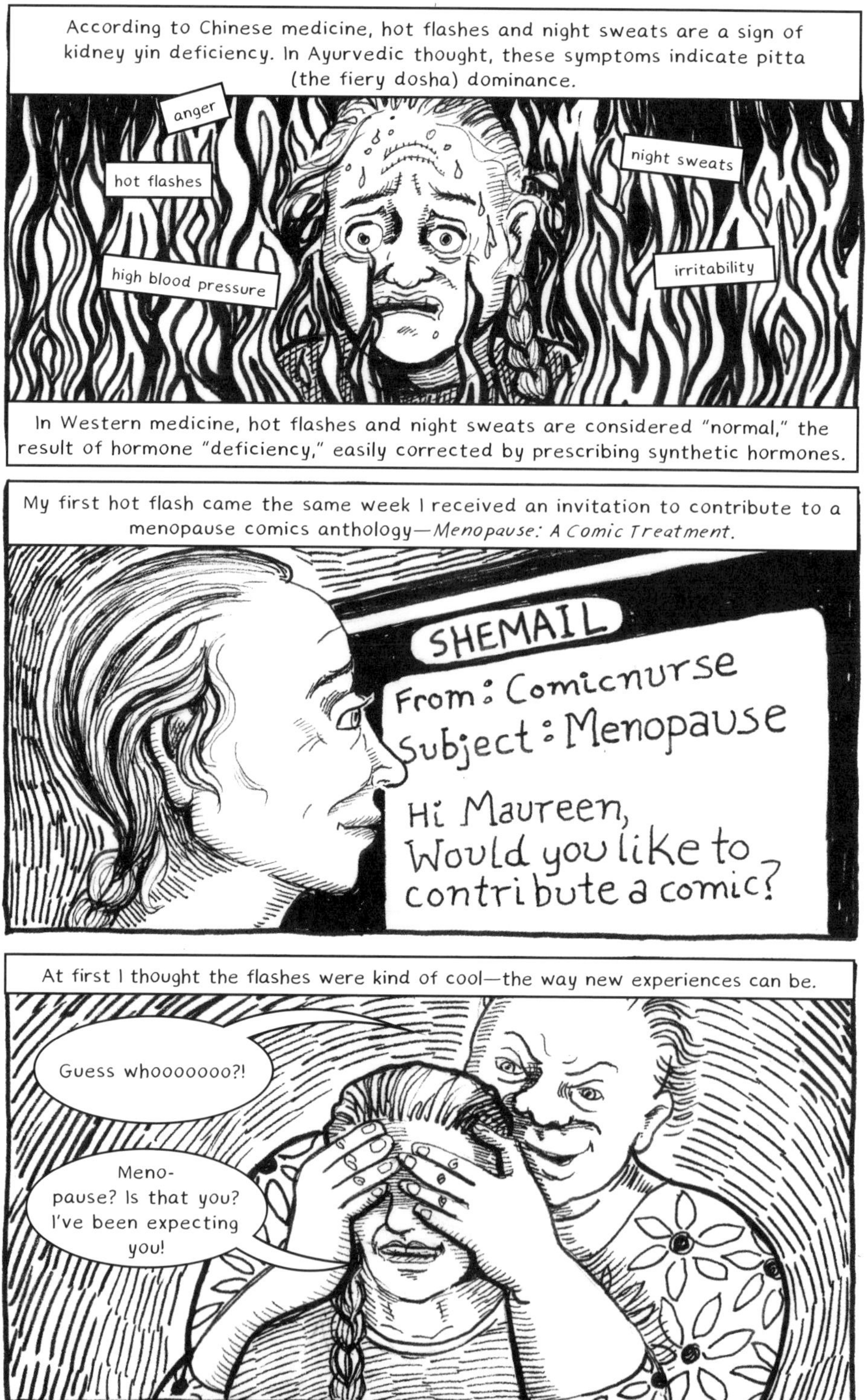
According to Chinese medicine, hot flashes and night sweats are a sign of kidney yin deficiency. In Ayurvedic thought, these symptoms indicate pitta (the fiery dosha) dominance.
anger
hot flashes
night sweats
high blood pressure
irritability
In Western medicine, hot flashes and night sweats are considered "normal," the result of hormone "deficiency," easily corrected by prescribing synthetic hormones.
My first hot flash came the same week I received an invitation to contribute to a menopause comics anthology—*Menopause: A Comic Treatment*.
SHEMAIL
From: Comicnurse
Subject: Menopause
Hi Maureen,
Would you like to contribute a comic?
At first I thought the flashes were kind of cool—the way new experiences can be.
Guess whooooooo?!
Meno-pause? Is that you? I've been expecting you!

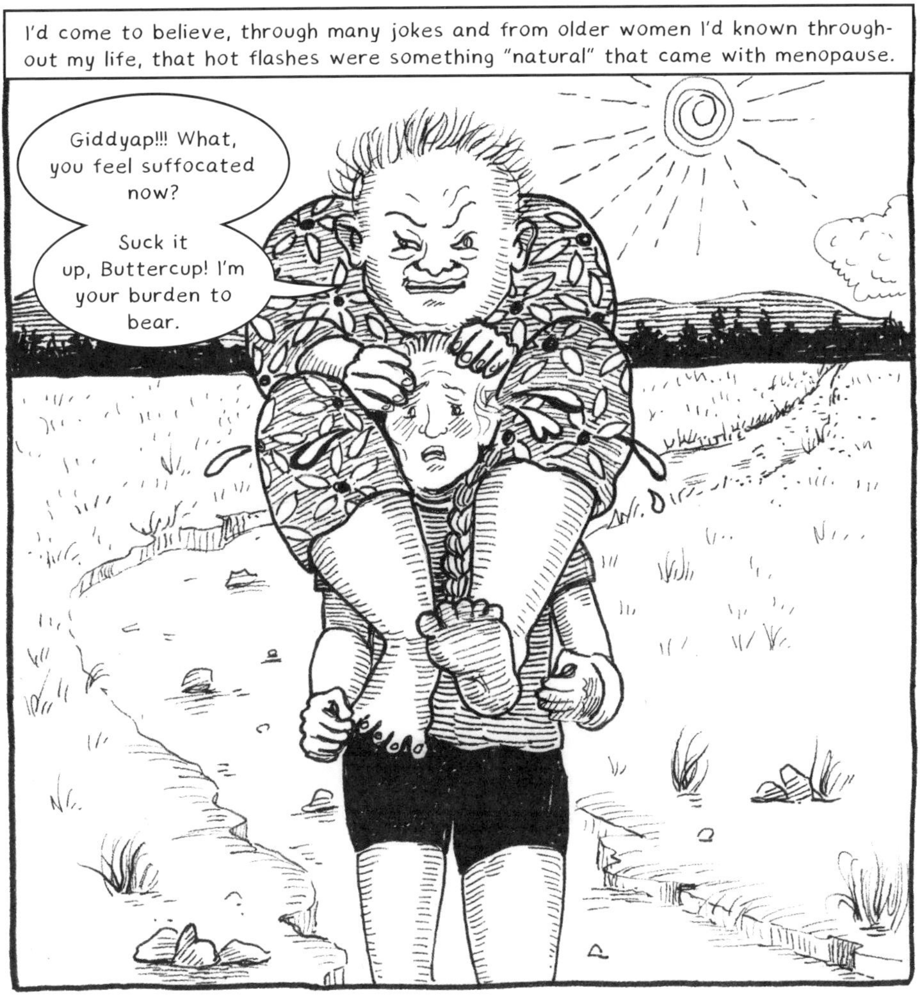
I'd come to believe, through many jokes and from older women I'd known throughout my life, that hot flashes were something "natural" that came with menopause.
Giddyap!!! What, you feel suffocated now?
Suck it up, Buttercup! I'm your burden to bear.

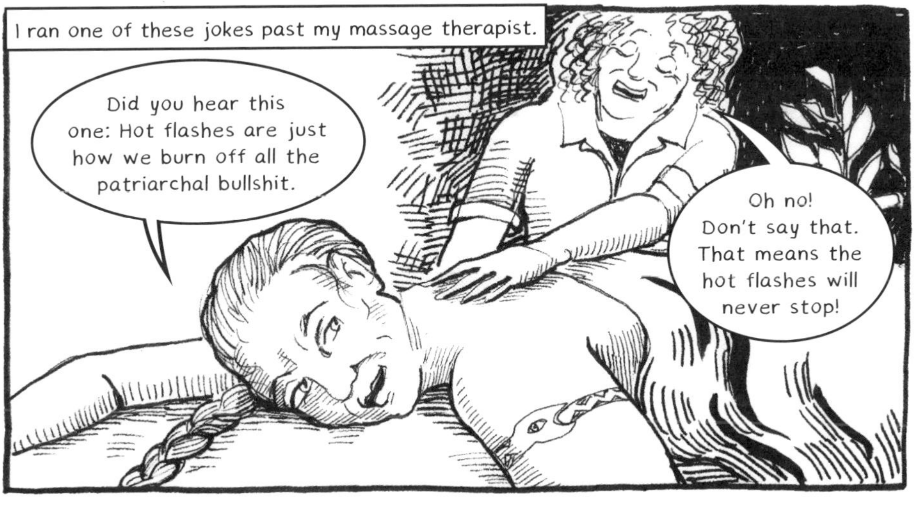
I ran one of these jokes past my massage therapist.
Did you hear this one: Hot flashes are just how we burn off all the patriarchal bullshit.
Oh no! Don't say that. That means the hot flashes will never stop!

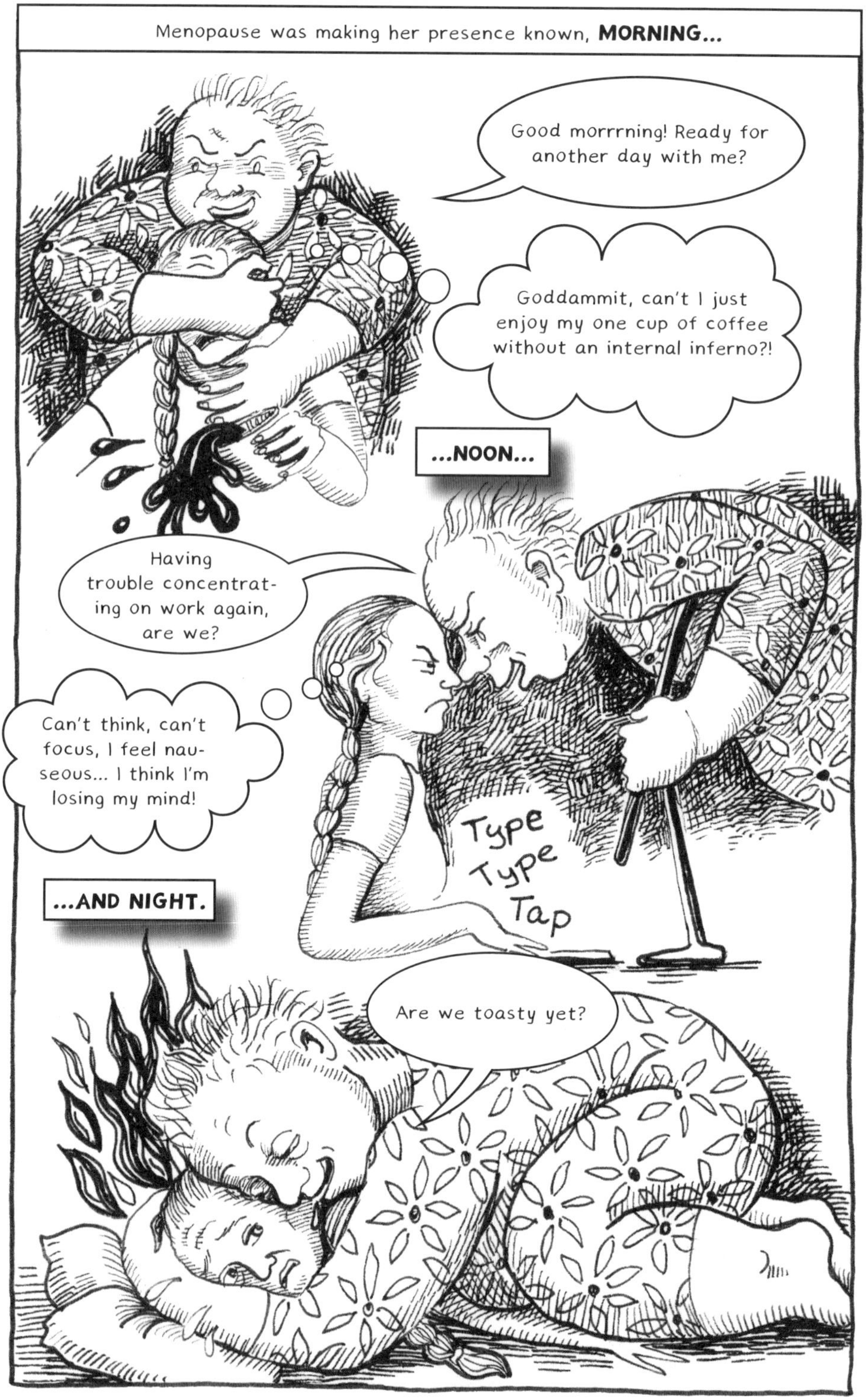
Menopause was making her presence known, **MORNING...**
Good morrrning! Ready for another day with me?
Goddammit, can't I just enjoy my one cup of coffee without an internal inferno?!
...NOON...
Having trouble concentrating on work again, are we?
Can't think, can't focus, I feel nauseous... I think I'm losing my mind!
Type Type Tap
...AND NIGHT.
Are we toasty yet?

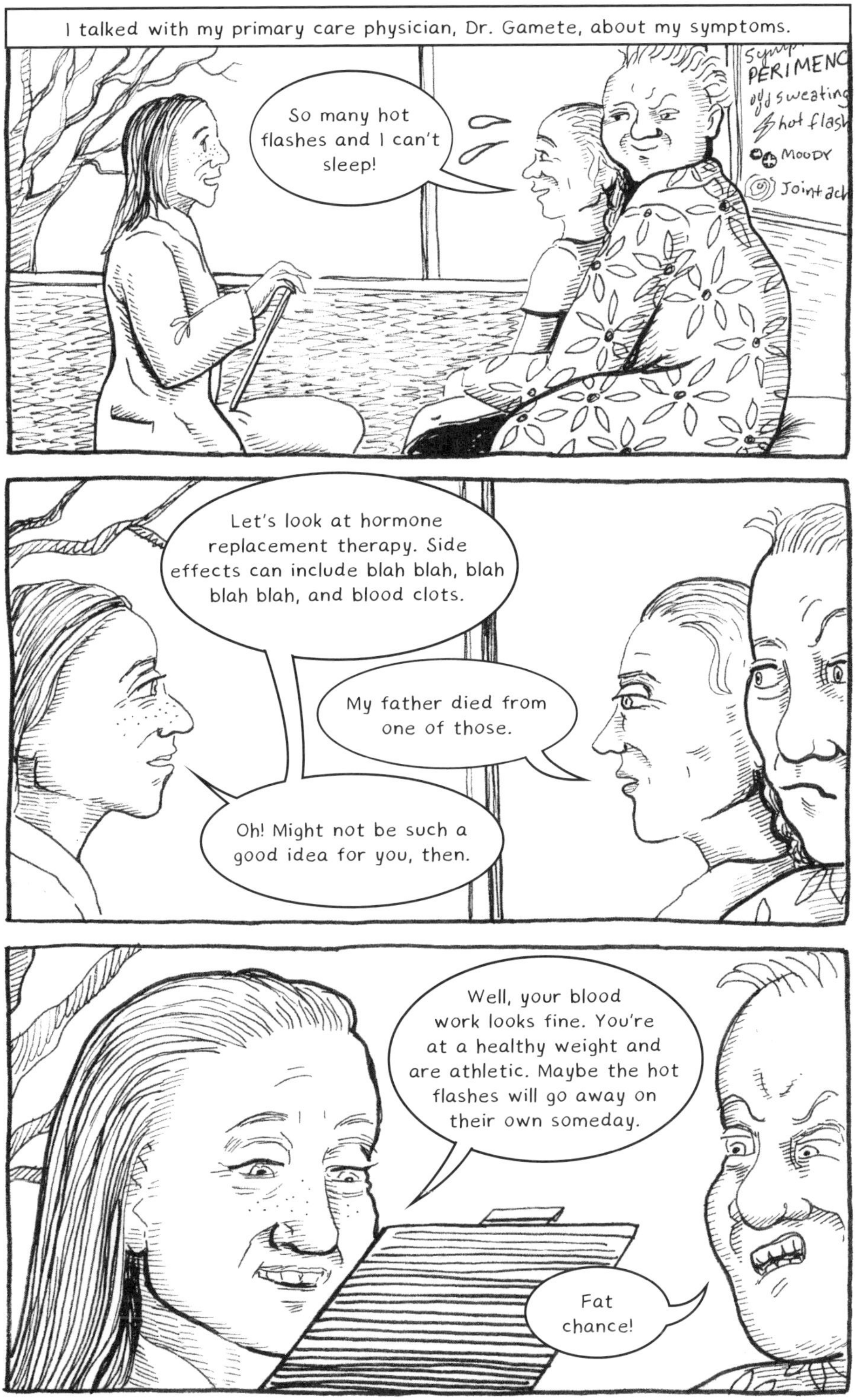
I talked with my primary care physician, Dr. Gamete, about my symptoms.
So many hot flashes and I can't sleep!
sweating
MOODY
Let's look at hormone replacement therapy. Side effects can include blah blah, blah blah blah, and blood clots.
My father died from one of those.
Oh! Might not be such a good idea for you, then.
Well, your blood work looks fine. You're at a healthy weight and are athletic. Maybe the hot flashes will go away on their own someday.
Fat chance!

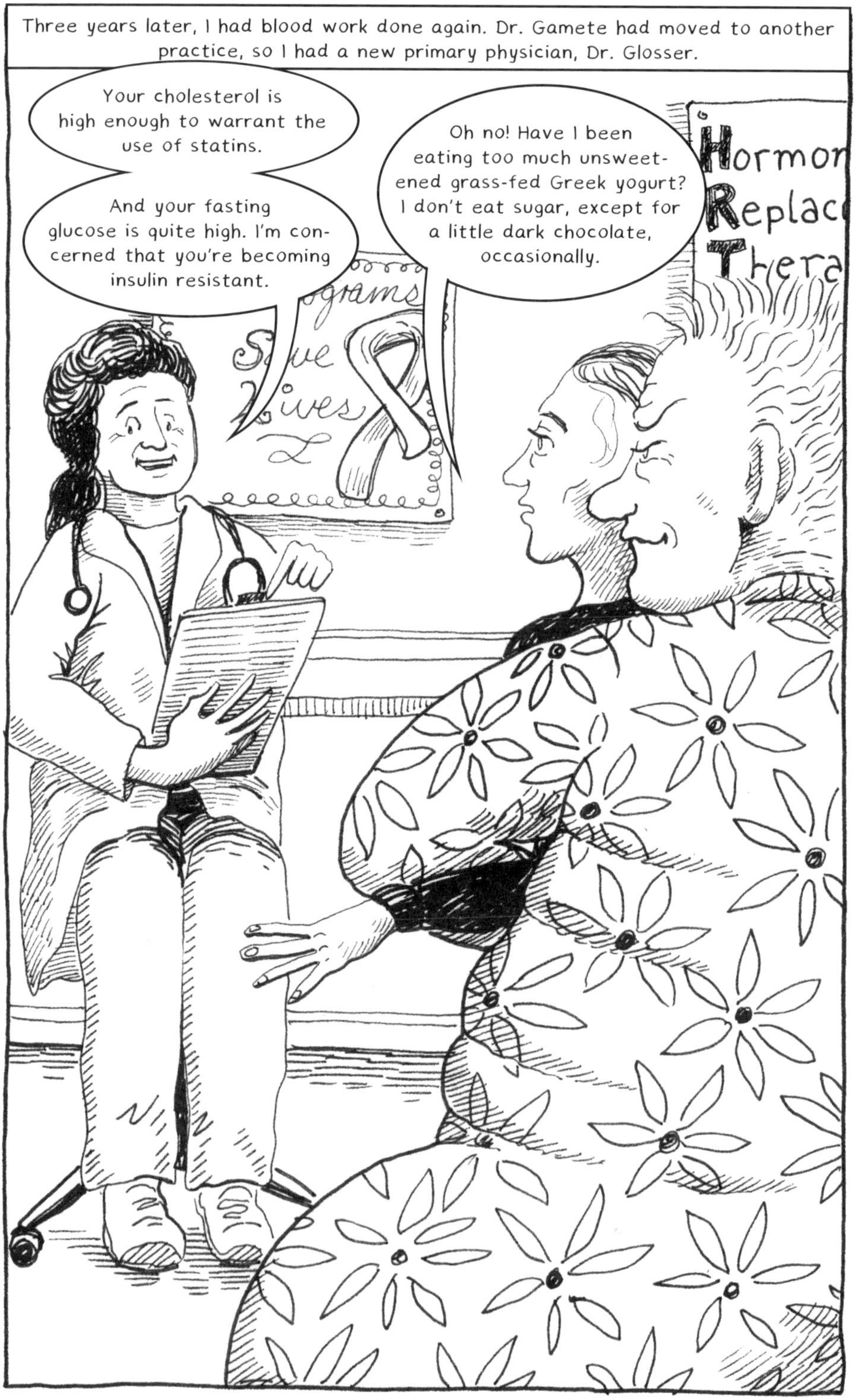
Three years later, I had blood work done again. Dr. Gamete had moved to another practice, so I had a new primary physician, Dr. Glosser.
Your cholesterol is high enough to warrant the use of statins.
And your fasting glucose is quite high. I'm concerned that you're becoming insulin resistant.
Oh no! Have I been eating too much unsweetened grass-fed Greek yogurt? I don't eat sugar, except for a little dark chocolate, occasionally.

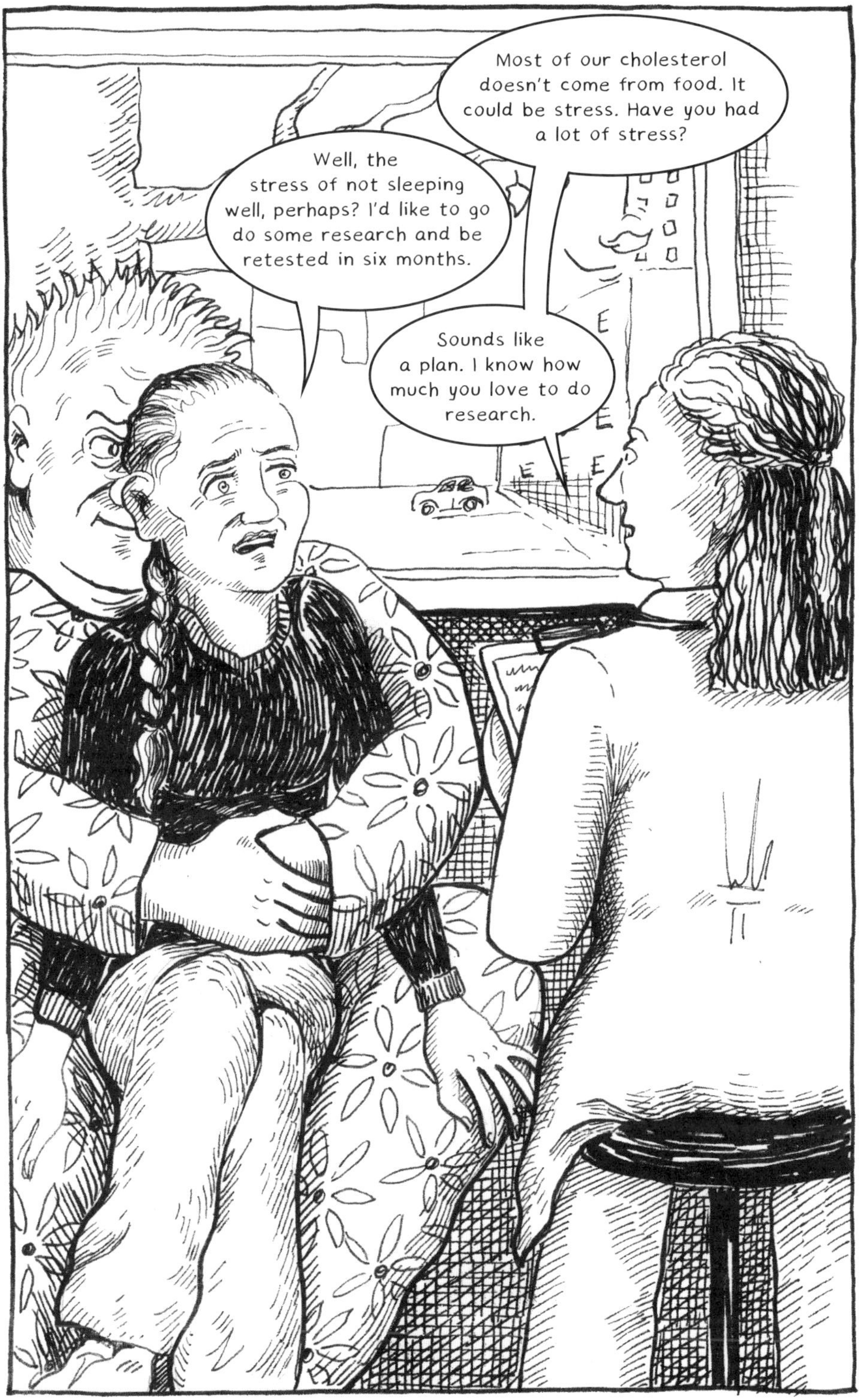

Most of our cholesterol doesn't come from food. It could be stress. Have you had a lot of stress?
Well, the stress of not sleeping well, perhaps? I'd like to go do some research and be retested in six months.
Sounds like a plan. I know how much you love to do research.

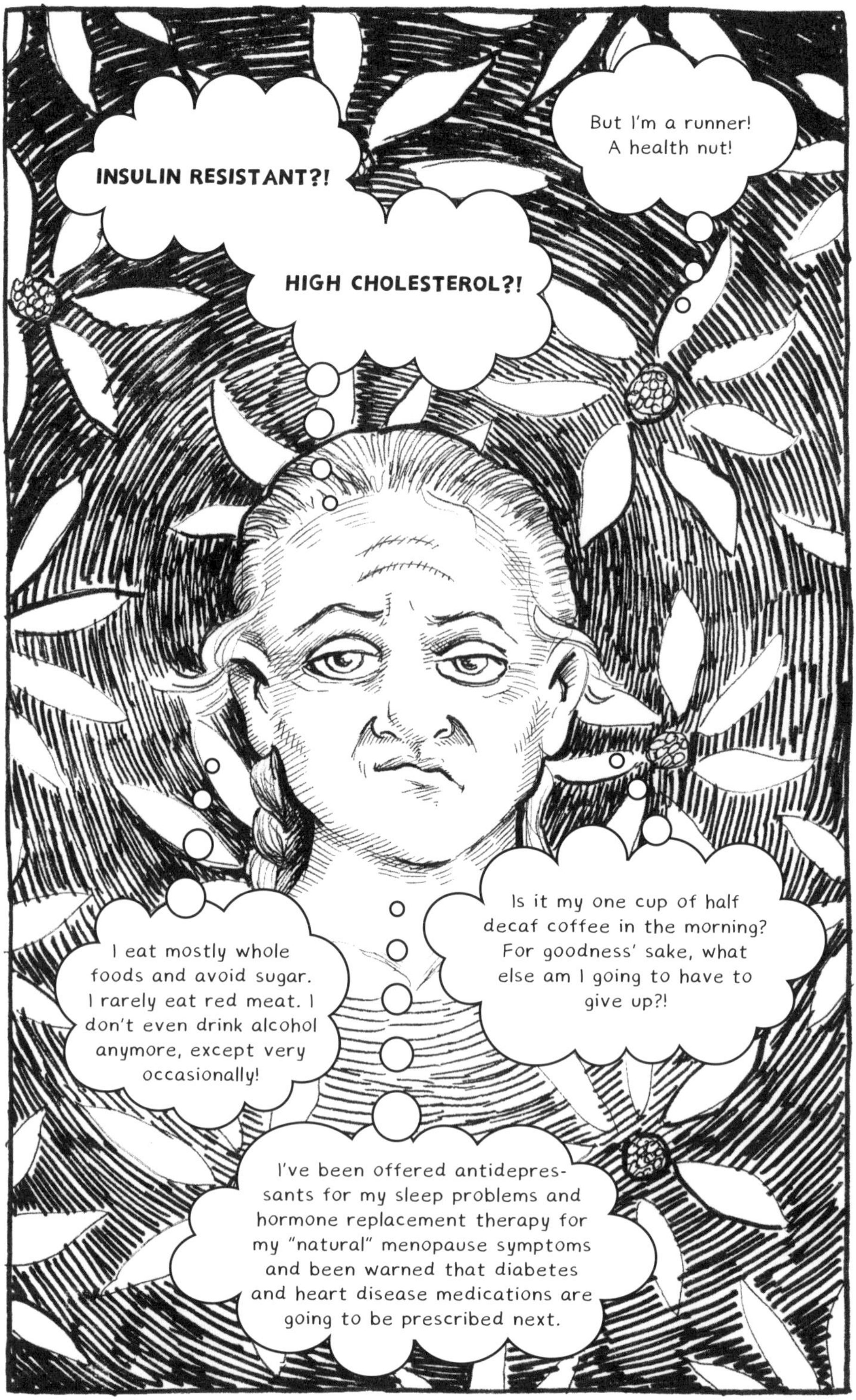
INSULIN RESISTANT?!
But I'm a runner! A health nut!
HIGH CHOLESTEROL?!
I eat mostly whole foods and avoid sugar. I rarely eat red meat. I don't even drink alcohol anymore, except very occasionally!
Is it my one cup of half decaf coffee in the morning? For goodness' sake, what else am I going to have to give up?!
I've been offered antidepressants for my sleep problems and hormone replacement therapy for my "natural" menopause symptoms and been warned that diabetes and heart disease medications are going to be prescribed next.

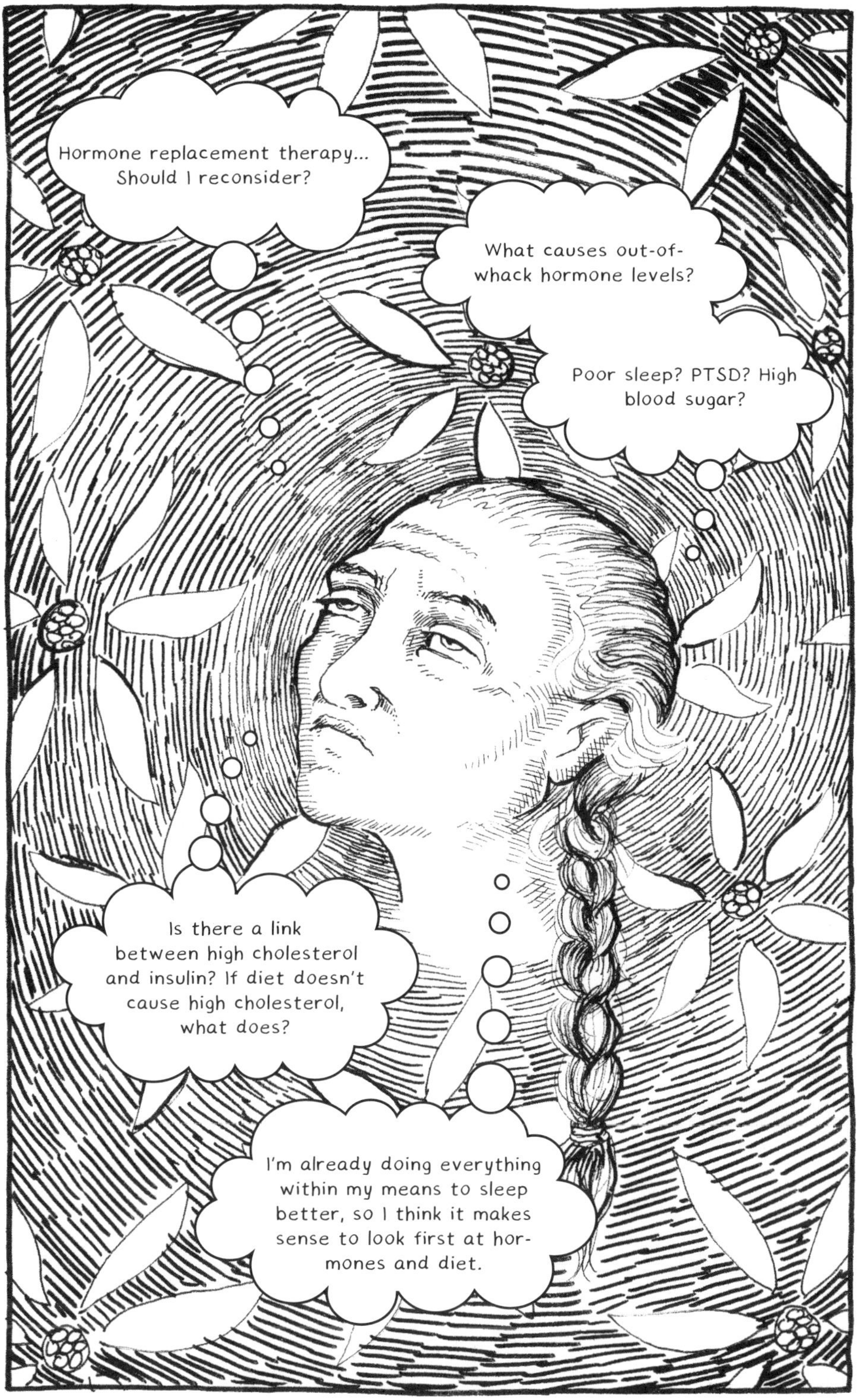
Hormone replacement therapy... Should I reconsider?
What causes out-of-whack hormone levels?
Poor sleep? PTSD? High blood sugar?
Is there a link between high cholesterol and insulin? If diet doesn't cause high cholesterol, what does?
I'm already doing everything within my means to sleep better, so I think it makes sense to look first at hormones and diet.

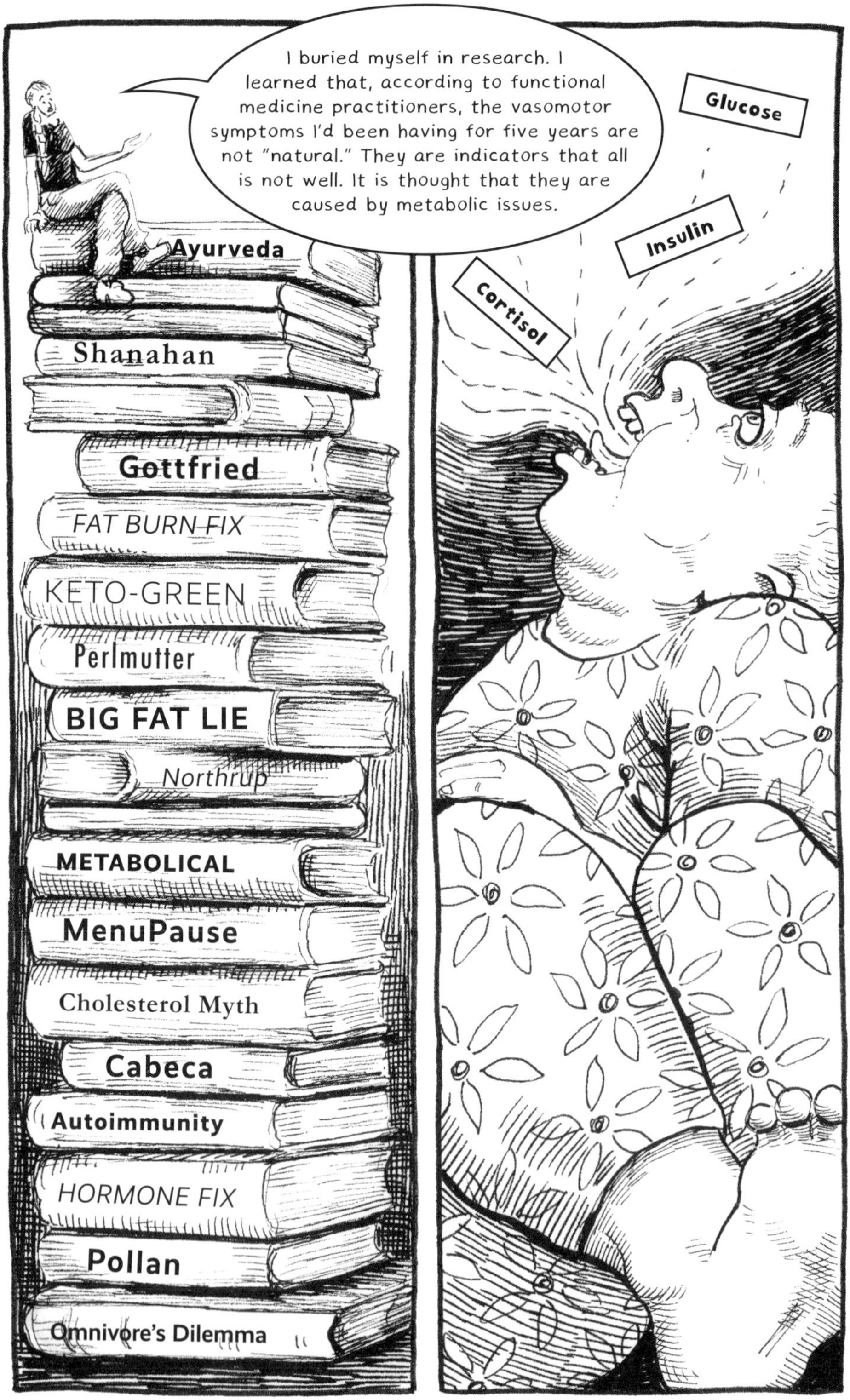
I buried myself in research. I learned that, according to functional medicine practitioners, the vasomotor symptoms I'd been having for five years are not "natural." They are indicators that all is not well. It is thought that they are caused by metabolic issues.
Ayurveda
Shanahan
Gottfried
FAT BURN FIX
KETO-GREEN
Perlmutter
BIG FAT LIE
Northrup
METABOLICAL
MenuPause
Cholesterol Myth
Cabeca
Autoimmunity
HORMONE FIX
Pollan
Omnivore's Dilemma
Glucose
Insulin
Cortisol

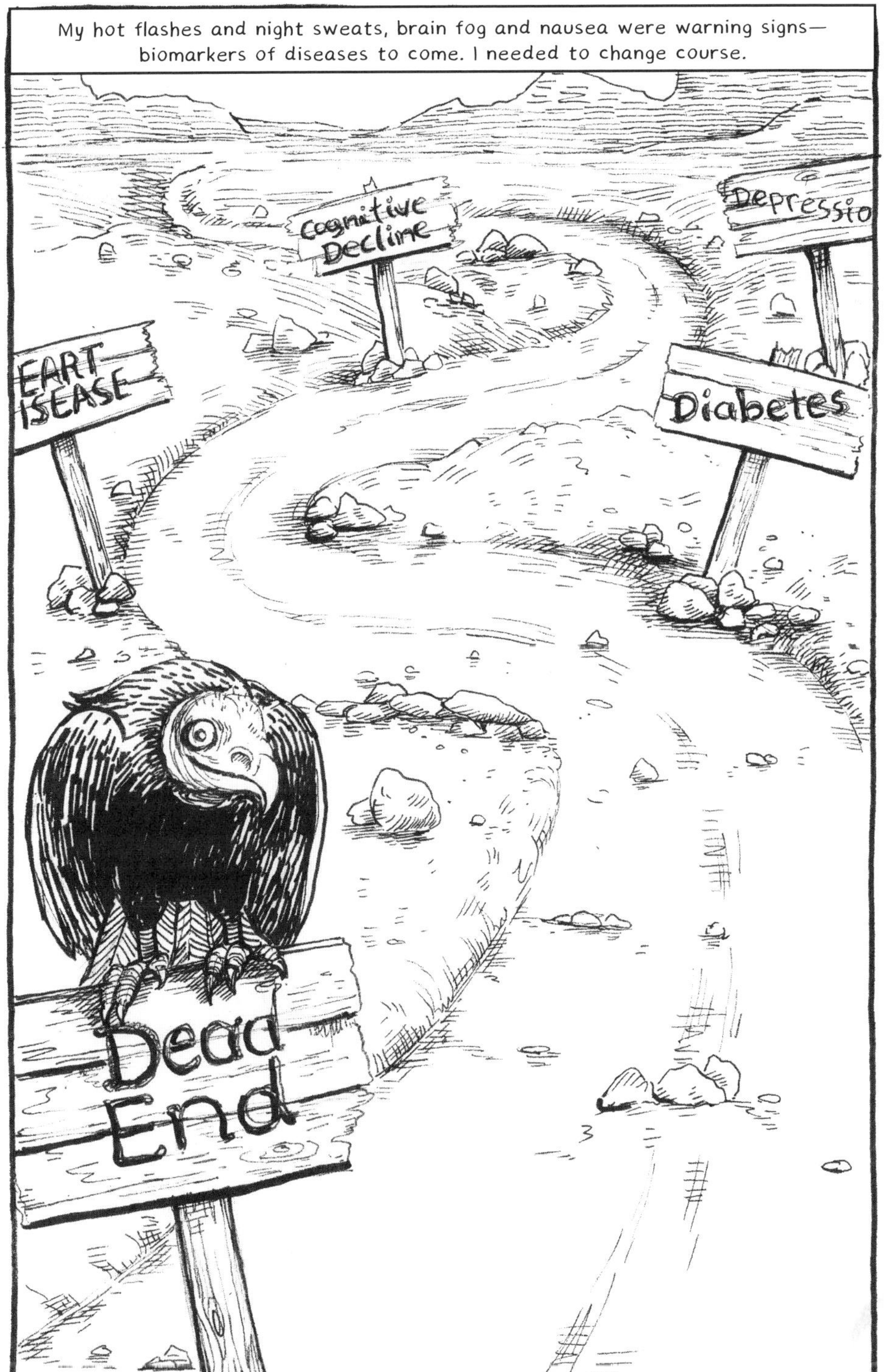
My hot flashes and night sweats, brain fog and nausea were warning signs—biomarkers of diseases to come. I needed to change course.
Cognitive Decline
Depressio
EART ISEASE
Diabetes
Dead End

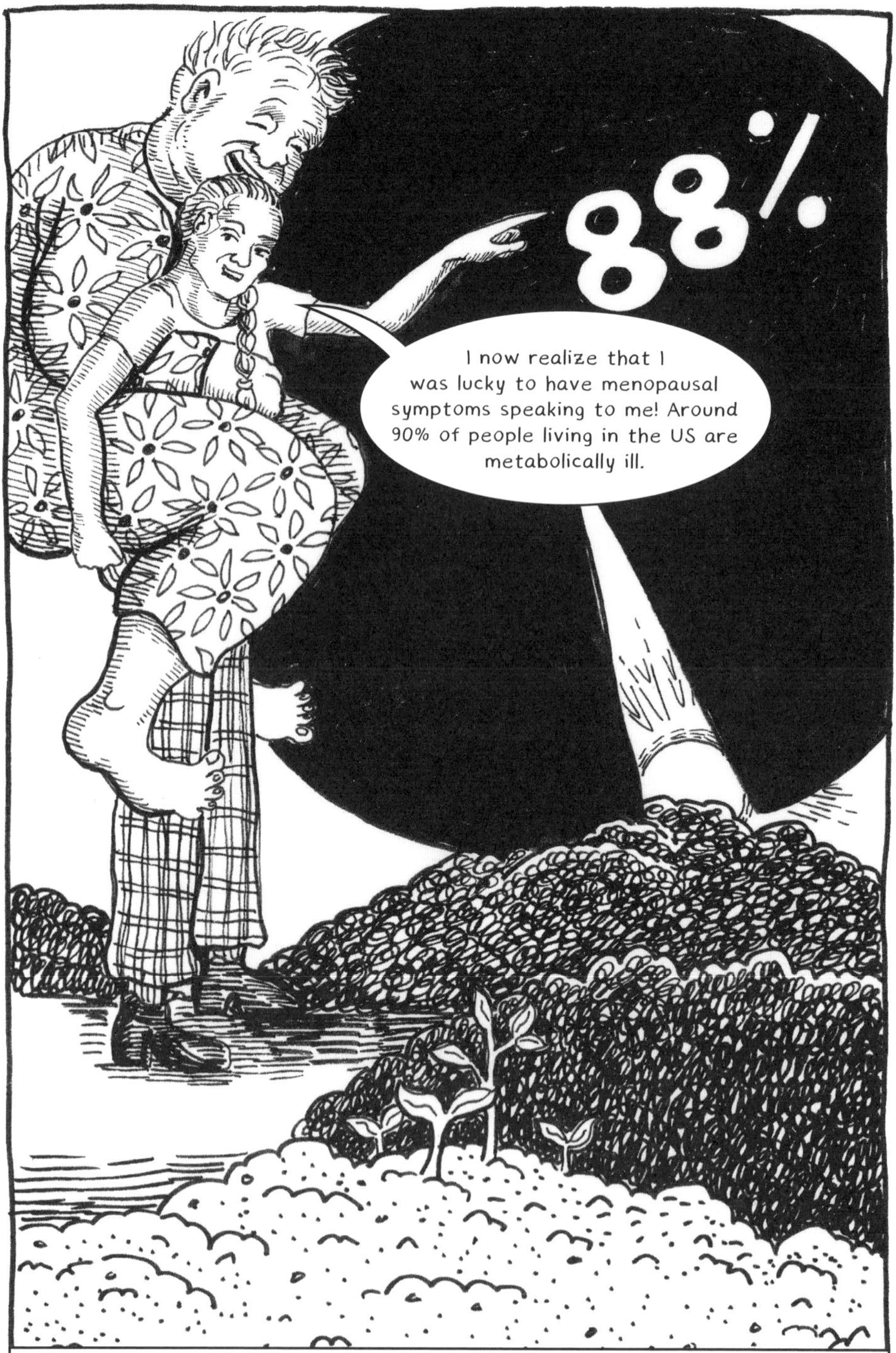
88%
I now realize that I was lucky to have menopausal symptoms speaking to me! Around 90% of people living in the US are metabolically ill.

Metabolism comes from the Greek *metabole*, a change. A healthy metabolism means the ability to transform food into energy. It means the ability to adapt to the availability of different foods, and varying quantities of foods, due to seasonal and other shifts.

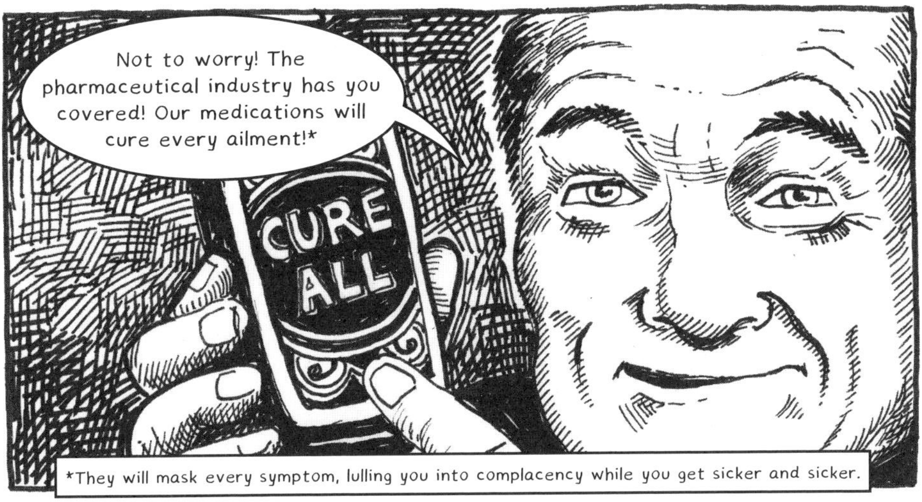
Not to worry! The pharmaceutical industry has you covered! Our medications will cure every ailment!*
CURE ALL
*They will mask every symptom, lulling you into complacency while you get sicker and sicker.

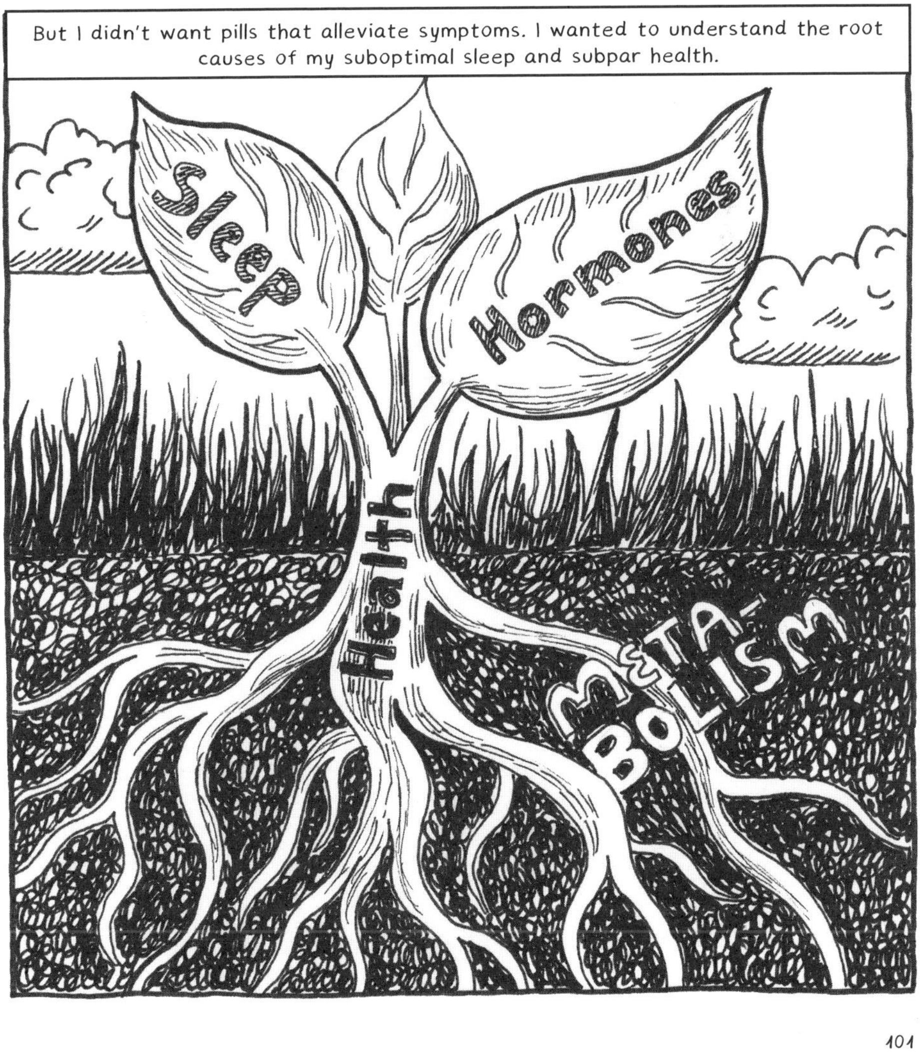
But I didn't want pills that alleviate symptoms. I wanted to understand the root causes of my suboptimal sleep and subpar health.
Sleep
Hormones
Health
META-BOLISM

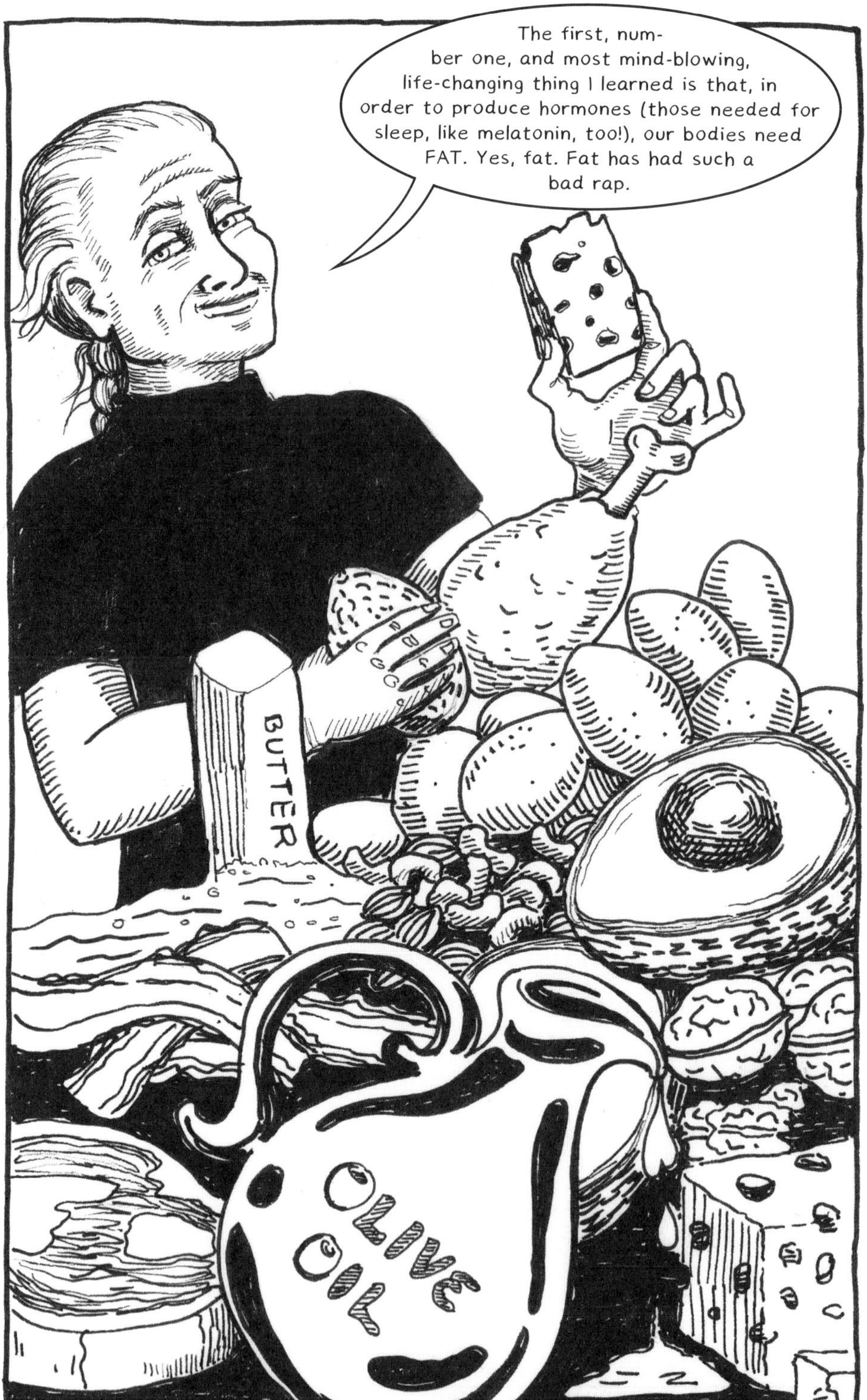
The first, number one, and most mind-blowing, life-changing thing I learned is that, in order to produce hormones (those needed for sleep, like melatonin, too!), our bodies need FAT. Yes, fat. Fat has had such a bad rap.
BUTTER
OLIVE OIL

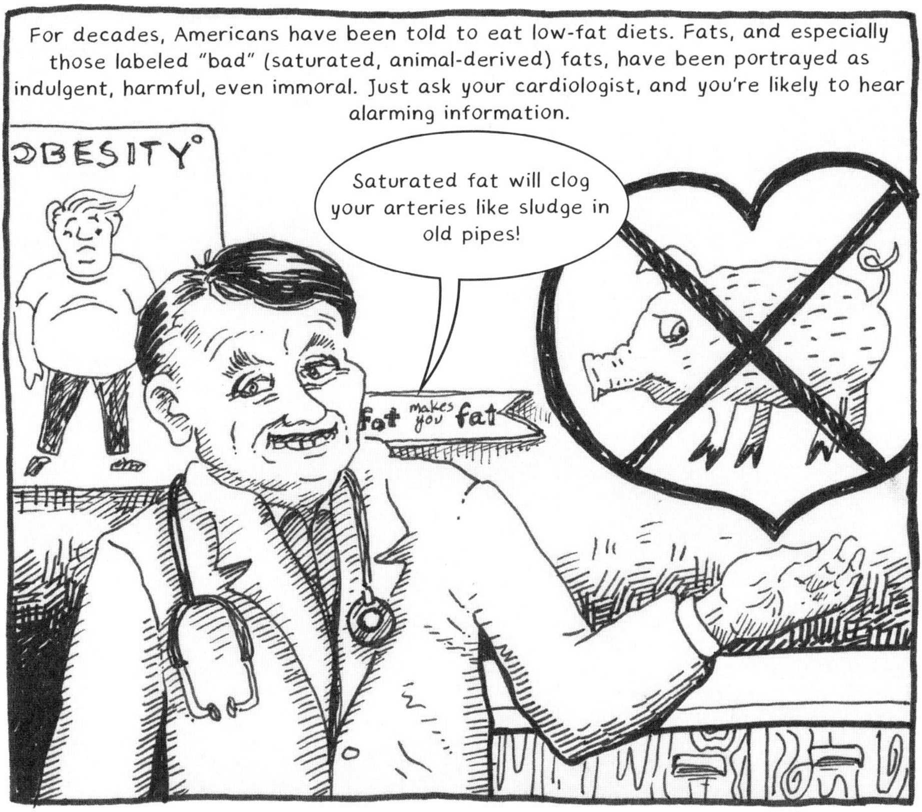
For decades, Americans have been told to eat low-fat diets. Fats, and especially those labeled "bad" (saturated, animal-derived) fats, have been portrayed as indulgent, harmful, even immoral. Just ask your cardiologist, and you're likely to hear alarming information.
OBESITY
Saturated fat will clog your arteries like sludge in old pipes!
fat makes you fat

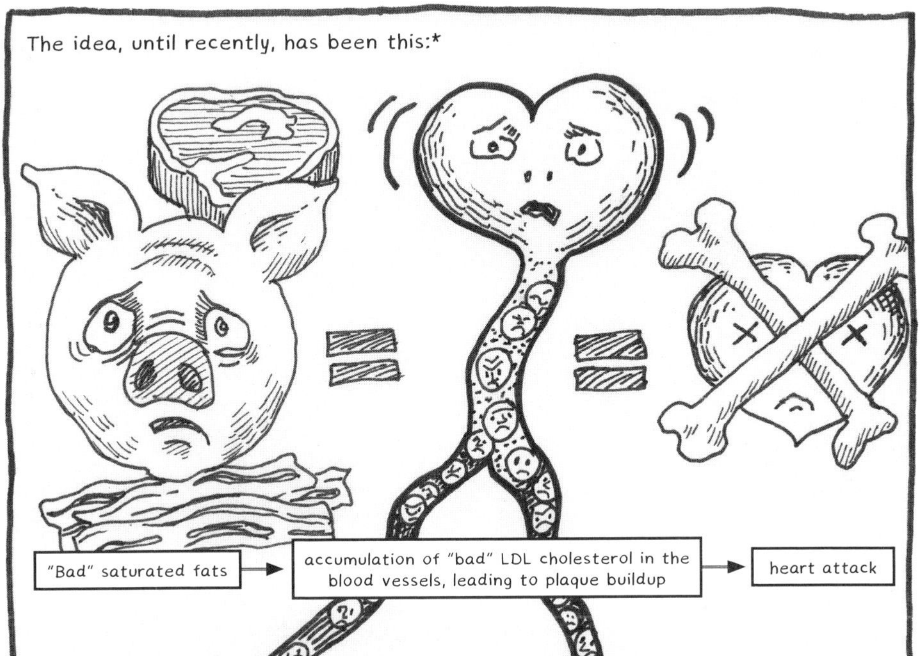
The idea, until recently, has been this:*
"Bad" saturated fats
accumulation of "bad" LDL cholesterol in the blood vessels, leading to plaque buildup
heart attack

*We are beginning to experience a paradigm shift as previous research and biases behind fats, cholesterol, and cardiovascular health are being scrutinized.

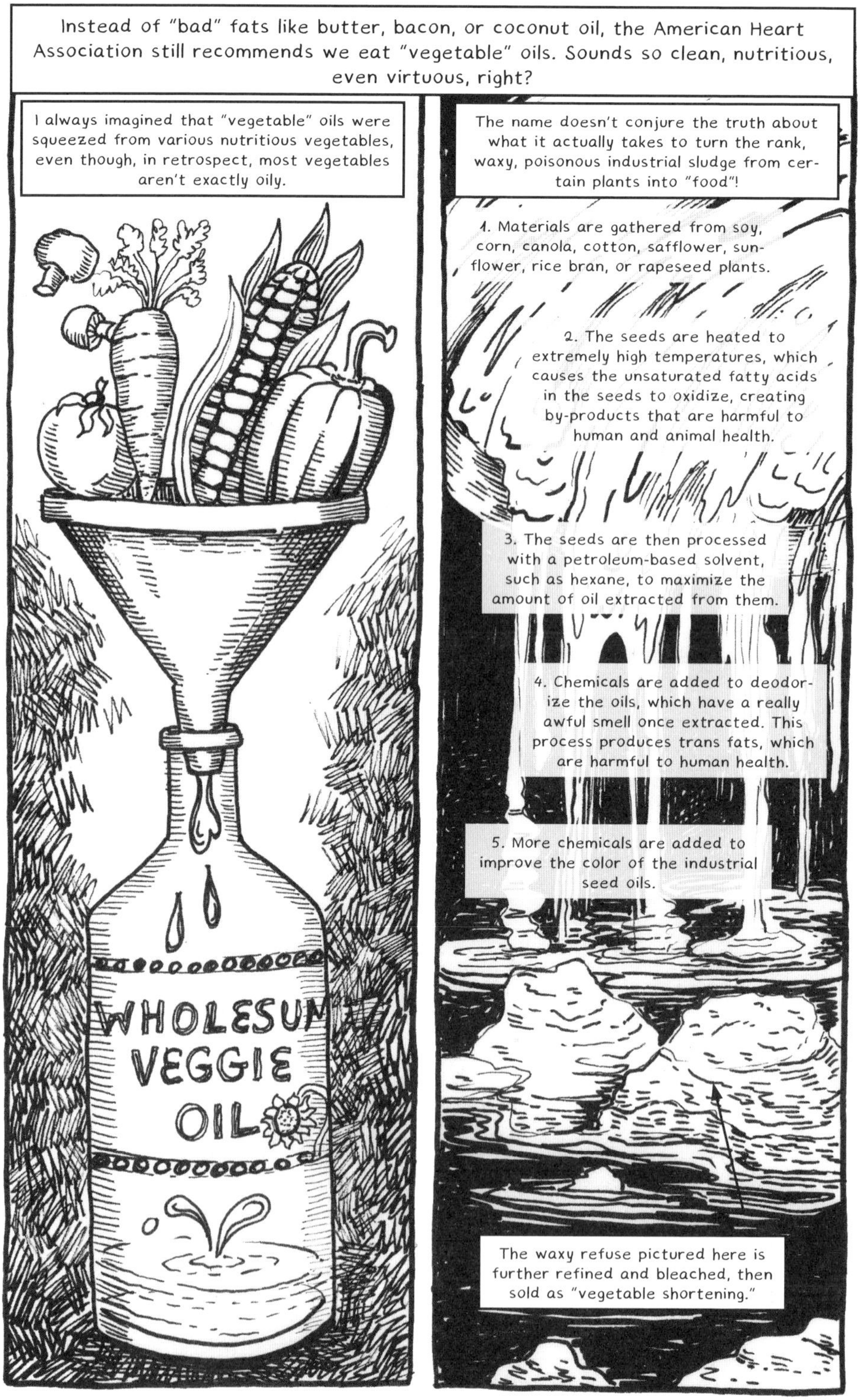
Instead of "bad" fats like butter, bacon, or coconut oil, the American Heart Association still recommends we eat "vegetable" oils. Sounds so clean, nutritious, even virtuous, right?
I always imagined that "vegetable" oils were squeezed from various nutritious vegetables, even though, in retrospect, most vegetables aren't exactly oily.
WHOLESUM VEGGIE OIL
The name doesn't conjure the truth about what it actually takes to turn the rank, waxy, poisonous industrial sludge from certain plants into "food"!
1. Materials are gathered from soy, corn, canola, cotton, safflower, sunflower, rice bran, or rapeseed plants.
2. The seeds are heated to extremely high temperatures, which causes the unsaturated fatty acids in the seeds to oxidize, creating by-products that are harmful to human and animal health.
3. The seeds are then processed with a petroleum-based solvent, such as hexane, to maximize the amount of oil extracted from them.
4. Chemicals are added to deodorize the oils, which have a really awful smell once extracted. This process produces trans fats, which are harmful to human health.
5. More chemicals are added to improve the color of the industrial seed oils.
The waxy refuse pictured here is further refined and bleached, then sold as "vegetable shortening."

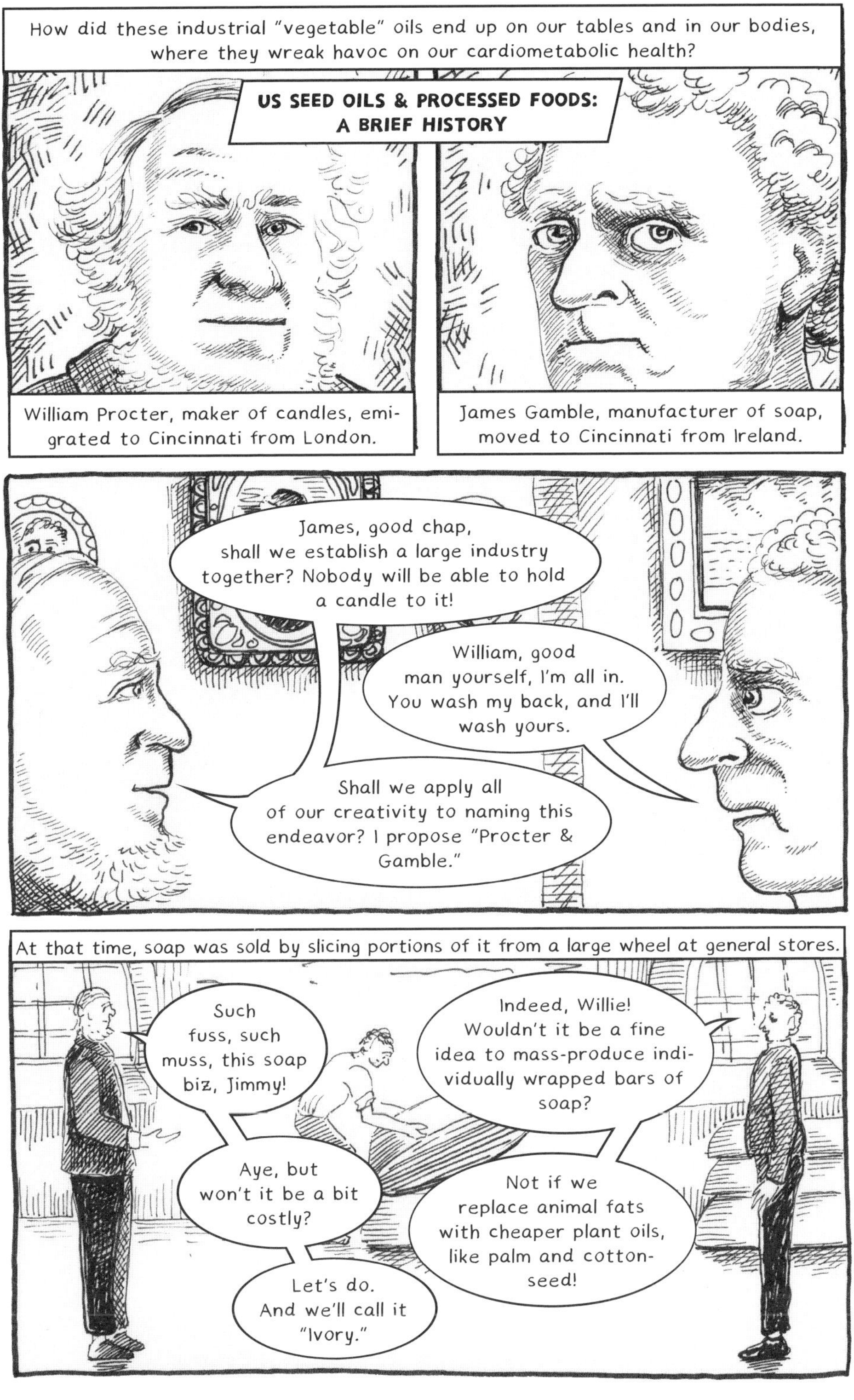
How did these industrial "vegetable" oils end up on our tables and in our bodies, where they wreak havoc on our cardiometabolic health?
US SEED OILS & PROCESSED FOODS: A BRIEF HISTORY
William Procter, maker of candles, emigrated to Cincinnati from London.
James Gamble, manufacturer of soap, moved to Cincinnati from Ireland.
James, good chap, shall we establish a large industry together? Nobody will be able to hold a candle to it!
William, good man yourself, I'm all in. You wash my back, and I'll wash yours.
Shall we apply all of our creativity to naming this endeavor? I propose "Procter & Gamble."
At that time, soap was sold by slicing portions of it from a large wheel at general stores.
Such fuss, such muss, this soap biz, Jimmy!
Indeed, Willie! Wouldn't it be a fine idea to mass-produce individually wrapped bars of soap?
Aye, but won't it be a bit costly?
Not if we replace animal fats with cheaper plant oils, like palm and cottonseed!
Let's do. And we'll call it "Ivory."

The refinement of cottonseed oil was key to this endeavor. Cotton was an enormous industry in the US in the 1800s. The demand for land to grow it meant intensified annihilation and displacement of Native Americans during the country's period of so-called westward expansion.

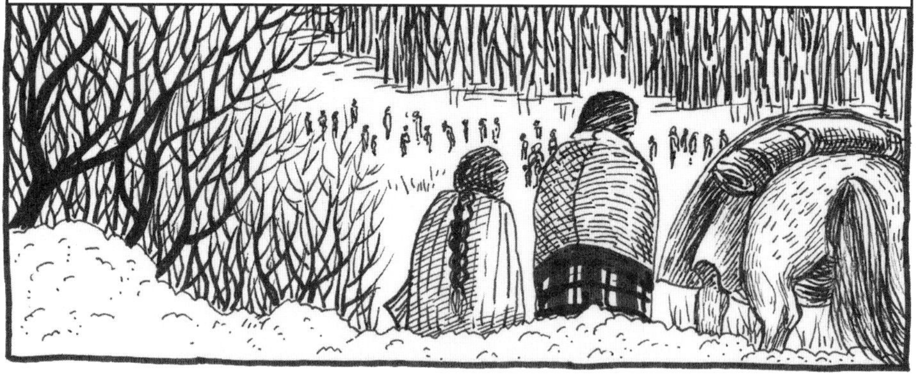

Greed for cheap labor escalated the slave trade. In 1790, there had been 6 slave states. By 1860, largely due to the heavy labor required on cotton plantations, there were 15!

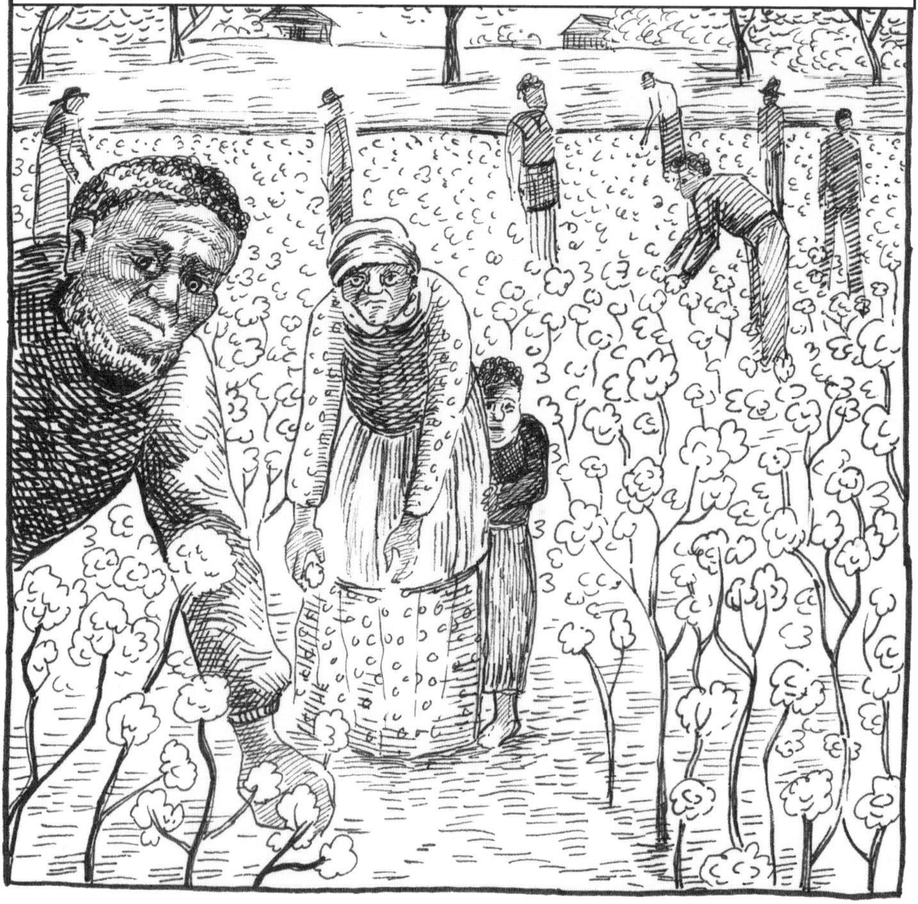

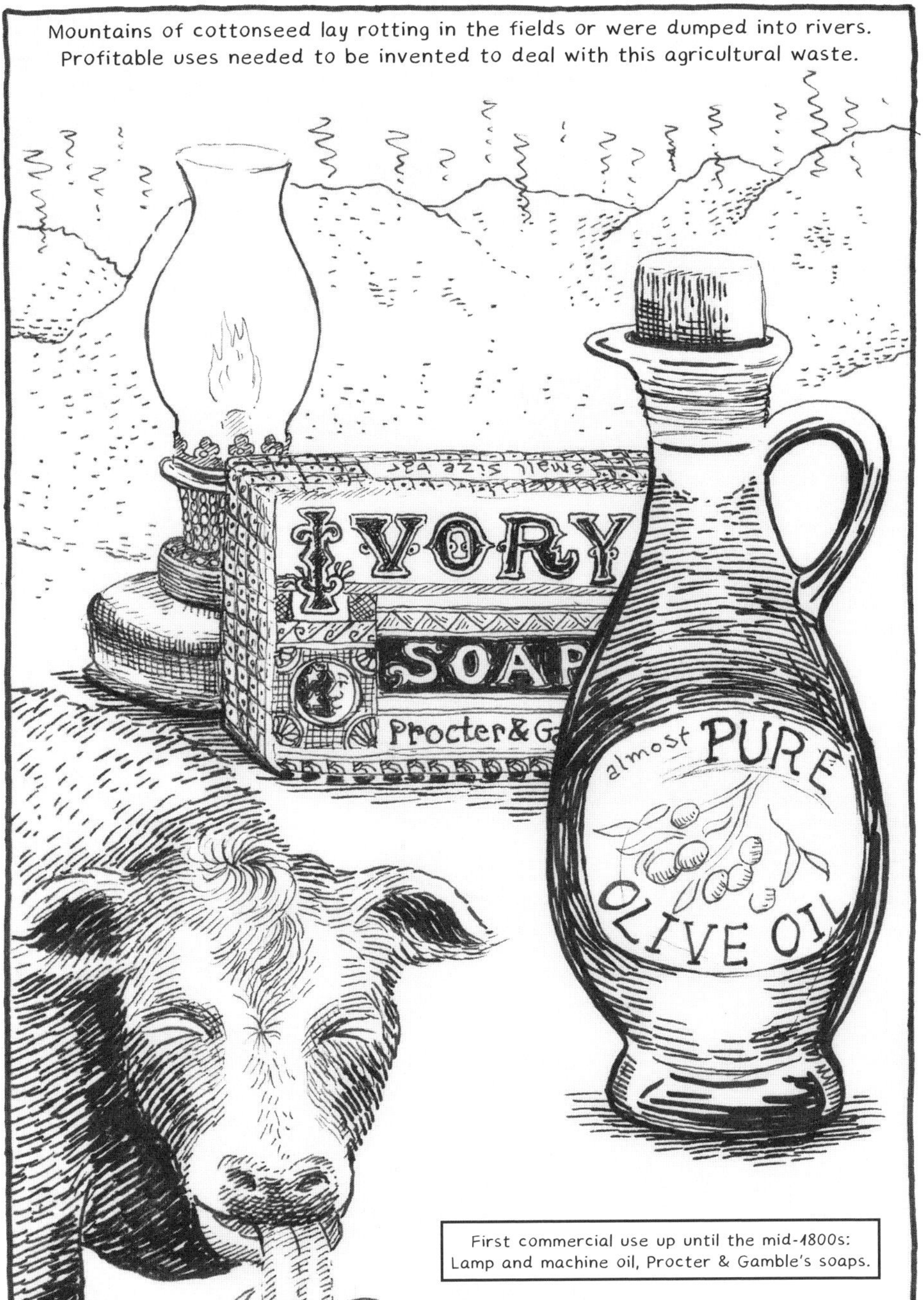
Mountains of cottonseed lay rotting in the fields or were dumped into rivers. Profitable uses needed to be invented to deal with this agricultural waste.
IVORY
SOAP
Procter&Ga
almost PURE
OLIVE OIL
First commercial use up until the mid-1800s: Lamp and machine oil, Procter & Gamble's soaps.
1870s: Used as fertilizer and to dilute olive oil to cheapen production.
1880s: Added to cattle feed.

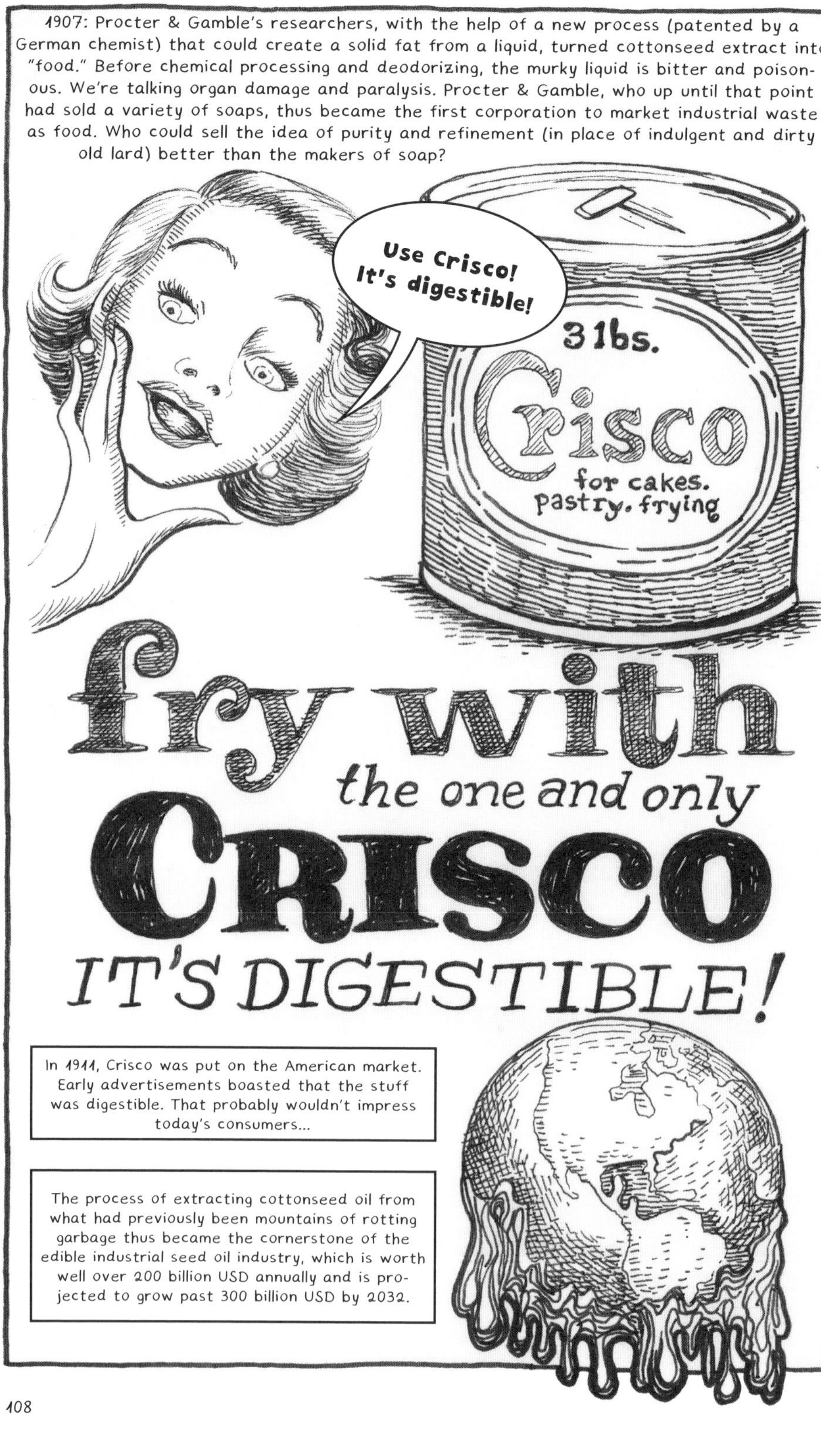

1907: Procter & Gamble's researchers, with the help of a new process (patented by a German chemist) that could create a solid fat from a liquid, turned cottonseed extract into "food." Before chemical processing and deodorizing, the murky liquid is bitter and poisonous. We're talking organ damage and paralysis. Procter & Gamble, who up until that point had sold a variety of soaps, thus became the first corporation to market industrial waste as food. Who could sell the idea of purity and refinement (in place of indulgent and dirty old lard) better than the makers of soap?

Use Crisco! It's digestible!

3 lbs.

Crisco
for cakes. pastry. frying

fry with
the one and only
CRISCO
IT'S DIGESTIBLE!

In 1911, Crisco was put on the American market. Early advertisements boasted that the stuff was digestible. That probably wouldn't impress today's consumers...

The process of extracting cottonseed oil from what had previously been mountains of rotting garbage thus became the cornerstone of the edible industrial seed oil industry, which is worth well over 200 billion USD annually and is projected to grow past 300 billion USD by 2032.

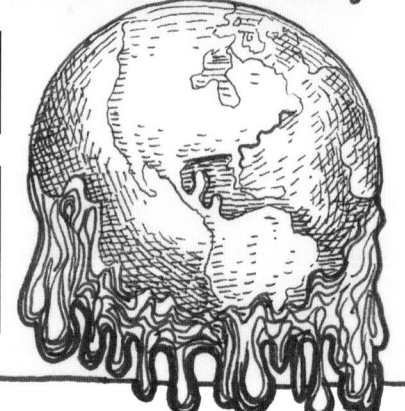

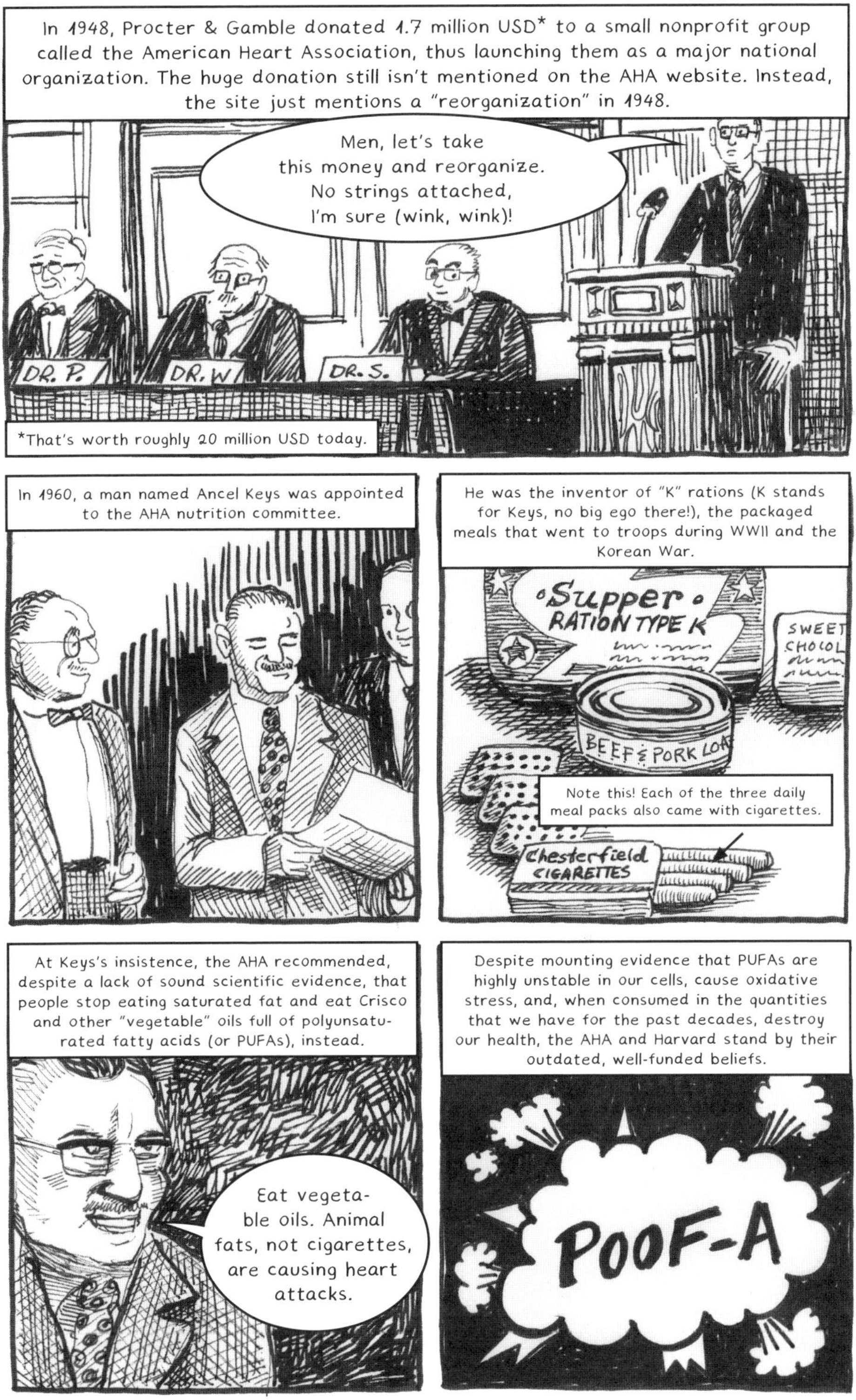
In 1948, Procter & Gamble donated 1.7 million USD* to a small nonprofit group called the American Heart Association, thus launching them as a major national organization. The huge donation still isn't mentioned on the AHA website. Instead, the site just mentions a "reorganization" in 1948.
Men, let's take this money and reorganize. No strings attached, I'm sure (wink, wink)!
DR. P.
DR. W
DR. S.
*That's worth roughly 20 million USD today.
In 1960, a man named Ancel Keys was appointed to the AHA nutrition committee.
He was the inventor of "K" rations (K stands for Keys, no big ego there!), the packaged meals that went to troops during WWII and the Korean War.
Supper
RATION TYPE K
SWEET
CHOCOL
BEEF & PORK LOA
Note this! Each of the three daily meal packs also came with cigarettes.
Chesterfield
CIGARETTES
At Keys's insistence, the AHA recommended, despite a lack of sound scientific evidence, that people stop eating saturated fat and eat Crisco and other "vegetable" oils full of polyunsaturated fatty acids (or PUFAs), instead.
Eat vegetable oils. Animal fats, not cigarettes, are causing heart attacks.
Despite mounting evidence that PUFAs are highly unstable in our cells, cause oxidative stress, and, when consumed in the quantities that we have for the past decades, destroy our health, the AHA and Harvard stand by their outdated, well-funded beliefs.
POOF-A

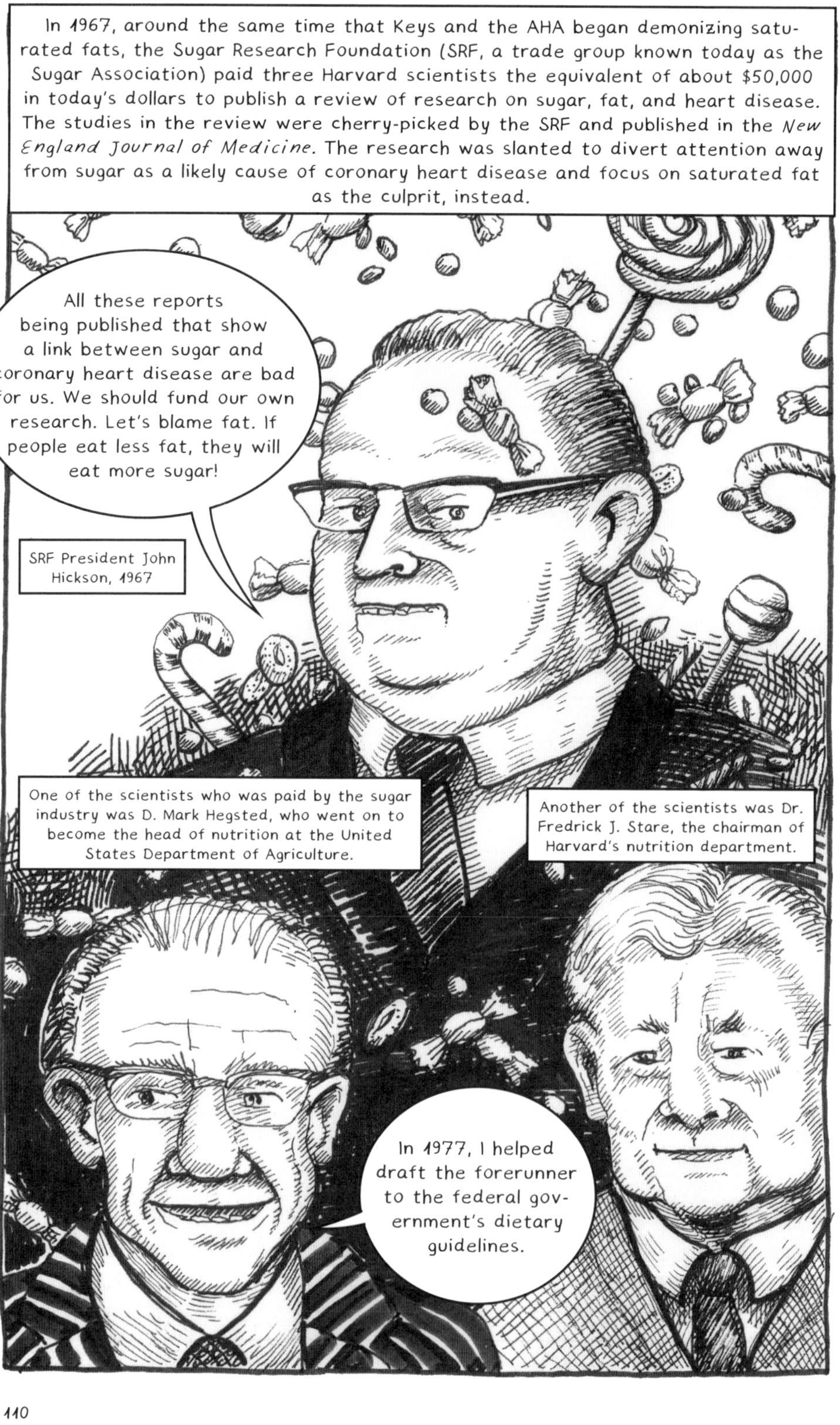
In 1967, around the same time that Keys and the AHA began demonizing saturated fats, the Sugar Research Foundation (SRF, a trade group known today as the Sugar Association) paid three Harvard scientists the equivalent of about $50,000 in today's dollars to publish a review of research on sugar, fat, and heart disease. The studies in the review were cherry-picked by the SRF and published in the *New England Journal of Medicine*. The research was slanted to divert attention away from sugar as a likely cause of coronary heart disease and focus on saturated fat as the culprit, instead.
All these reports being published that show a link between sugar and coronary heart disease are bad for us. We should fund our own research. Let's blame fat. If people eat less fat, they will eat more sugar!
SRF President John Hickson, 1967
One of the scientists who was paid by the sugar industry was D. Mark Hegsted, who went on to become the head of nutrition at the United States Department of Agriculture.
Another of the scientists was Dr. Fredrick J. Stare, the chairman of Harvard's nutrition department.
In 1977, I helped draft the forerunner to the federal government's dietary guidelines.

In 1977, a Senate committee led by George McGovern published its "Dietary Goals for the United States," urging people to eat less meat, eggs, and dairy in favor of carbohydrates.

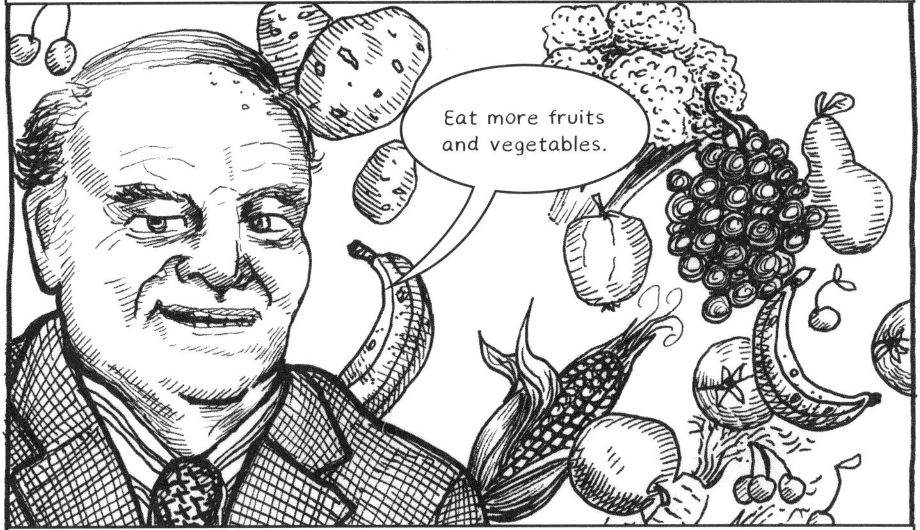
Eat more fruits and vegetables.

While eating more vegetables (instead of ultra-processed junk) is probably a good idea for most Americans, the advice should be to eat more vegetables and a small amount of seasonal organic whole fruit. Non-starchy vegetables such as leafy greens (grown in healthy soil, not sprayed with pesticides) should take center stage. But most Americans favor things like fruit and fruit juices (and fruit loops) to a spinach salad.

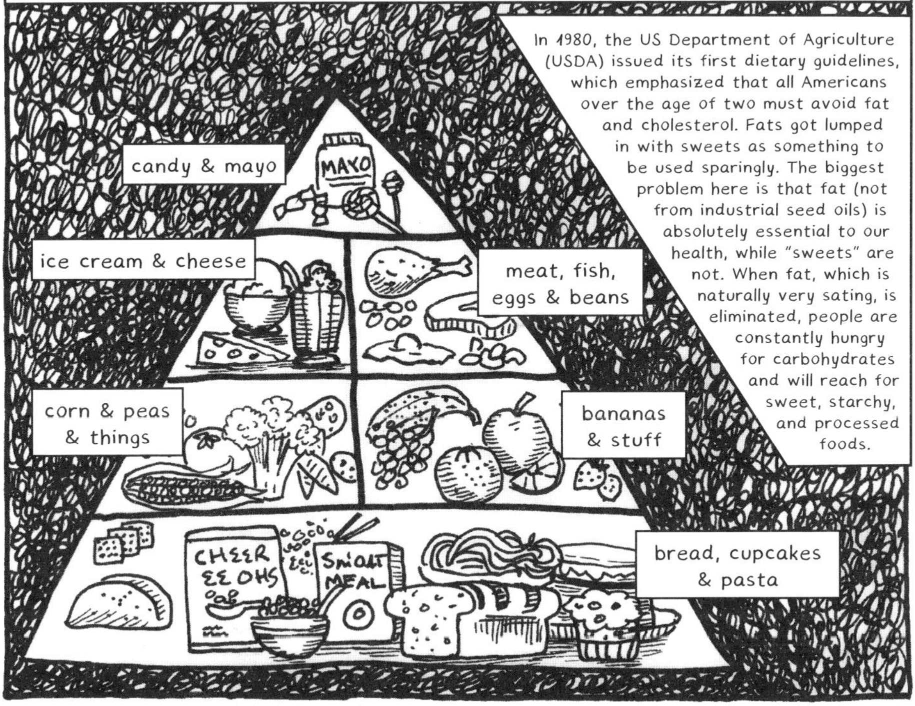
In 1980, the US Department of Agriculture (USDA) issued its first dietary guidelines, which emphasized that all Americans over the age of two must avoid fat and cholesterol. Fats got lumped in with sweets as something to be used sparingly. The biggest problem here is that fat (not from industrial seed oils) is absolutely essential to our health, while "sweets" are not. When fat, which is naturally very sating, is eliminated, people are constantly hungry for carbohydrates and will reach for sweet, starchy, and processed foods.
candy & mayo
MAYO
ice cream & cheese
meat, fish, eggs & beans
corn & peas & things
bananas & stuff
bread, cupcakes & pasta
CHEER EE OHS
SNOAT MEAL

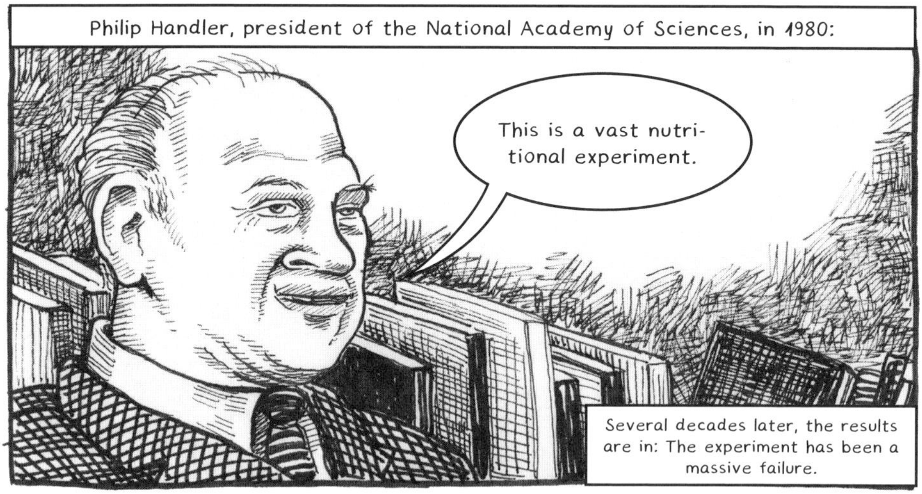
Philip Handler, president of the National Academy of Sciences, in 1980:
This is a vast nutritional experiment.
Several decades later, the results are in: The experiment has been a massive failure.

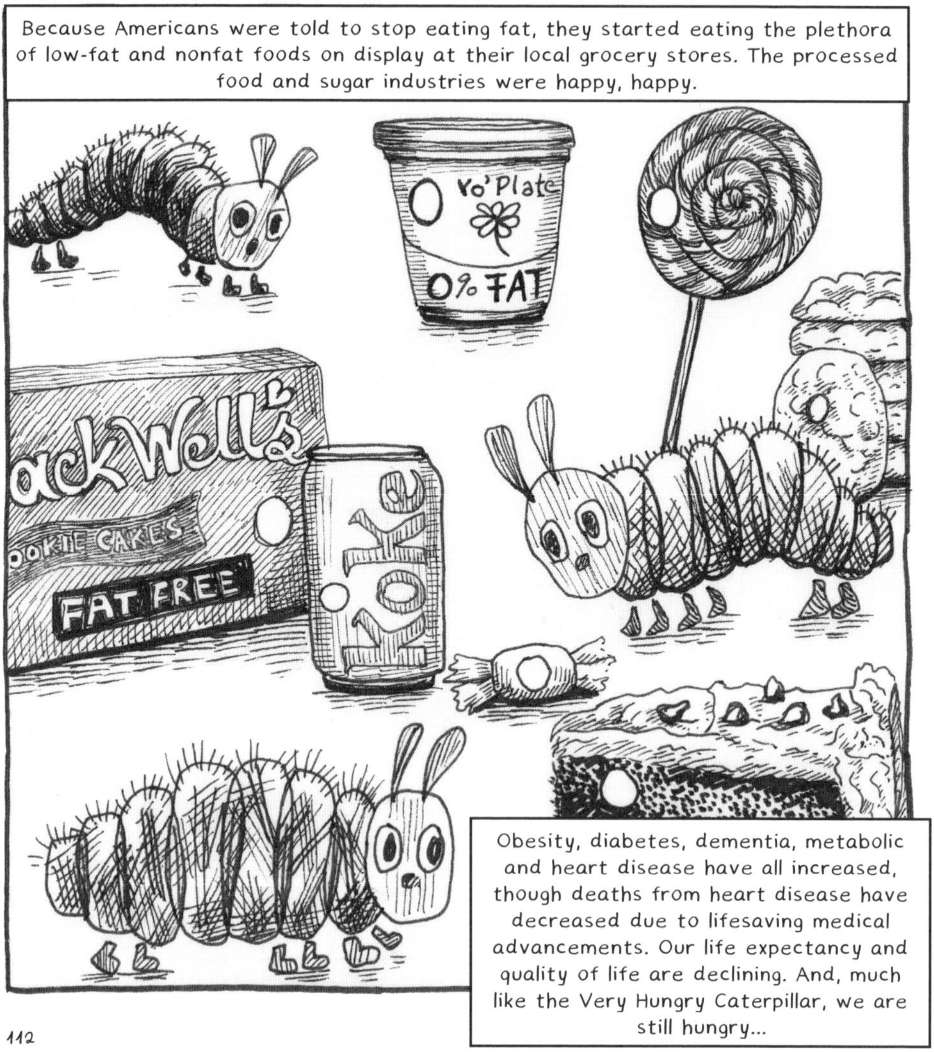
Because Americans were told to stop eating fat, they started eating the plethora of low-fat and nonfat foods on display at their local grocery stores. The processed food and sugar industries were happy, happy.
Yo'Plate
0% FAT
ackWell's
OOKIE CAKES
FAT FREE
Koke
Obesity, diabetes, dementia, metabolic and heart disease have all increased, though deaths from heart disease have decreased due to lifesaving medical advancements. Our life expectancy and quality of life are declining. And, much like the Very Hungry Caterpillar, we are still hungry...

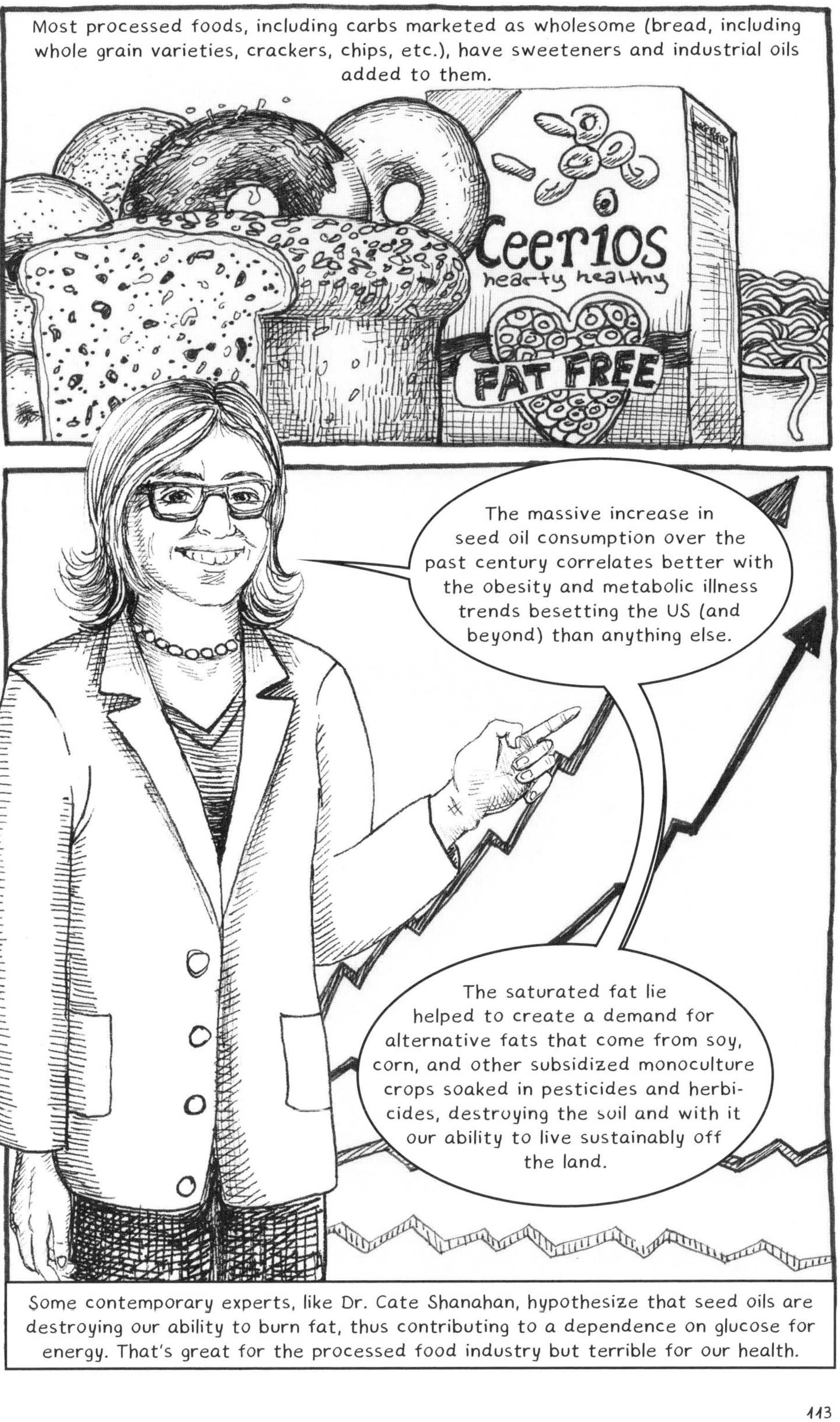
Most processed foods, including carbs marketed as wholesome (bread, including whole grain varieties, crackers, chips, etc.), have sweeteners and industrial oils added to them.
Ceerios
hearty healthy
FAT FREE
The massive increase in seed oil consumption over the past century correlates better with the obesity and metabolic illness trends besetting the US (and beyond) than anything else.
The saturated fat lie helped to create a demand for alternative fats that come from soy, corn, and other subsidized monoculture crops soaked in pesticides and herbicides, destroying the soil and with it our ability to live sustainably off the land.
Some contemporary experts, like Dr. Cate Shanahan, hypothesize that seed oils are destroying our ability to burn fat, thus contributing to a dependence on glucose for energy. That's great for the processed food industry but terrible for our health.

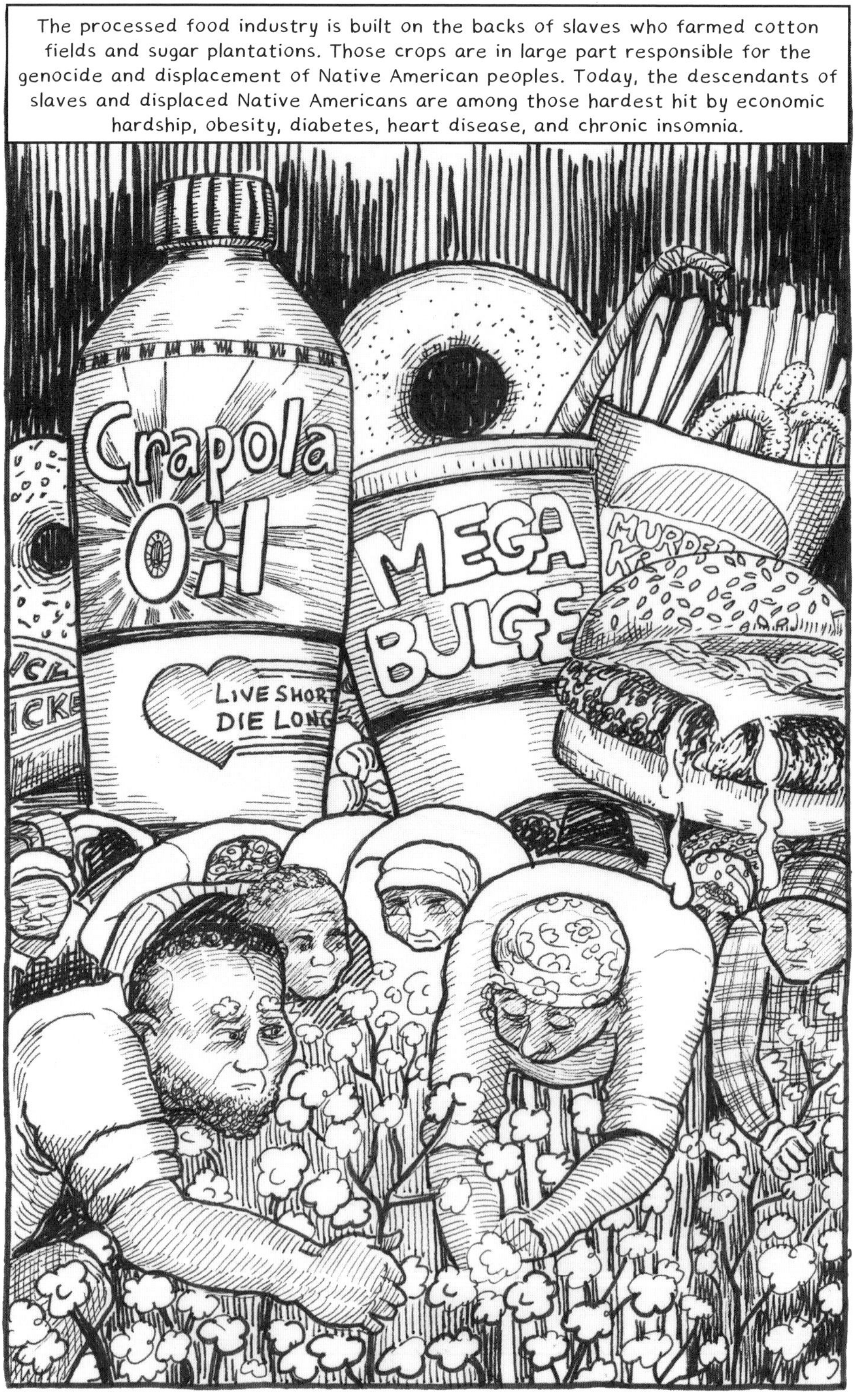
The processed food industry is built on the backs of slaves who farmed cotton fields and sugar plantations. Those crops are in large part responsible for the genocide and displacement of Native American peoples. Today, the descendants of slaves and displaced Native Americans are among those hardest hit by economic hardship, obesity, diabetes, heart disease, and chronic insomnia.
Crapola
Oil
LIVE SHORT
DIE LONG
MEGA
BULGE

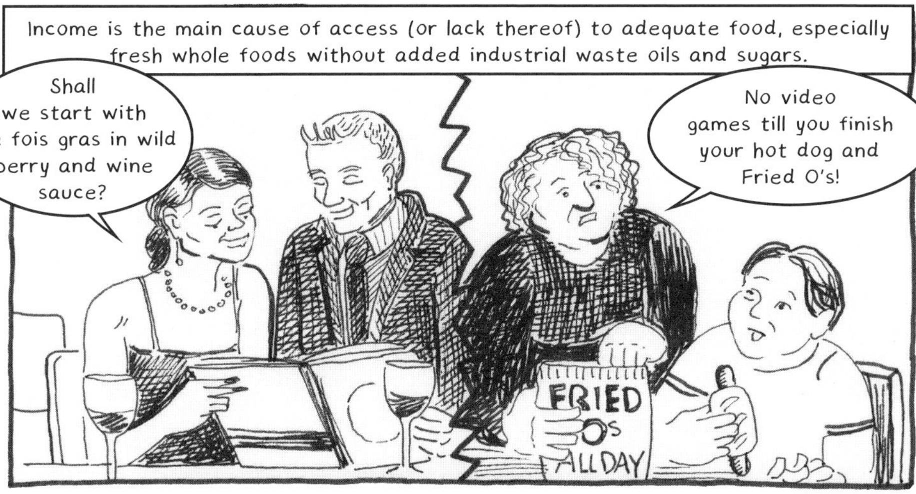
Income is the main cause of access (or lack thereof) to adequate food, especially fresh whole foods without added industrial waste oils and sugars.
Shall we start with the fois gras in wild berry and wine sauce?
No video games till you finish your hot dog and Fried O's!
FRIED O's ALL DAY

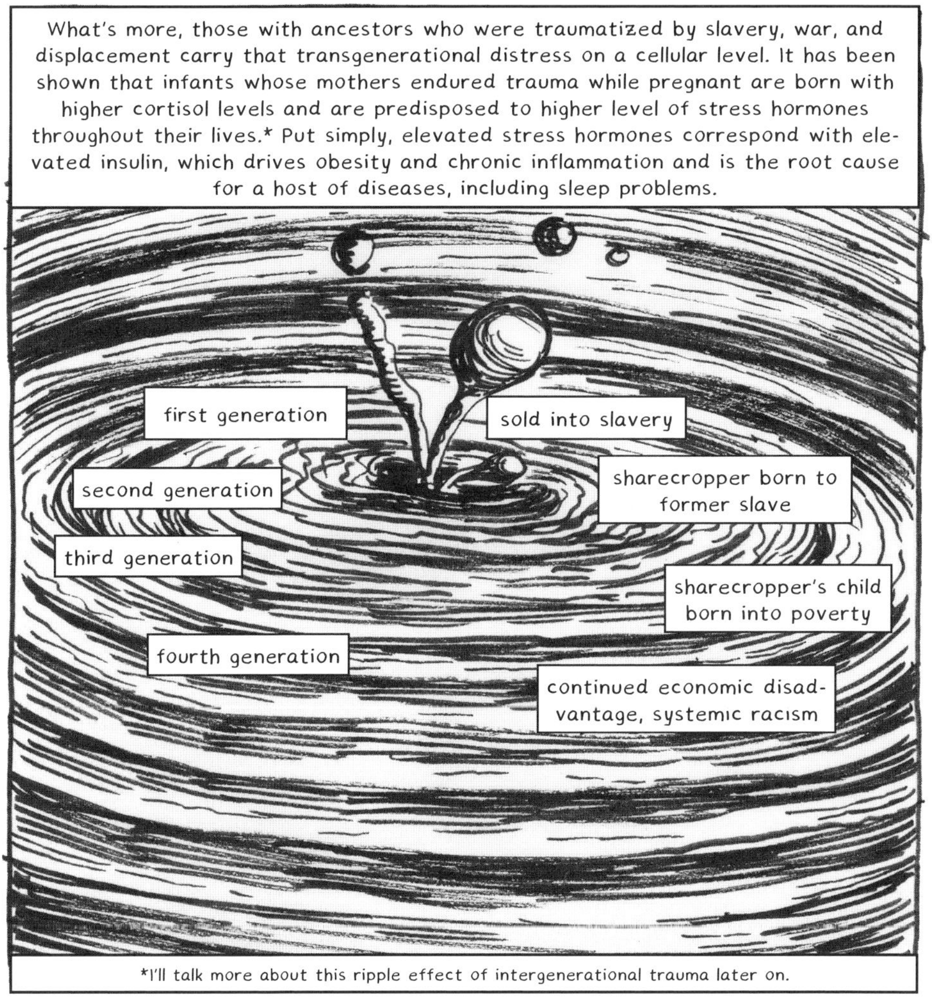
What's more, those with ancestors who were traumatized by slavery, war, and displacement carry that transgenerational distress on a cellular level. It has been shown that infants whose mothers endured trauma while pregnant are born with higher cortisol levels and are predisposed to higher level of stress hormones throughout their lives.* Put simply, elevated stress hormones correspond with elevated insulin, which drives obesity and chronic inflammation and is the root cause for a host of diseases, including sleep problems.
first generation
sold into slavery
second generation
sharecropper born to former slave
third generation
sharecropper's child born into poverty
fourth generation
continued economic disadvantage, systemic racism
*I'll talk more about this ripple effect of intergenerational trauma later on.

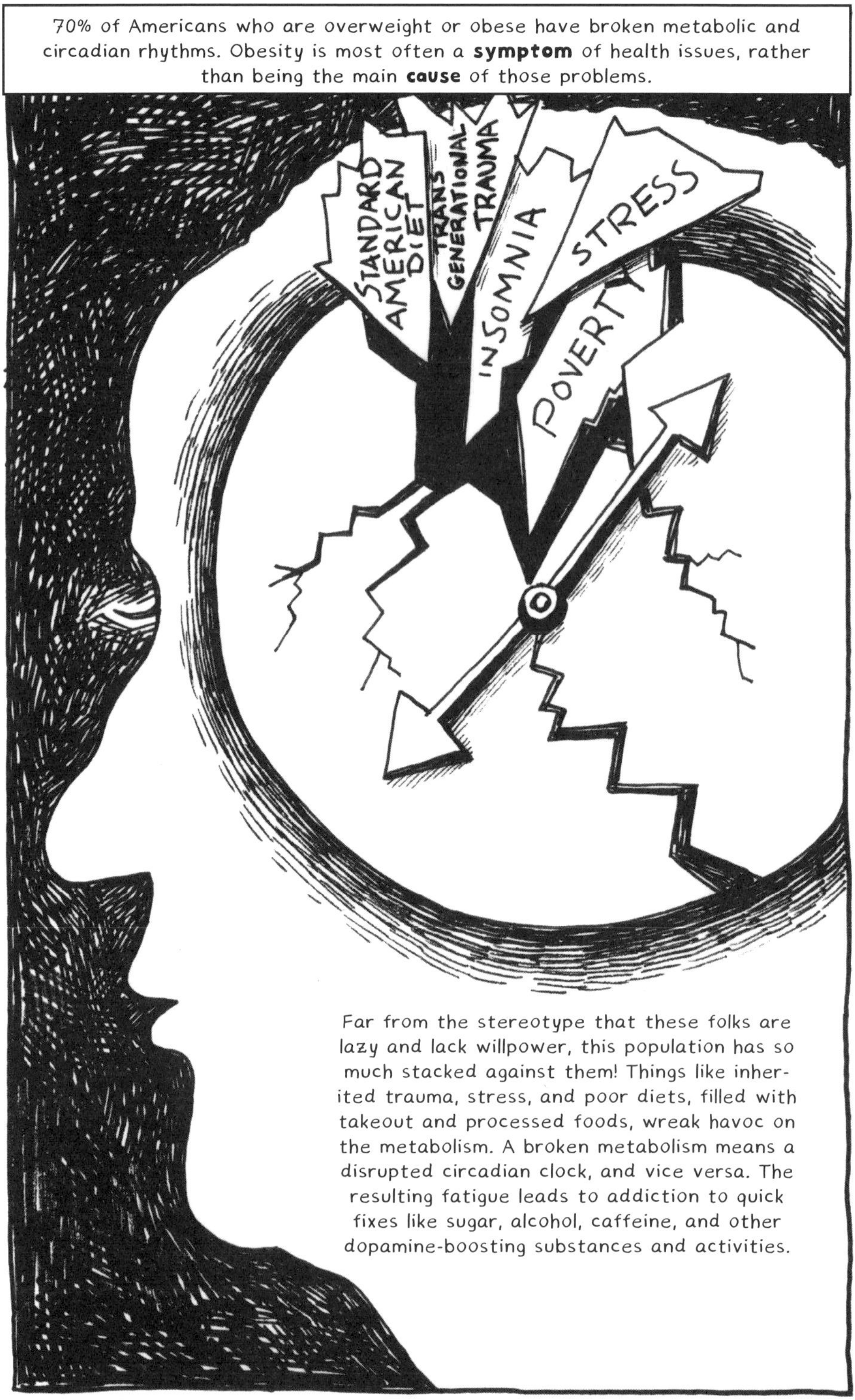
70% of Americans who are overweight or obese have broken metabolic and circadian rhythms. Obesity is most often a **symptom** of health issues, rather than being the main **cause** of those problems.
STANDARD AMERICAN DIET
TRANS GENERATIONAL TRAUMA
INSOMNIA
STRESS
POVERTY
Far from the stereotype that these folks are lazy and lack willpower, this population has so much stacked against them! Things like inherited trauma, stress, and poor diets, filled with takeout and processed foods, wreak havoc on the metabolism. A broken metabolism means a disrupted circadian clock, and vice versa. The resulting fatigue leads to addiction to quick fixes like sugar, alcohol, caffeine, and other dopamine-boosting substances and activities.

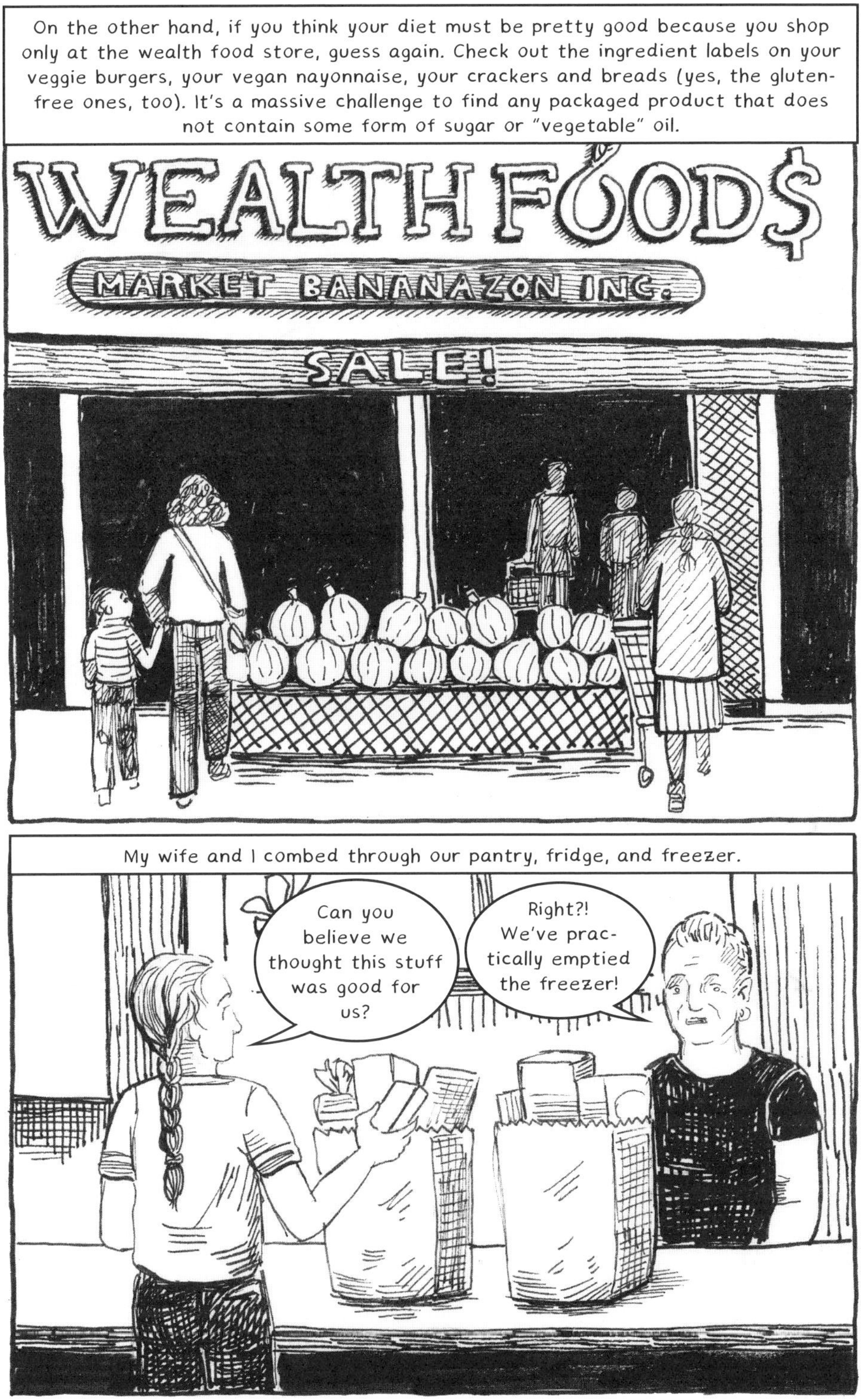

On the other hand, if you think your diet must be pretty good because you shop only at the wealth food store, guess again. Check out the ingredient labels on your veggie burgers, your vegan nayonnaise, your crackers and breads (yes, the gluten-free ones, too). It's a massive challenge to find any packaged product that does not contain some form of sugar or "vegetable" oil.
WEALTH FOOD$
MARKET BANANAZON INC.
SALE!
My wife and I combed through our pantry, fridge, and freezer.
Can you believe we thought this stuff was good for us?
Right?! We've practically emptied the freezer!

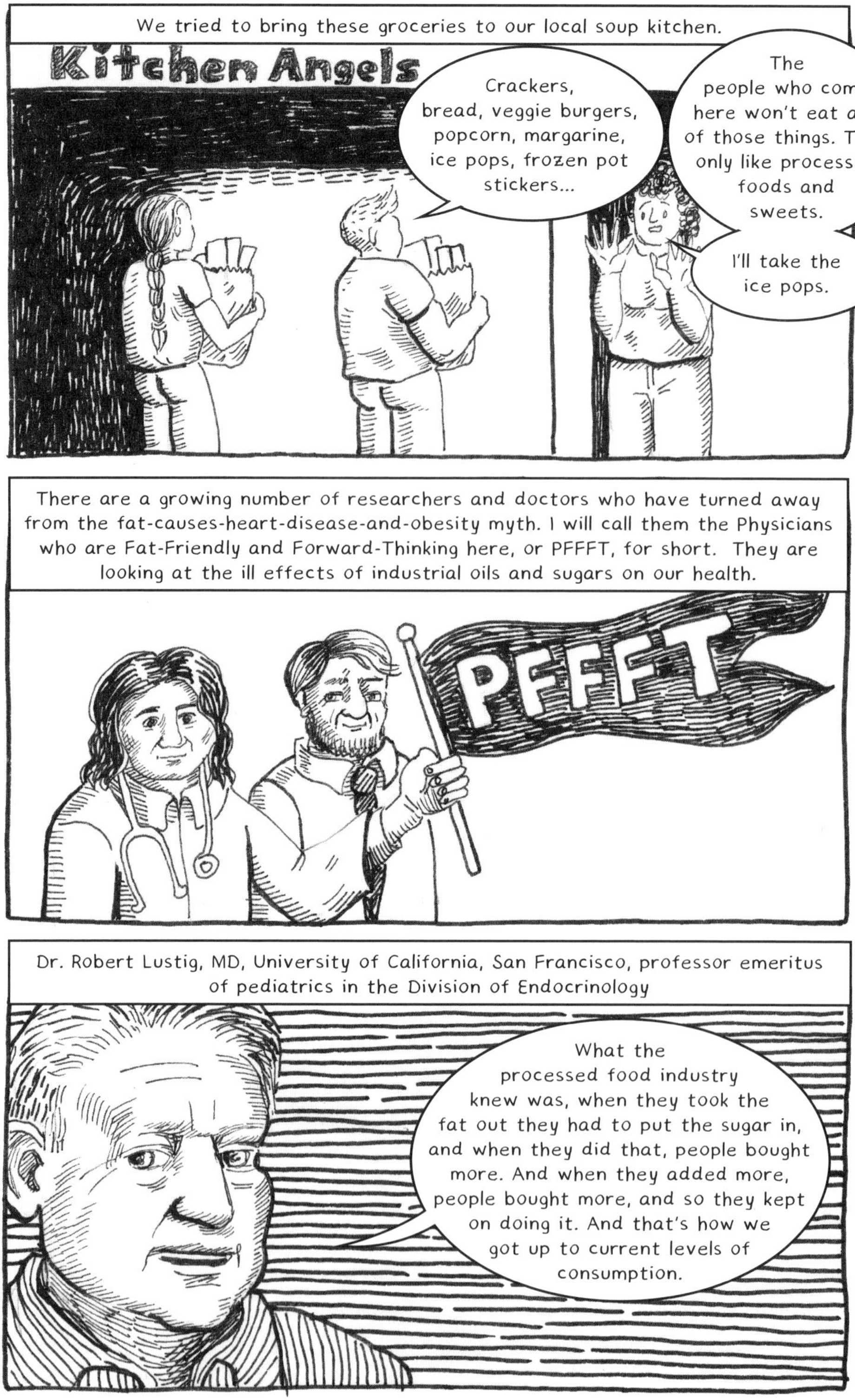
We tried to bring these groceries to our local soup kitchen.
Kitchen Angels
Crackers, bread, veggie burgers, popcorn, margarine, ice pops, frozen pot stickers...
The people who come here won't eat any of those things. They only like processed foods and sweets.
I'll take the ice pops.
There are a growing number of researchers and doctors who have turned away from the fat-causes-heart-disease-and-obesity myth. I will call them the Physicians who are Fat-Friendly and Forward-Thinking here, or PFFFT, for short. They are looking at the ill effects of industrial oils and sugars on our health.
PFFFT
Dr. Robert Lustig, MD, University of California, San Francisco, professor emeritus of pediatrics in the Division of Endocrinology
What the processed food industry knew was, when they took the fat out they had to put the sugar in, and when they did that, people bought more. And when they added more, people bought more, and so they kept on doing it. And that's how we got up to current levels of consumption.

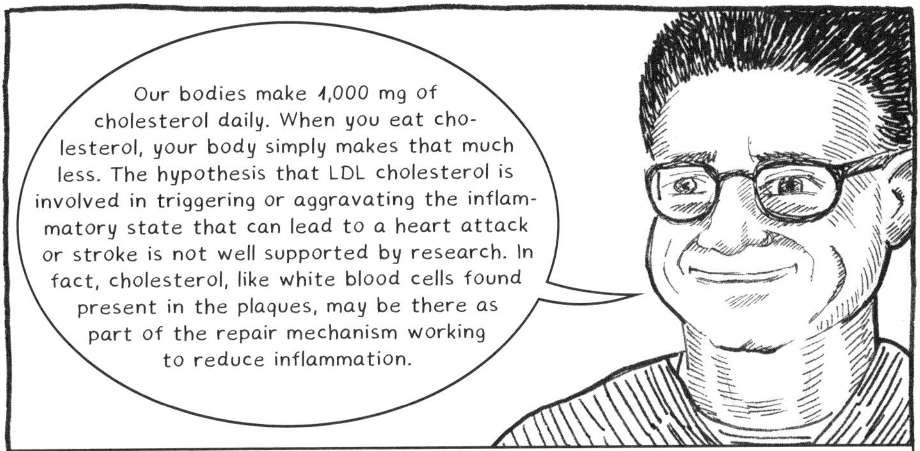
Our bodies make 1,000 mg of cholesterol daily. When you eat cholesterol, your body simply makes that much less. The hypothesis that LDL cholesterol is involved in triggering or aggravating the inflammatory state that can lead to a heart attack or stroke is not well supported by research. In fact, cholesterol, like white blood cells found present in the plaques, may be there as part of the repair mechanism working to reduce inflammation.

Dr. Nadir Ali, MD, cardiologist

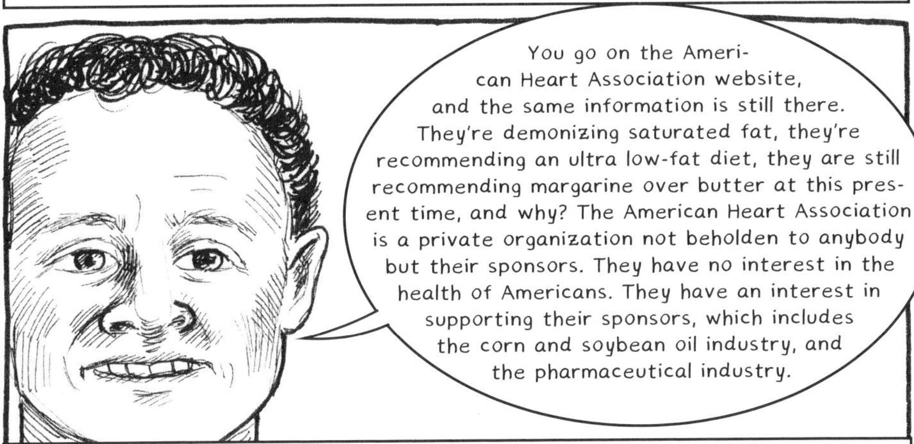
You go on the American Heart Association website, and the same information is still there. They're demonizing saturated fat, they're recommending an ultra low-fat diet, they are still recommending margarine over butter at this present time, and why? The American Heart Association is a private organization not beholden to anybody but their sponsors. They have no interest in the health of Americans. They have an interest in supporting their sponsors, which includes the corn and soybean oil industry, and the pharmaceutical industry.

David Diamond, University of South Florida professor of psychology, molecular pharmacology, and physiology and director of the USF Neuroscience Collaborative

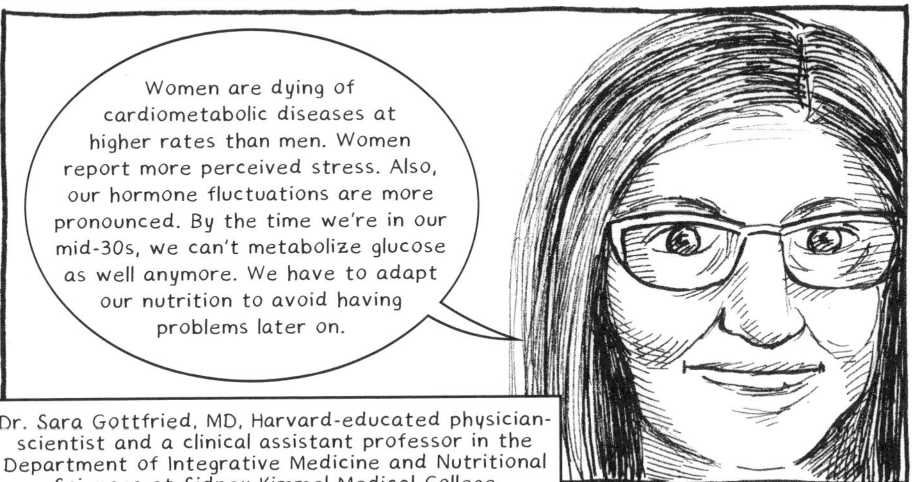
Women are dying of cardiometabolic diseases at higher rates than men. Women report more perceived stress. Also, our hormone fluctuations are more pronounced. By the time we're in our mid-30s, we can't metabolize glucose as well anymore. We have to adapt our nutrition to avoid having problems later on.

Dr. Sara Gottfried, MD, Harvard-educated physician-scientist and a clinical assistant professor in the Department of Integrative Medicine and Nutritional Sciences at Sidney Kimmel Medical College

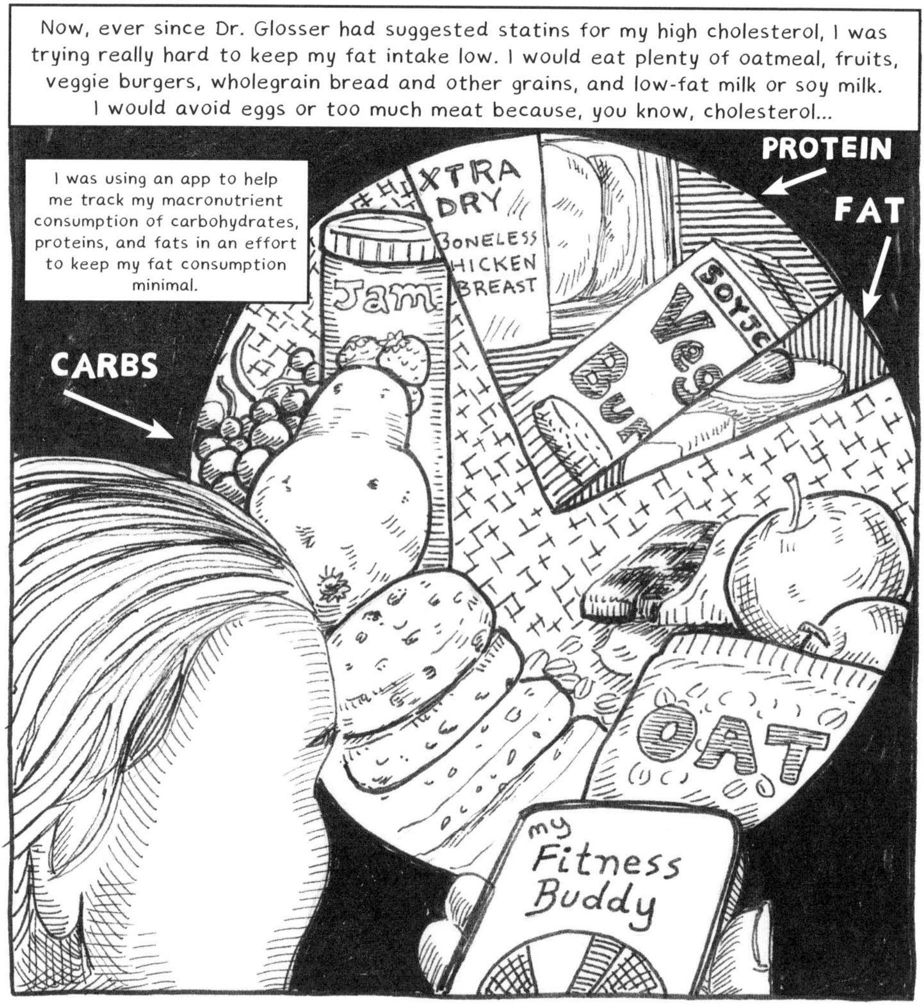
Now, ever since Dr. Glosser had suggested statins for my high cholesterol, I was trying really hard to keep my fat intake low. I would eat plenty of oatmeal, fruits, veggie burgers, wholegrain bread and other grains, and low-fat milk or soy milk. I would avoid eggs or too much meat because, you know, cholesterol...
I was using an app to help me track my macronutrient consumption of carbohydrates, proteins, and fats in an effort to keep my fat consumption minimal.
PROTEIN
FAT
CARBS
XTRA DRY
HICKEN
BREAST
Jam
SOYJC
OAT
my Fitness Buddy

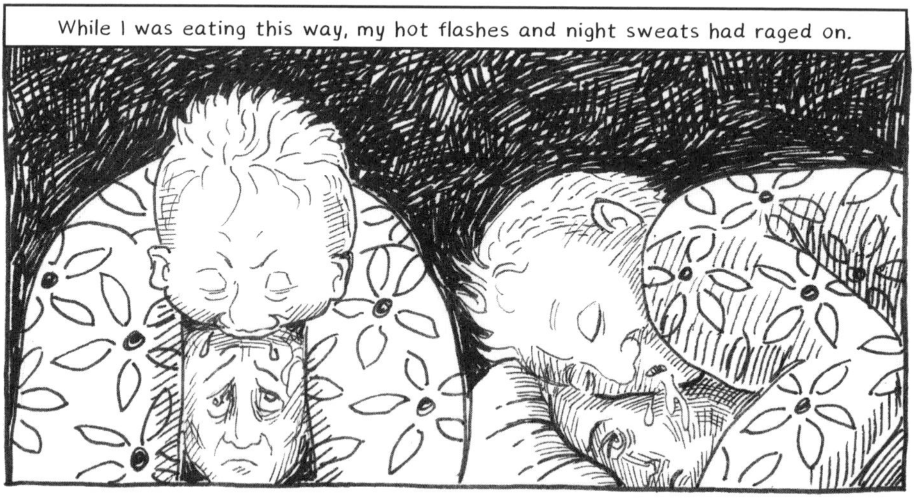
While I was eating this way, my hot flashes and night sweats had raged on.

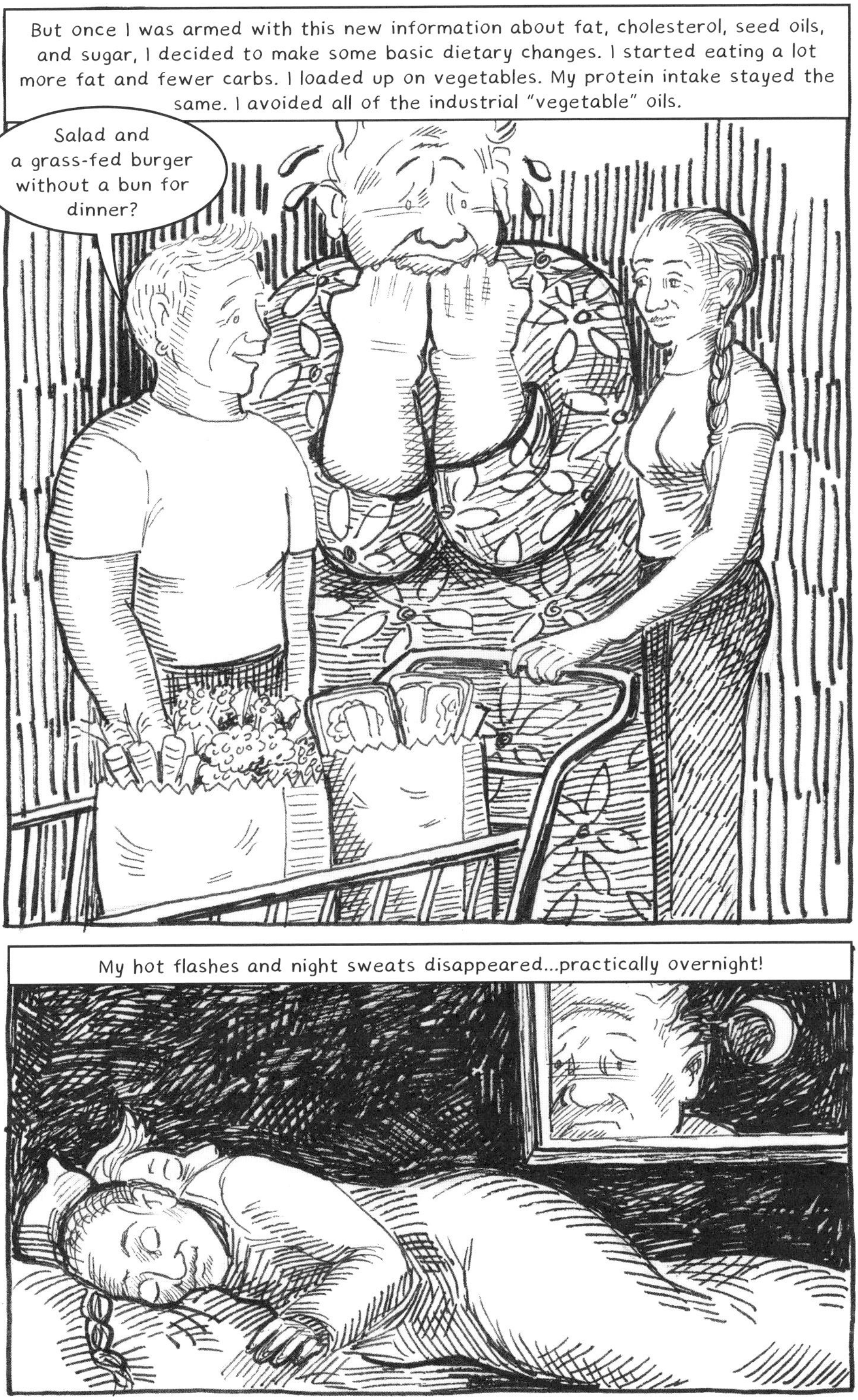
But once I was armed with this new information about fat, cholesterol, seed oils, and sugar, I decided to make some basic dietary changes. I started eating a lot more fat and fewer carbs. I loaded up on vegetables. My protein intake stayed the same. I avoided all of the industrial "vegetable" oils.
Salad and a grass-fed burger without a bun for dinner?
My hot flashes and night sweats disappeared...practically overnight!

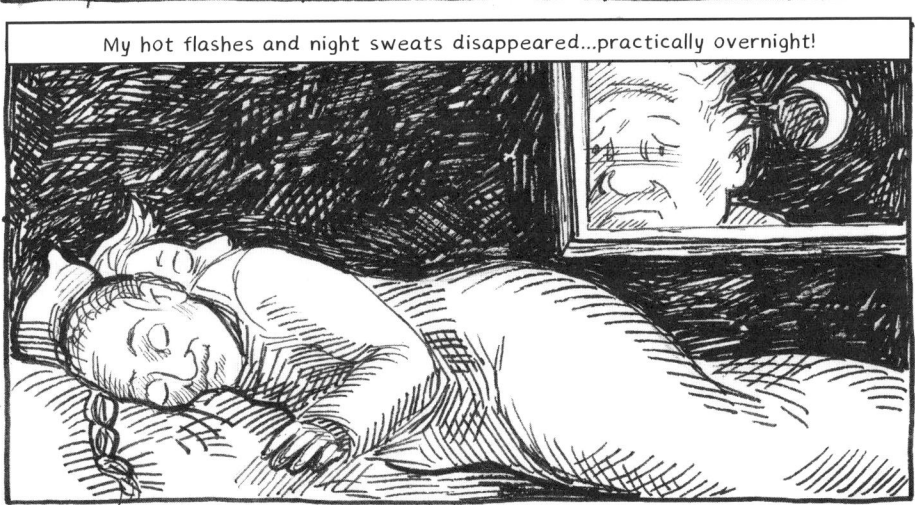

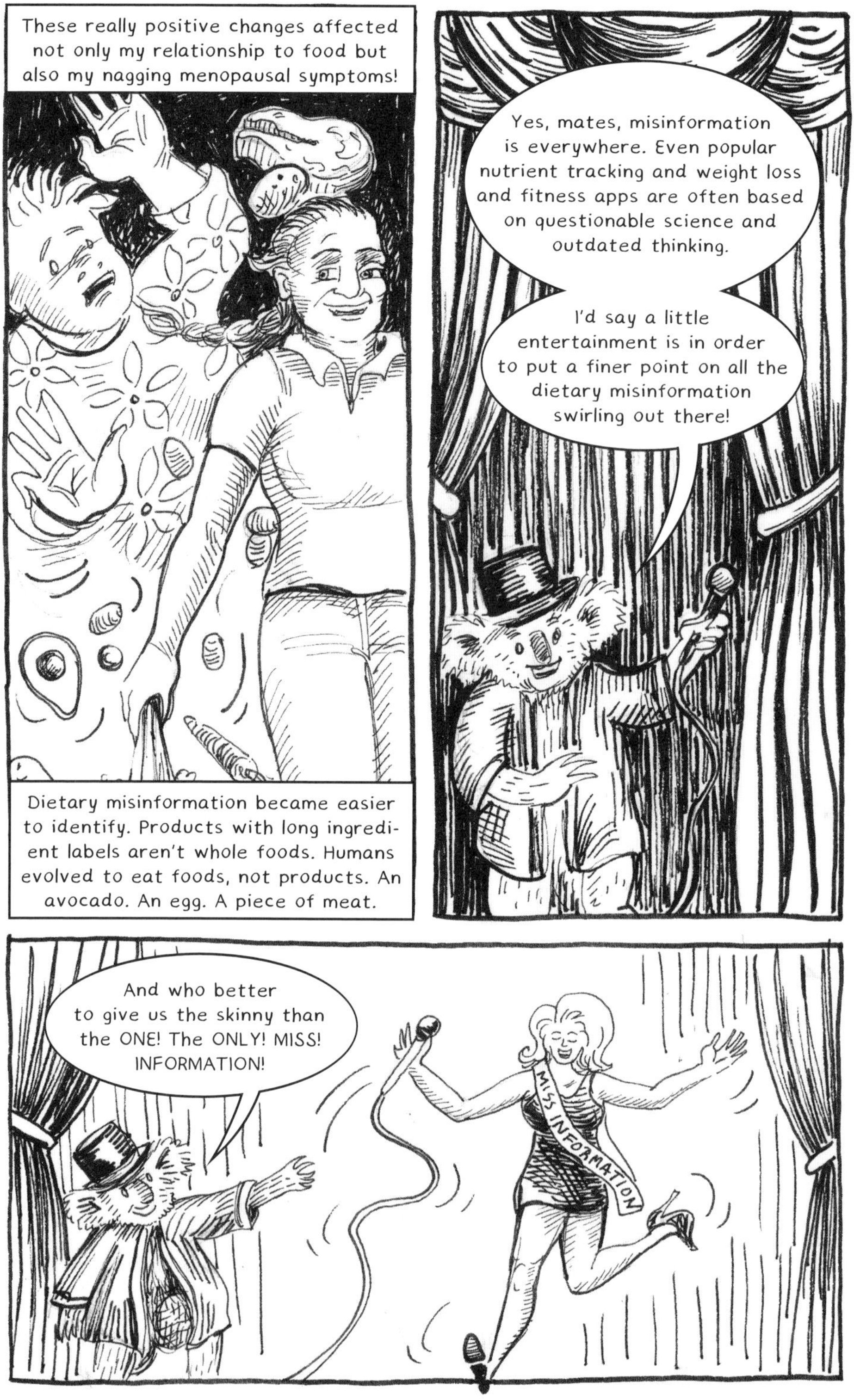
These really positive changes affected not only my relationship to food but also my nagging menopausal symptoms!
Dietary misinformation became easier to identify. Products with long ingredient labels aren't whole foods. Humans evolved to eat foods, not products. An avocado. An egg. A piece of meat.
Yes, mates, misinformation is everywhere. Even popular nutrient tracking and weight loss and fitness apps are often based on questionable science and outdated thinking.
I'd say a little entertainment is in order to put a finer point on all the dietary misinformation swirling out there!
And who better to give us the skinny than the ONE! The ONLY! MISS! INFORMATION!
MISS INFORMATION

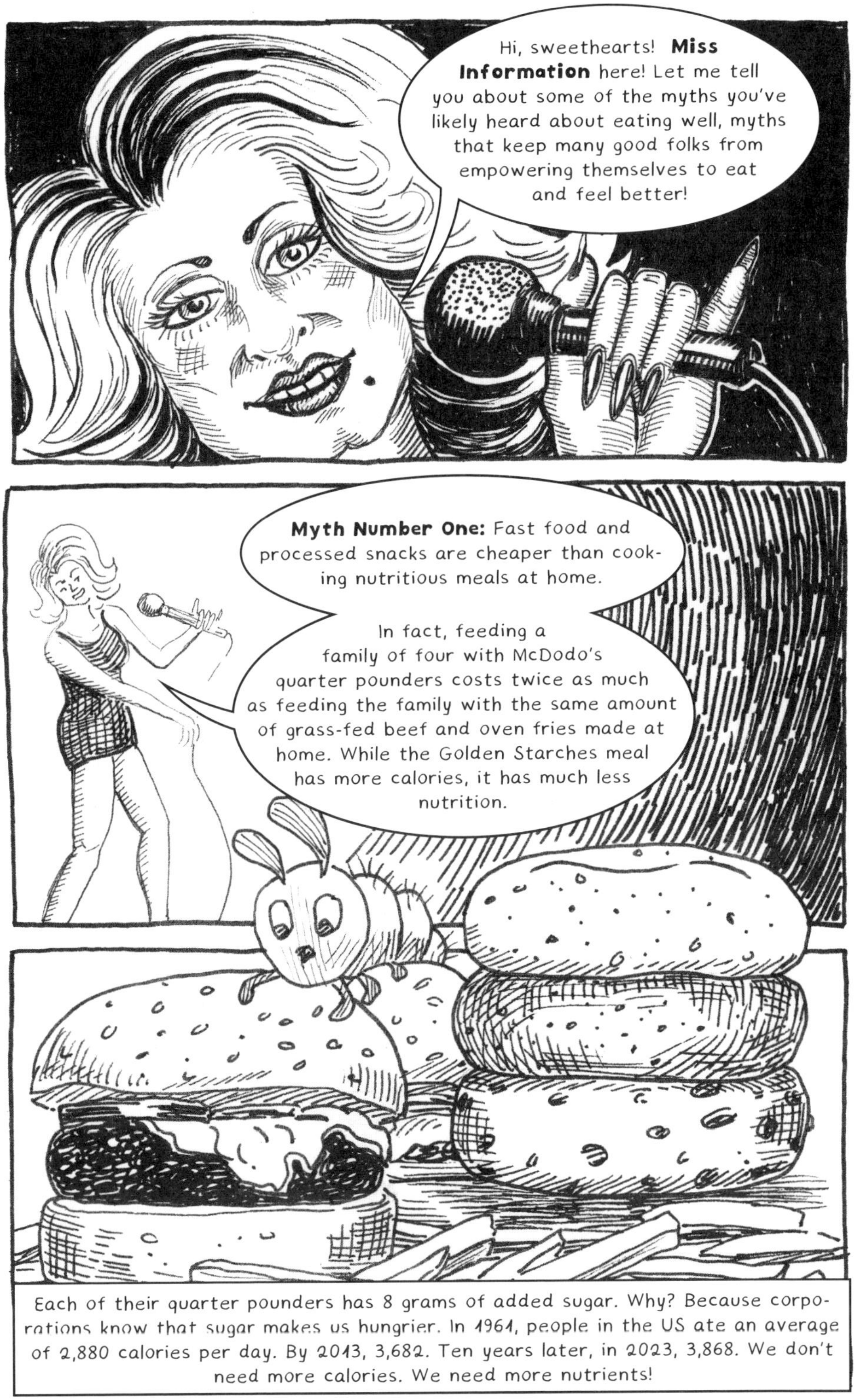
Hi, sweethearts! **Miss Information** here! Let me tell you about some of the myths you've likely heard about eating well, myths that keep many good folks from empowering themselves to eat and feel better!
Myth Number One: Fast food and processed snacks are cheaper than cooking nutritious meals at home.
In fact, feeding a family of four with McDodo's quarter pounders costs twice as much as feeding the family with the same amount of grass-fed beef and oven fries made at home. While the Golden Starches meal has more calories, it has much less nutrition.
Each of their quarter pounders has 8 grams of added sugar. Why? Because corporations know that sugar makes us hungrier. In 1961, people in the US ate an average of 2,880 calories per day. By 2013, 3,682. Ten years later, in 2023, 3,868. We don't need more calories. We need more nutrients!

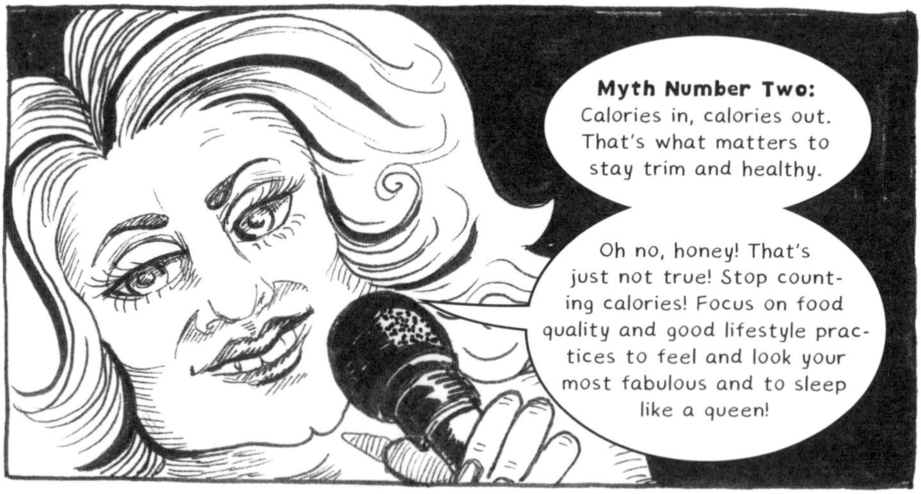
Myth Number Two: Calories in, calories out. That's what matters to stay trim and healthy.
Oh no, honey! That's just not true! Stop counting calories! Focus on food quality and good lifestyle practices to feel and look your most fabulous and to sleep like a queen!

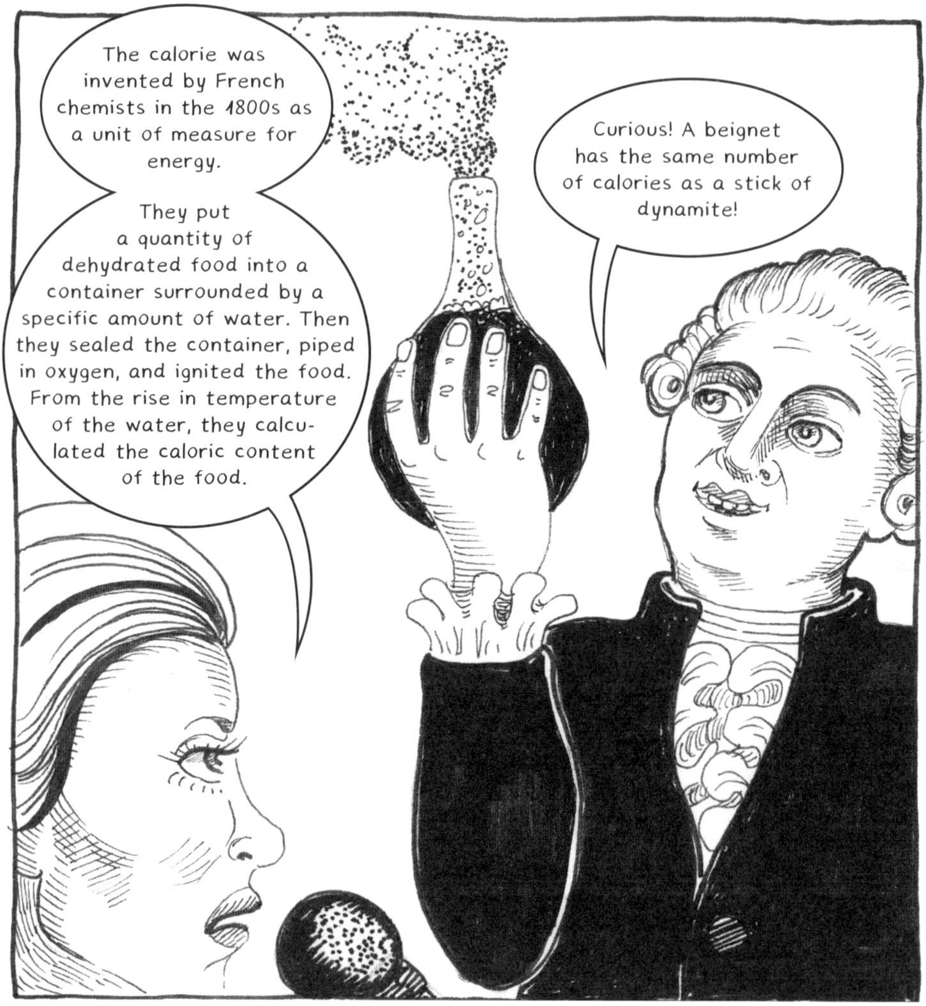
The calorie was invented by French chemists in the 1800s as a unit of measure for energy.
They put a quantity of dehydrated food into a container surrounded by a specific amount of water. Then they sealed the container, piped in oxygen, and ignited the food. From the rise in temperature of the water, they calculated the caloric content of the food.
Curious! A beignet has the same number of calories as a stick of dynamite!

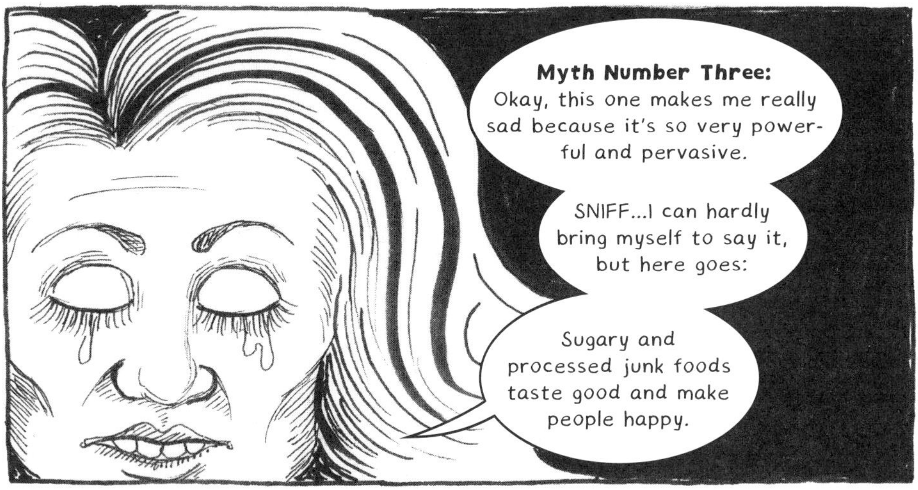
Myth Number Three:
Okay, this one makes me really sad because it's so very powerful and pervasive.
SNIFF...I can hardly bring myself to say it, but here goes:
Sugary and processed junk foods taste good and make people happy.

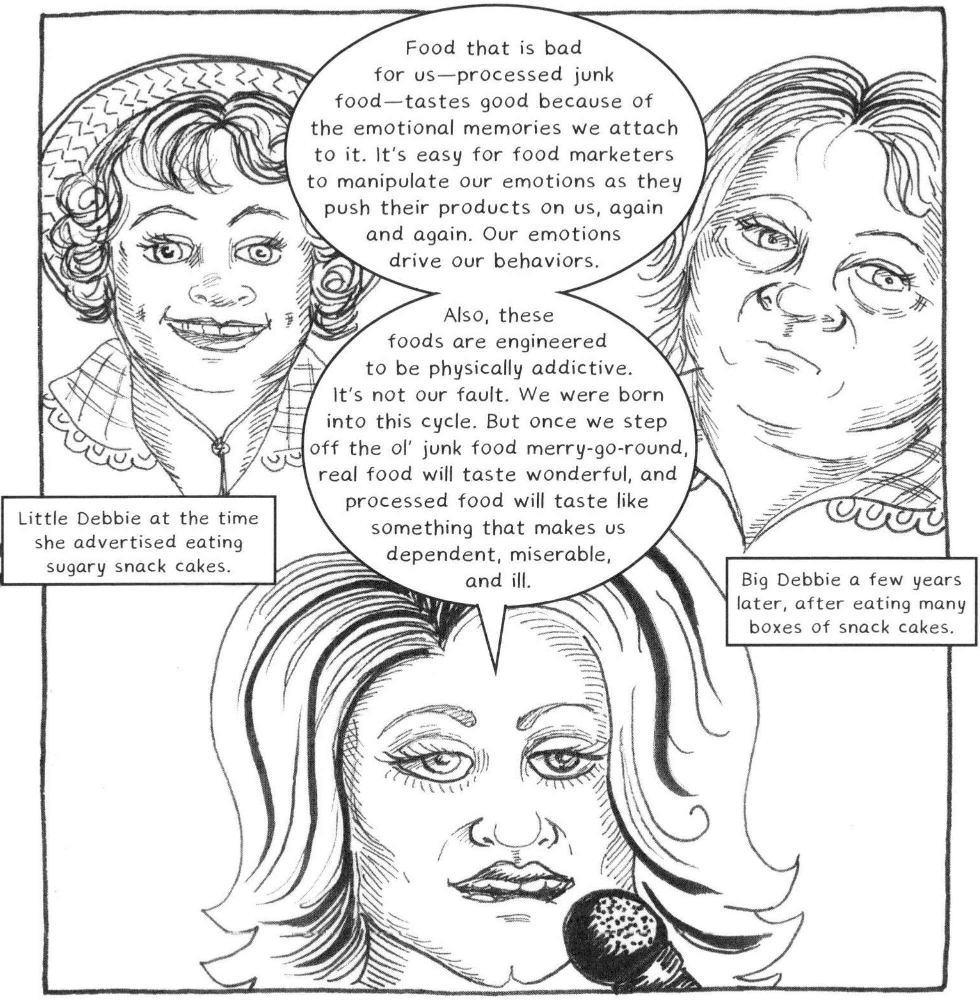
Food that is bad for us—processed junk food—tastes good because of the emotional memories we attach to it. It's easy for food marketers to manipulate our emotions as they push their products on us, again and again. Our emotions drive our behaviors.
Also, these foods are engineered to be physically addictive. It's not our fault. We were born into this cycle. But once we step off the ol' junk food merry-go-round, real food will taste wonderful, and processed food will taste like something that makes us dependent, miserable, and ill.
Little Debbie at the time she advertised eating sugary snack cakes.
Big Debbie a few years later, after eating many boxes of snack cakes.

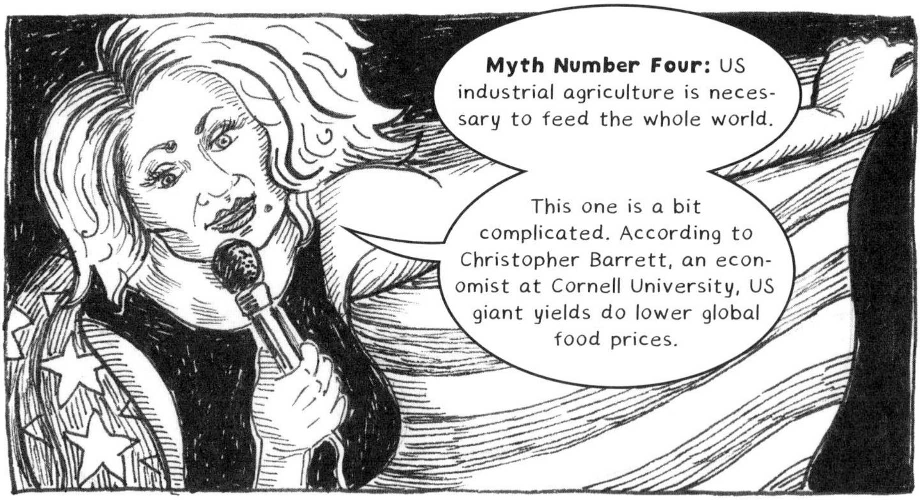
Myth Number Four: US industrial agriculture is neces-sary to feed the whole world.
This one is a bit complicated. According to Christopher Barrett, an econ-omist at Cornell University, US giant yields do lower global food prices.

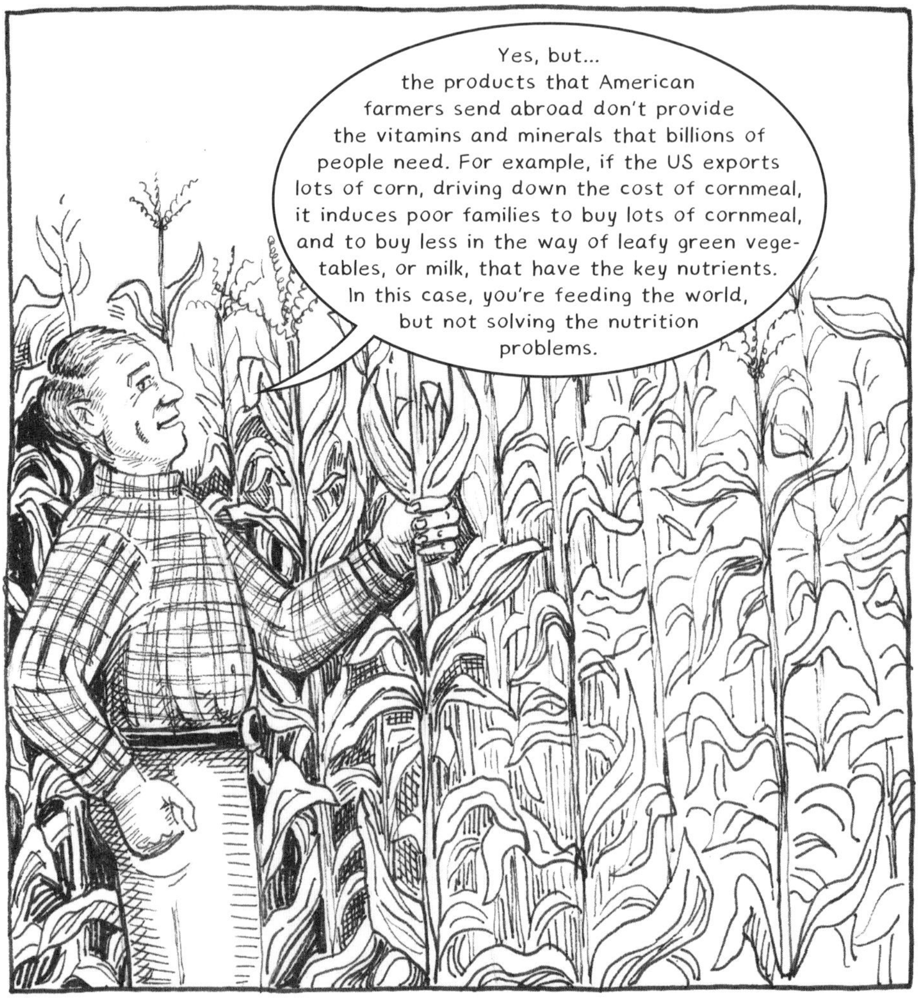
Yes, but... the products that American farmers send abroad don't provide the vitamins and minerals that billions of people need. For example, if the US exports lots of corn, driving down the cost of cornmeal, it induces poor families to buy lots of cornmeal, and to buy less in the way of leafy green vege-tables, or milk, that have the key nutrients. In this case, you're feeding the world, but not solving the nutrition problems.

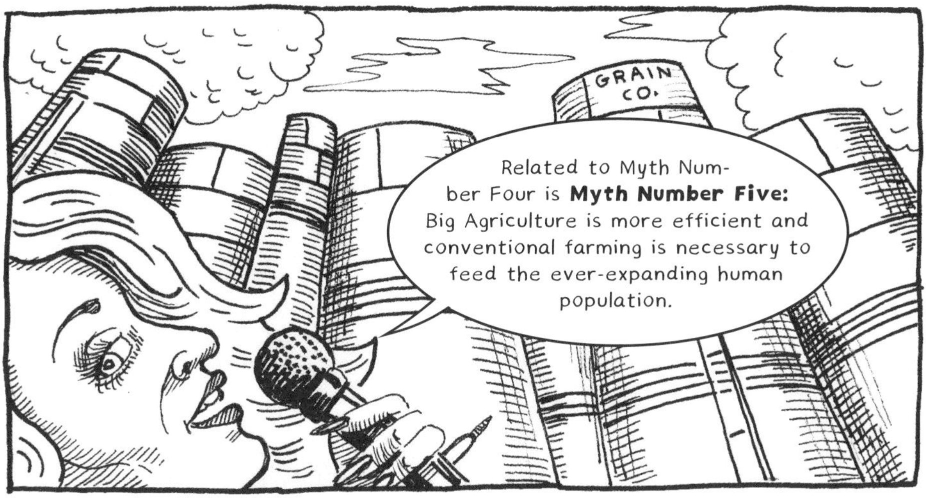
GRAIN CO.
Related to Myth Number Four is **Myth Number Five:** Big Agriculture is more efficient and conventional farming is necessary to feed the ever-expanding human population.

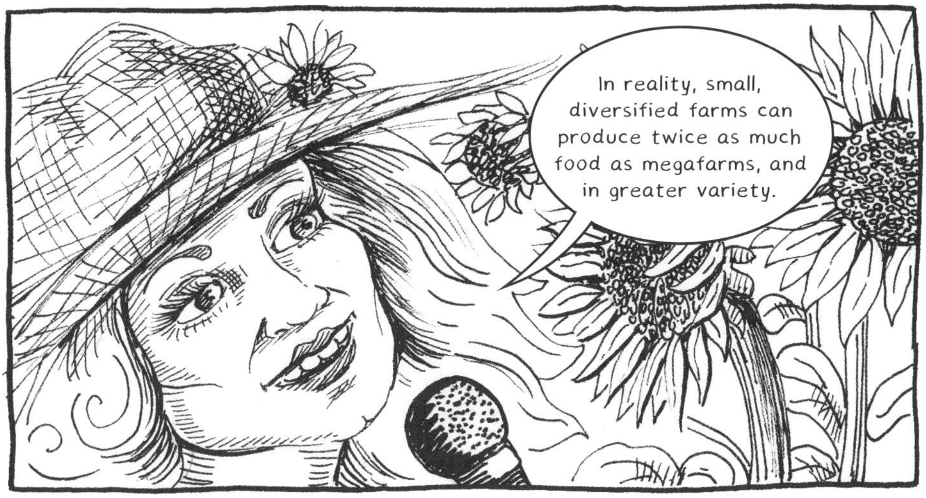
In reality, small, diversified farms can produce twice as much food as megafarms, and in greater variety.

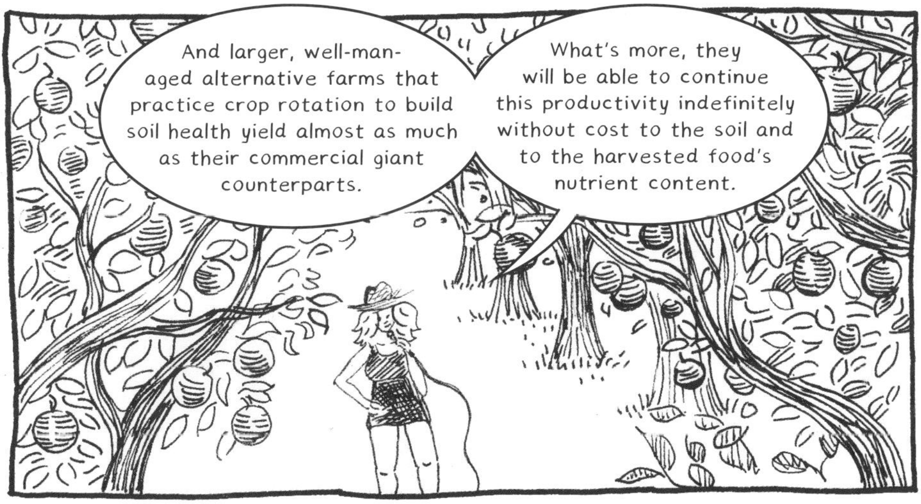
And larger, well-managed alternative farms that practice crop rotation to build soil health yield almost as much as their commercial giant counterparts.
What's more, they will be able to continue this productivity indefinitely without cost to the soil and to the harvested food's nutrient content.

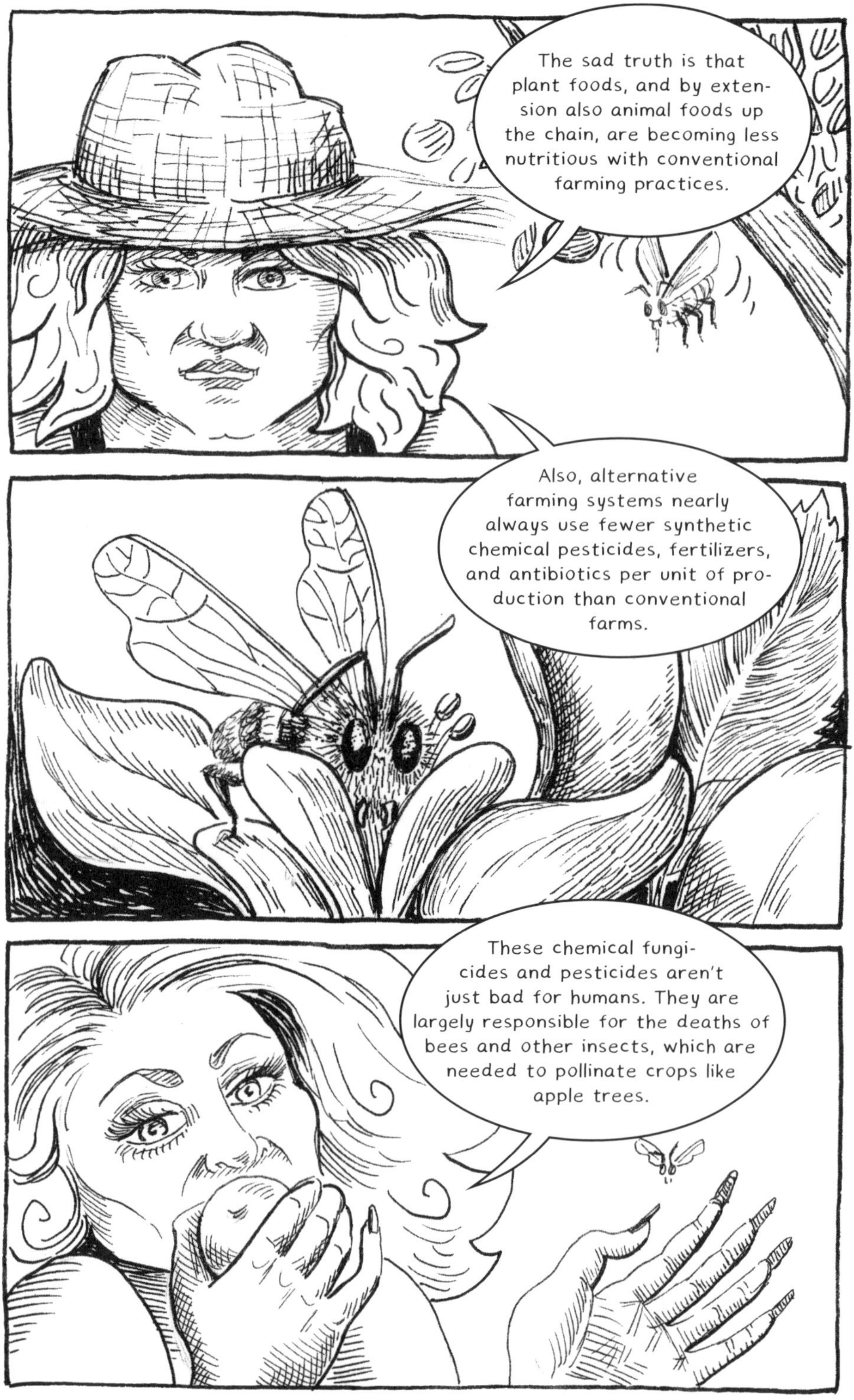
The sad truth is that plant foods, and by extension also animal foods up the chain, are becoming less nutritious with conventional farming practices.
Also, alternative farming systems nearly always use fewer synthetic chemical pesticides, fertilizers, and antibiotics per unit of production than conventional farms.
These chemical fungicides and pesticides aren't just bad for humans. They are largely responsible for the deaths of bees and other insects, which are needed to pollinate crops like apple trees.

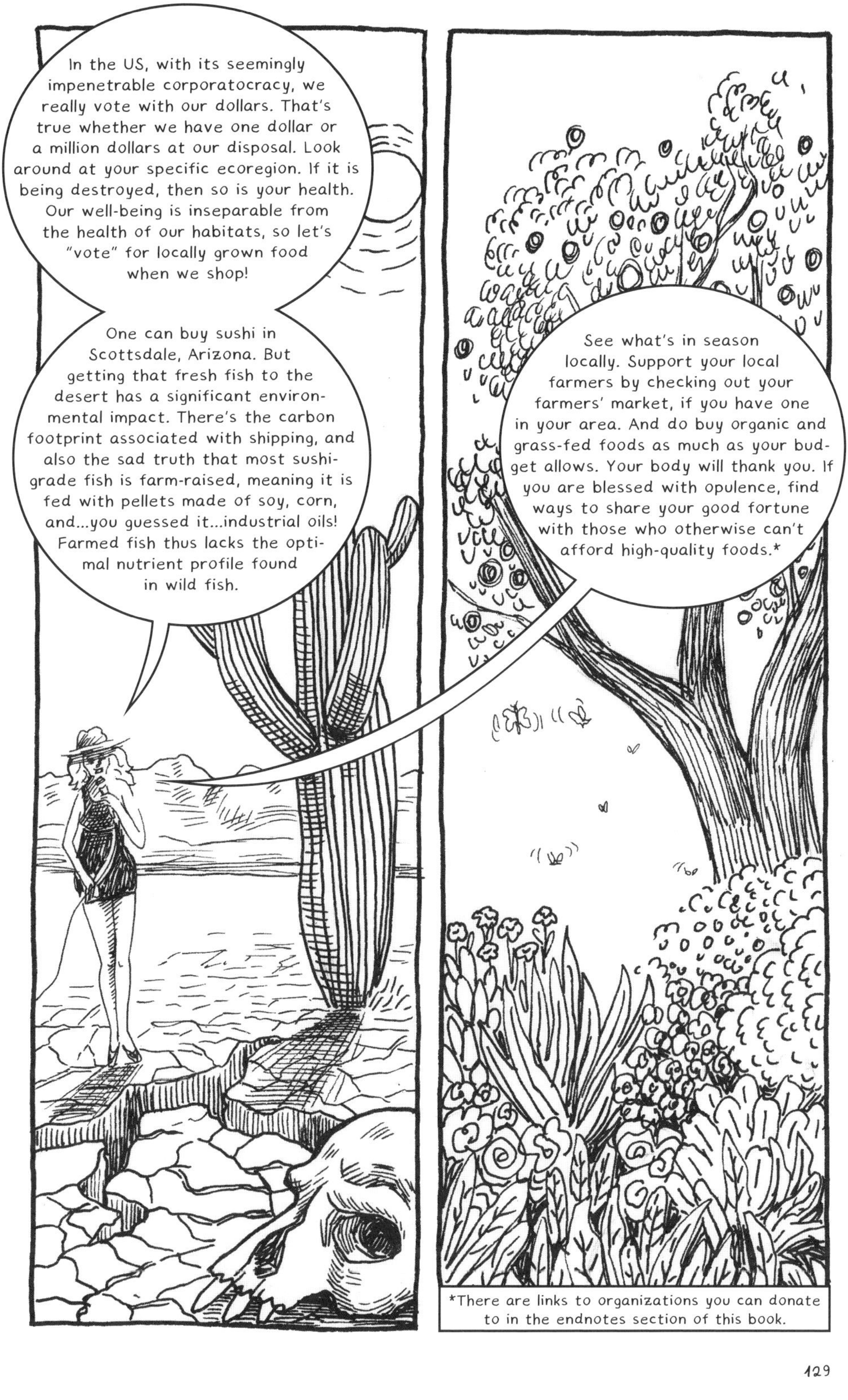
In the US, with its seemingly impenetrable corporatocracy, we really vote with our dollars. That's true whether we have one dollar or a million dollars at our disposal. Look around at your specific ecoregion. If it is being destroyed, then so is your health. Our well-being is inseparable from the health of our habitats, so let's "vote" for locally grown food when we shop!
One can buy sushi in Scottsdale, Arizona. But getting that fresh fish to the desert has a significant environmental impact. There's the carbon footprint associated with shipping, and also the sad truth that most sushi-grade fish is farm-raised, meaning it is fed with pellets made of soy, corn, and...you guessed it...industrial oils! Farmed fish thus lacks the optimal nutrient profile found in wild fish.
See what's in season locally. Support your local farmers by checking out your farmers' market, if you have one in your area. And do buy organic and grass-fed foods as much as your budget allows. Your body will thank you. If you are blessed with opulence, find ways to share your good fortune with those who otherwise can't afford high-quality foods.*
*There are links to organizations you can donate to in the endnotes section of this book.

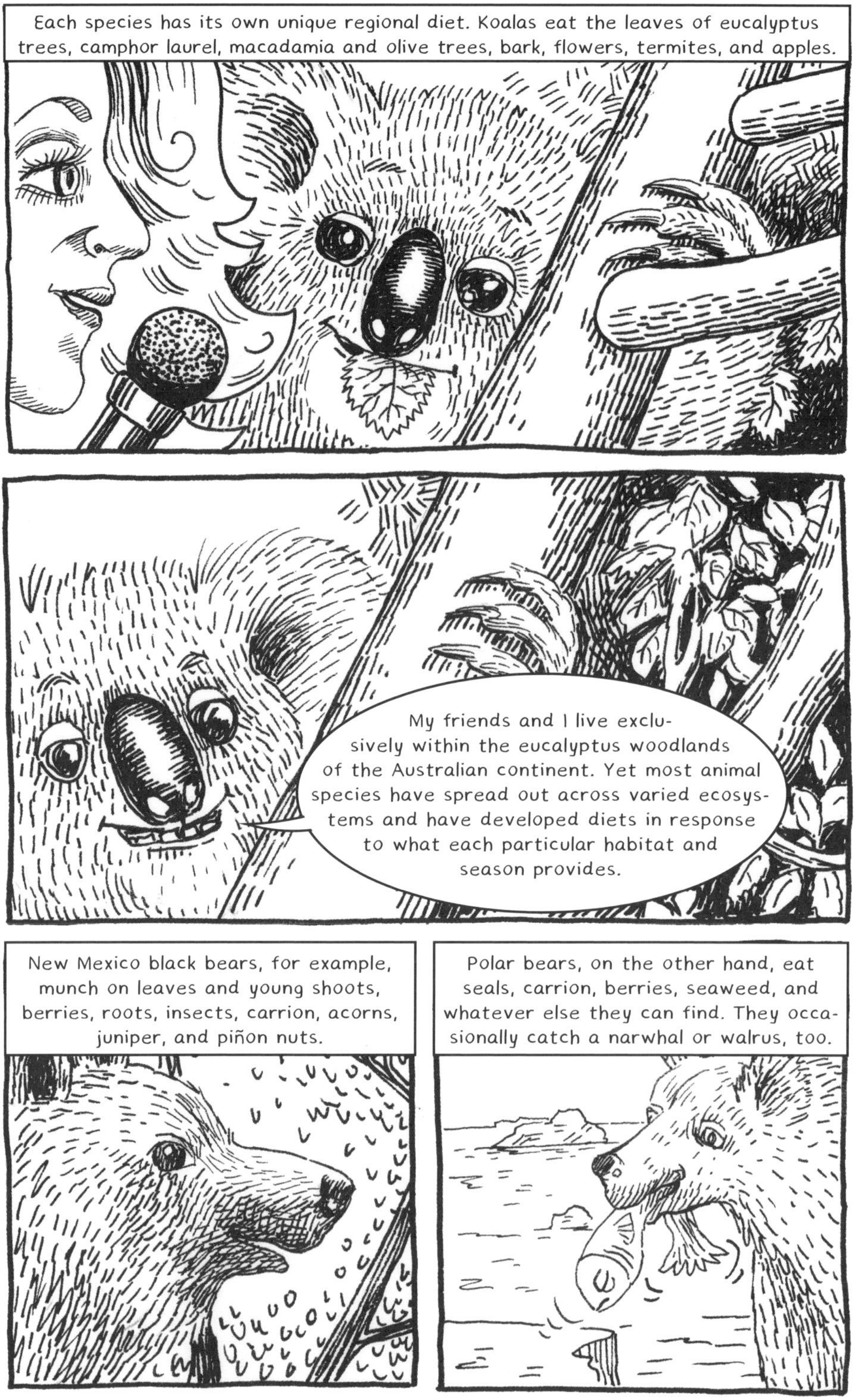
Each species has its own unique regional diet. Koalas eat the leaves of eucalyptus trees, camphor laurel, macadamia and olive trees, bark, flowers, termites, and apples.
My friends and I live exclusively within the eucalyptus woodlands of the Australian continent. Yet most animal species have spread out across varied ecosystems and have developed diets in response to what each particular habitat and season provides.
New Mexico black bears, for example, munch on leaves and young shoots, berries, roots, insects, carrion, acorns, juniper, and piñon nuts.
Polar bears, on the other hand, eat seals, carrion, berries, seaweed, and whatever else they can find. They occasionally catch a narwhal or walrus, too.

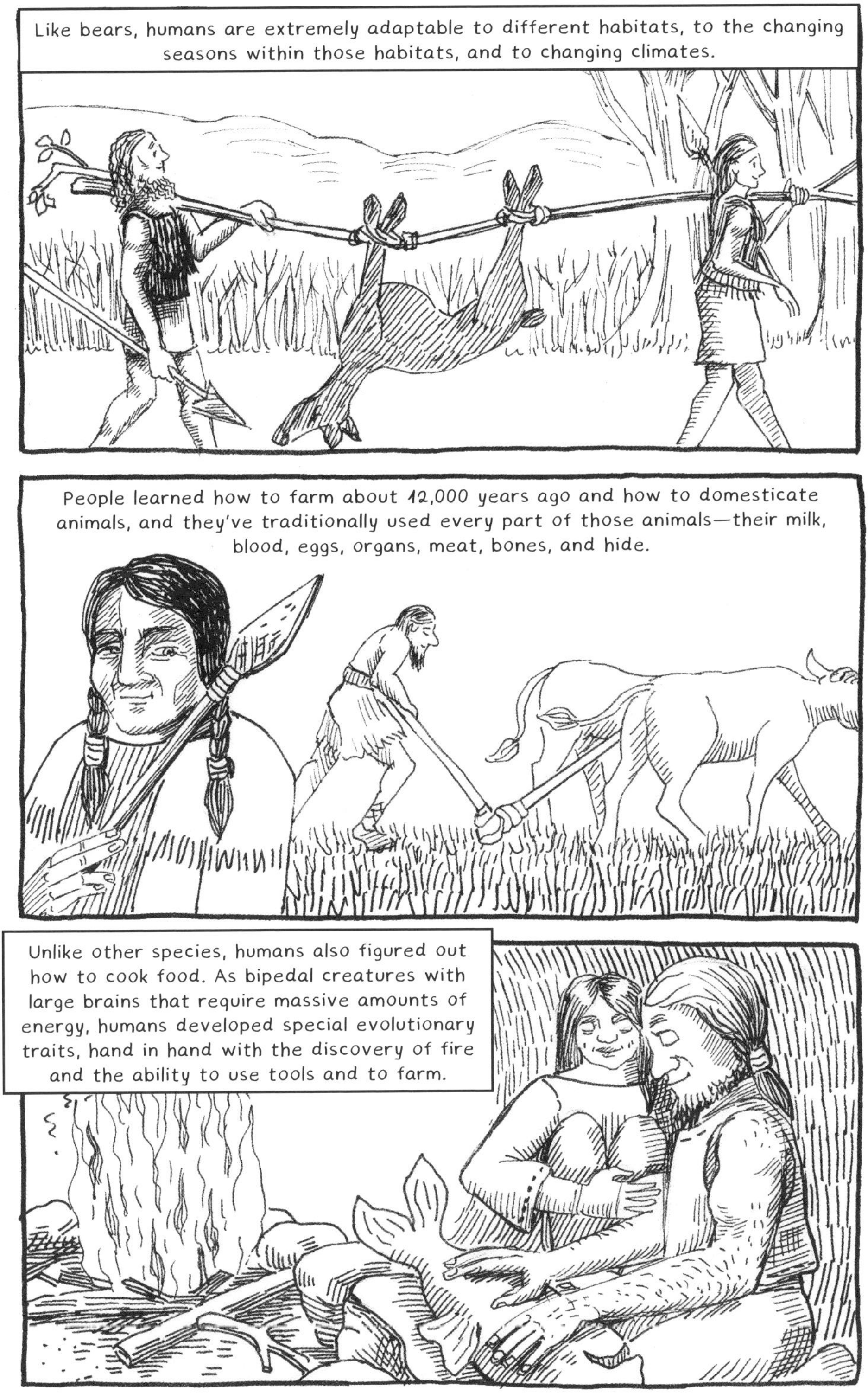
Like bears, humans are extremely adaptable to different habitats, to the changing seasons within those habitats, and to changing climates.
People learned how to farm about 12,000 years ago and how to domesticate animals, and they've traditionally used every part of those animals—their milk, blood, eggs, organs, meat, bones, and hide.
Unlike other species, humans also figured out how to cook food. As bipedal creatures with large brains that require massive amounts of energy, humans developed special evolutionary traits, hand in hand with the discovery of fire and the ability to use tools and to farm.

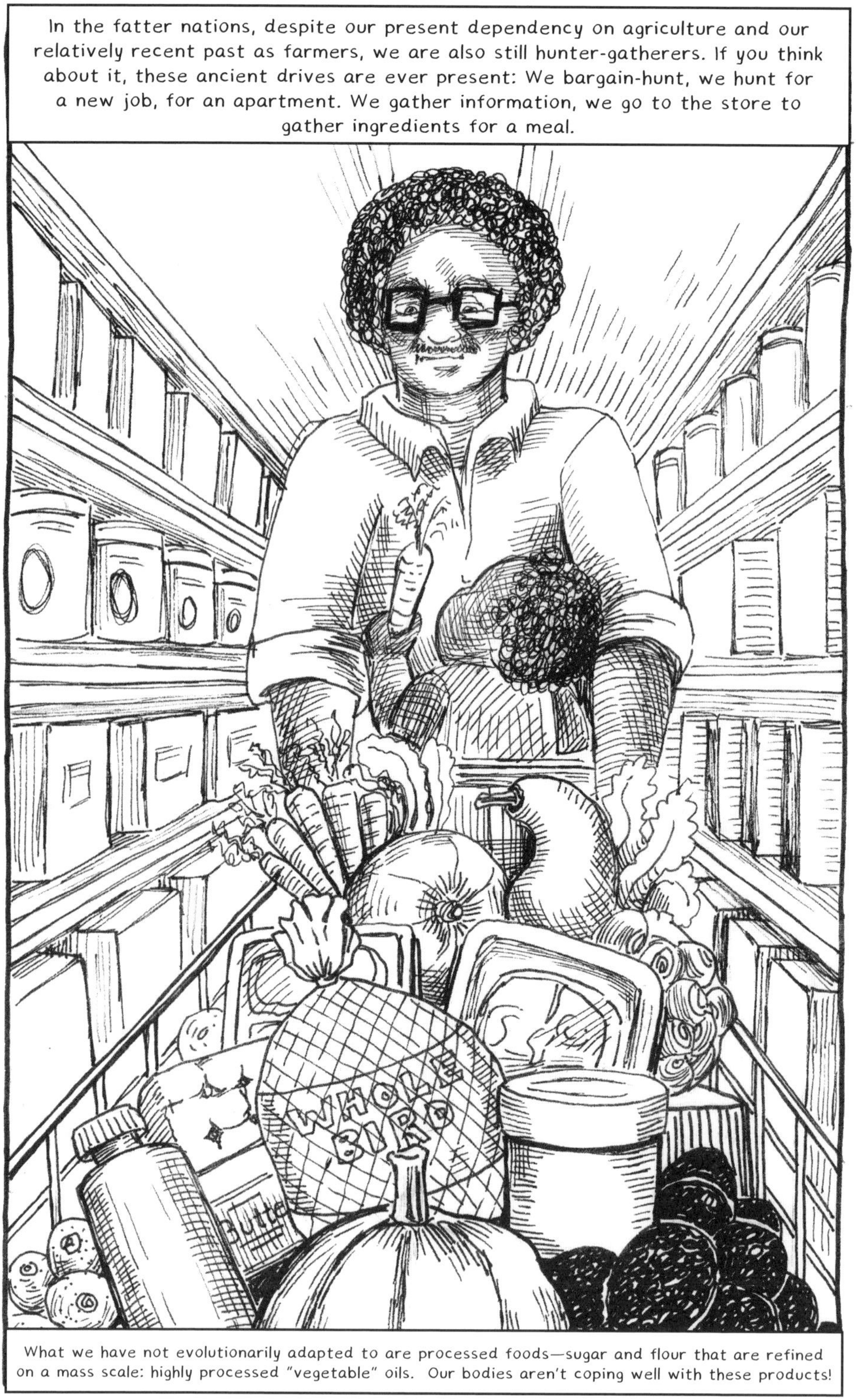

In the fatter nations, despite our present dependency on agriculture and our relatively recent past as farmers, we are also still hunter-gatherers. If you think about it, these ancient drives are ever present: We bargain-hunt, we hunt for a new job, for an apartment. We gather information, we go to the store to gather ingredients for a meal.
WHOLE BIRD
What we have not evolutionarily adapted to are processed foods—sugar and flour that are refined on a mass scale: highly processed "vegetable" oils. Our bodies aren't coping well with these products!

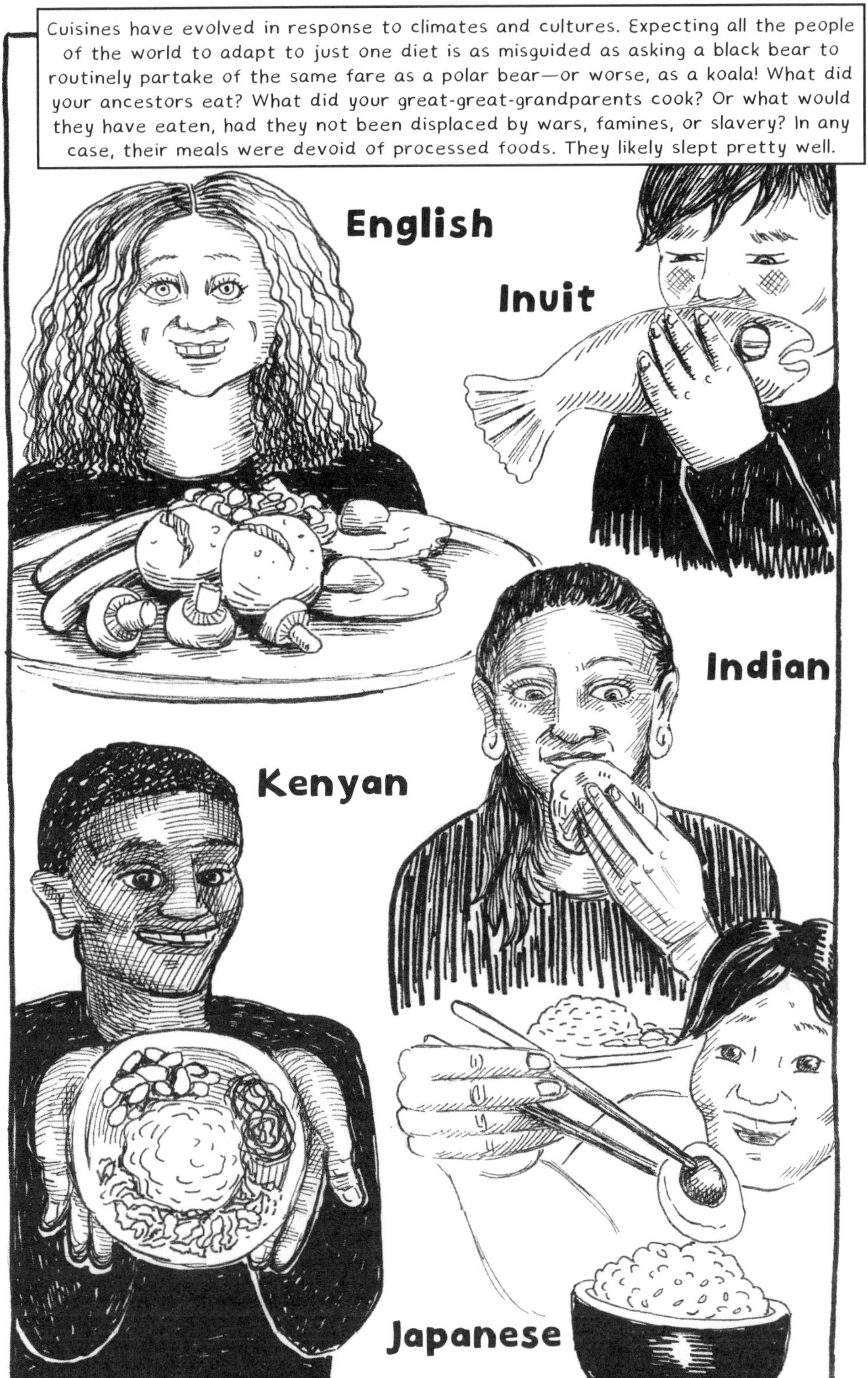
Cuisines have evolved in response to climates and cultures. Expecting all the people of the world to adapt to just one diet is as misguided as asking a black bear to routinely partake of the same fare as a polar bear—or worse, as a koala! What did your ancestors eat? What did your great-great-grandparents cook? Or what would they have eaten, had they not been displaced by wars, famines, or slavery? In any case, their meals were devoid of processed foods. They likely slept pretty well.
English
Inuit
Indian
Kenyan
Japanese

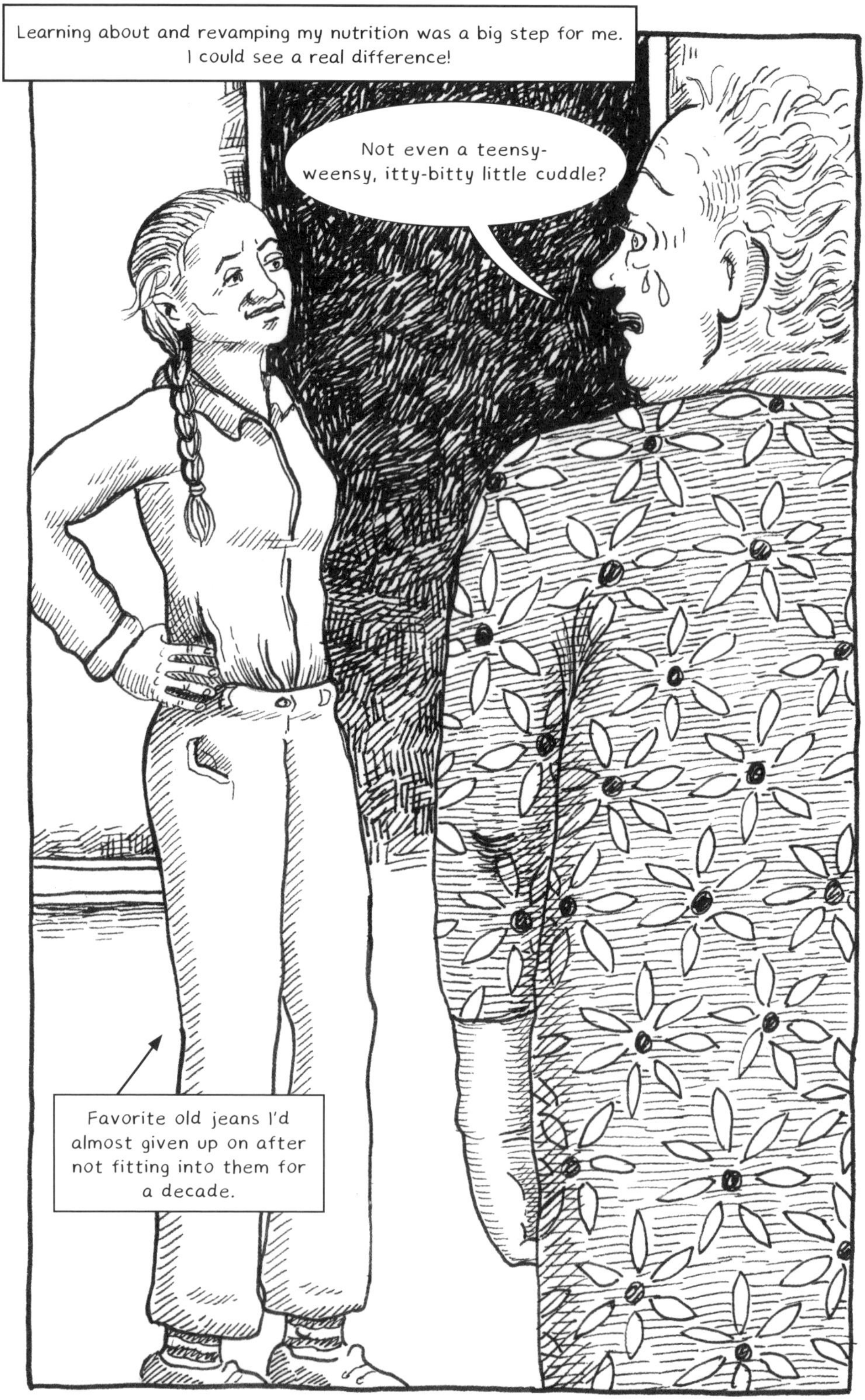
Learning about and revamping my nutrition was a big step for me. I could see a real difference!
Not even a teensy-weensy, itty-bitty little cuddle?
Favorite old jeans I'd almost given up on after not fitting into them for a decade.

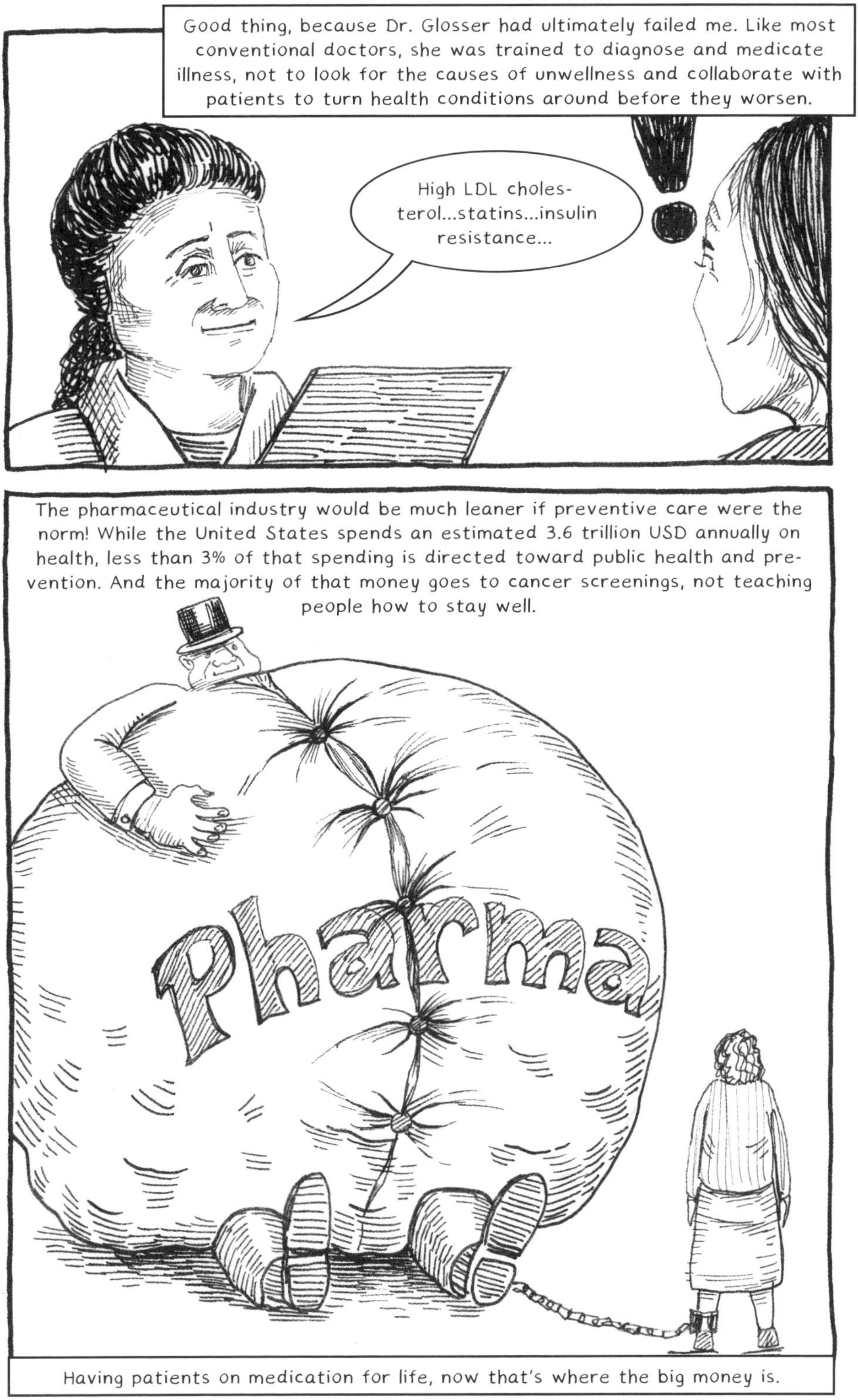
Good thing, because Dr. Glosser had ultimately failed me. Like most conventional doctors, she was trained to diagnose and medicate illness, not to look for the causes of unwellness and collaborate with patients to turn health conditions around before they worsen.
High LDL choles-terol...statins...insulin resistance...
!
The pharmaceutical industry would be much leaner if preventive care were the norm! While the United States spends an estimated 3.6 trillion USD annually on health, less than 3% of that spending is directed toward public health and prevention. And the majority of that money goes to cancer screenings, not teaching people how to stay well.
Pharma
Having patients on medication for life, now that's where the big money is.

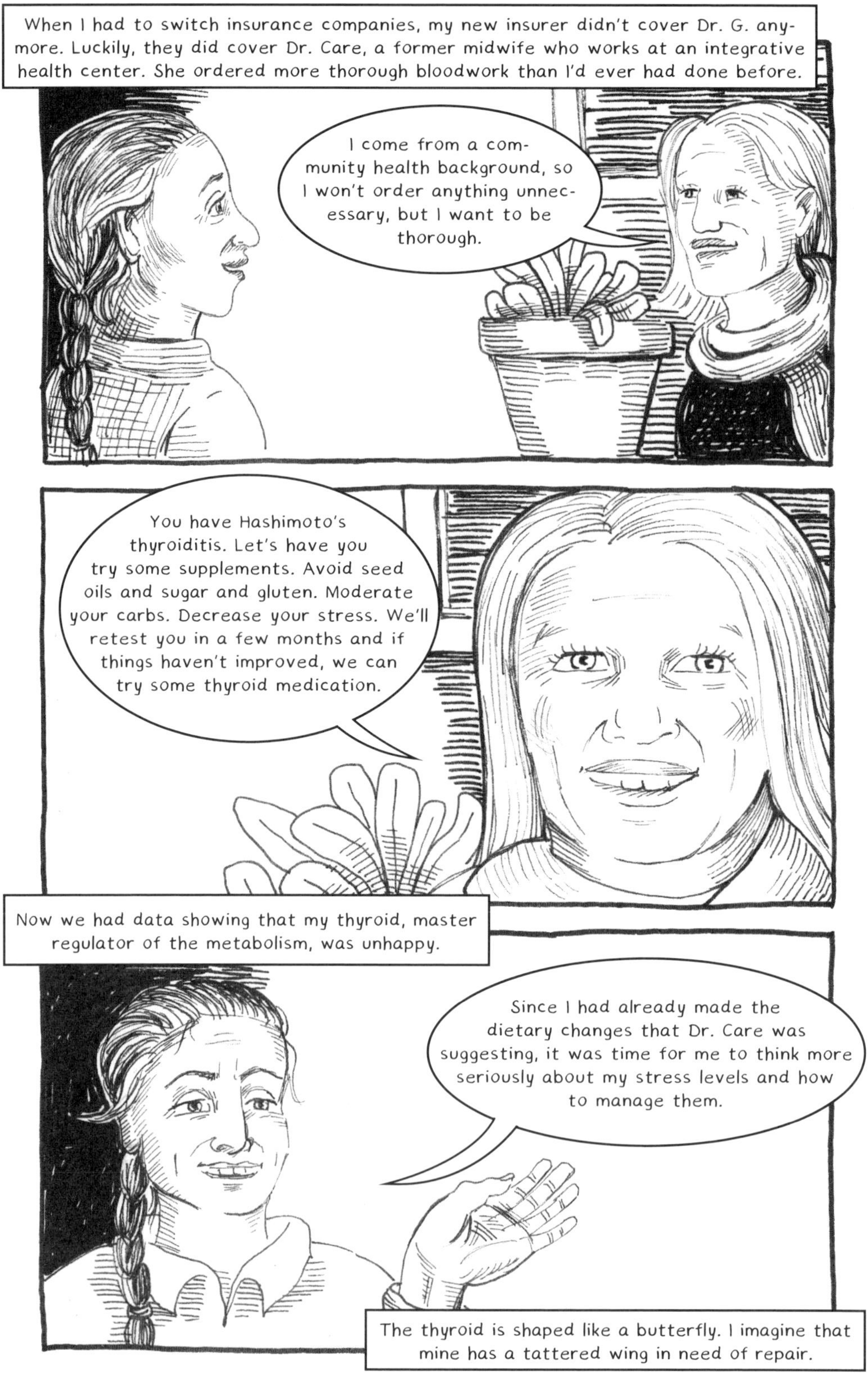
When I had to switch insurance companies, my new insurer didn't cover Dr. G. anymore. Luckily, they did cover Dr. Care, a former midwife who works at an integrative health center. She ordered more thorough bloodwork than I'd ever had done before.
I come from a community health background, so I won't order anything unnecessary, but I want to be thorough.
You have Hashimoto's thyroiditis. Let's have you try some supplements. Avoid seed oils and sugar and gluten. Moderate your carbs. Decrease your stress. We'll retest you in a few months and if things haven't improved, we can try some thyroid medication.
Now we had data showing that my thyroid, master regulator of the metabolism, was unhappy.
Since I had already made the dietary changes that Dr. Care was suggesting, it was time for me to think more seriously about my stress levels and how to manage them.
The thyroid is shaped like a butterfly. I imagine that mine has a tattered wing in need of repair.

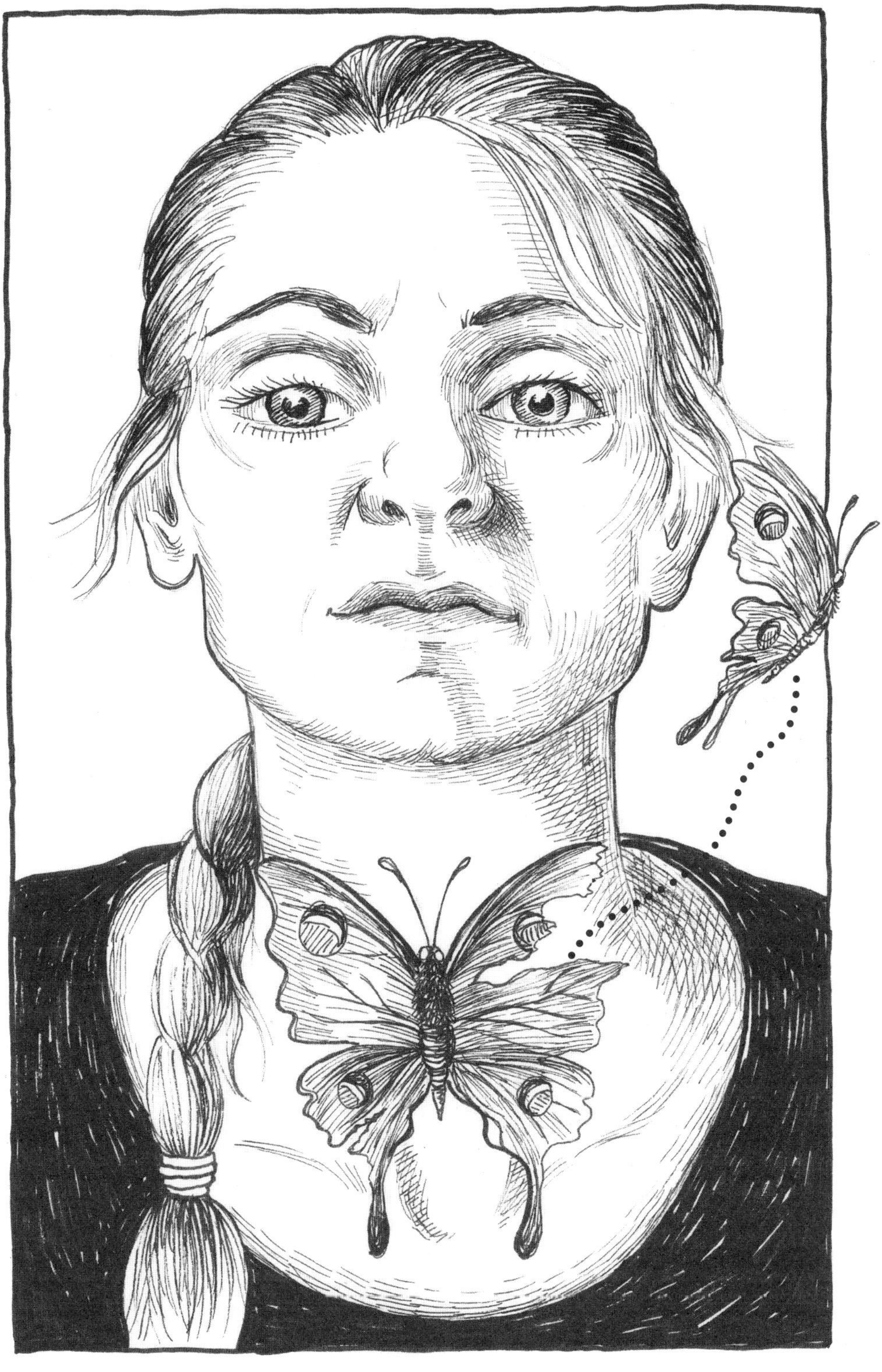

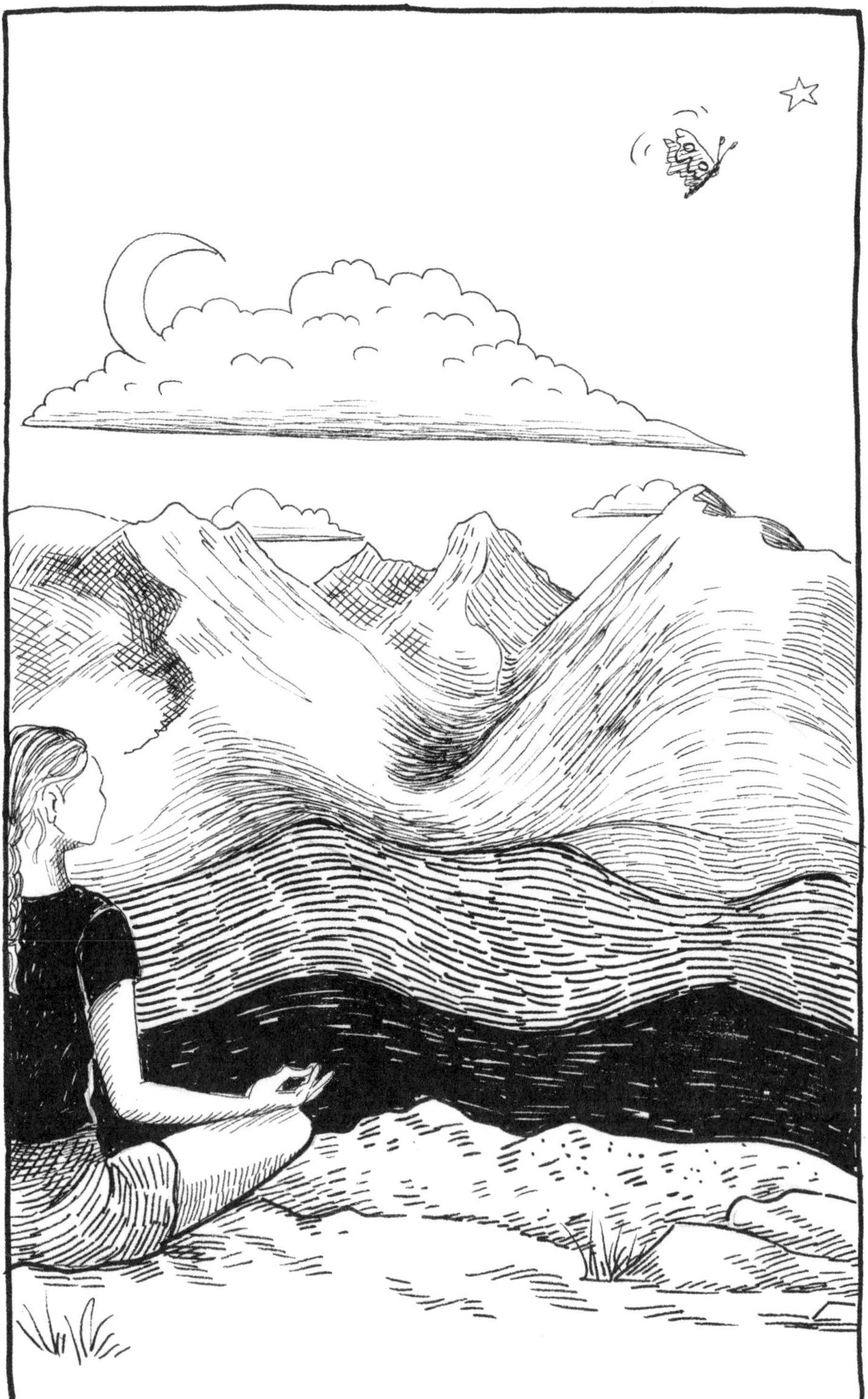

PART THREE: EARTH

Circadian Rhythms

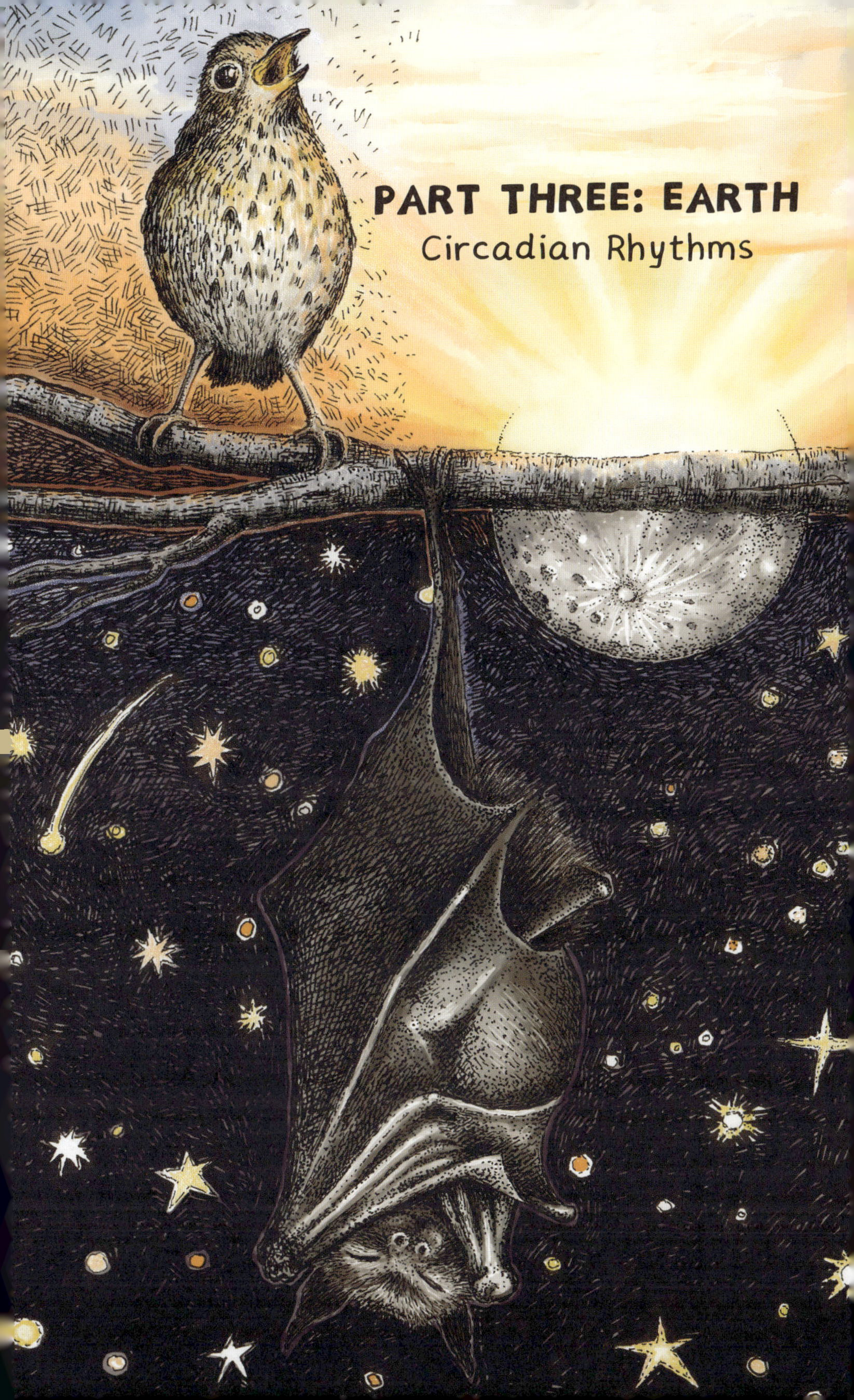

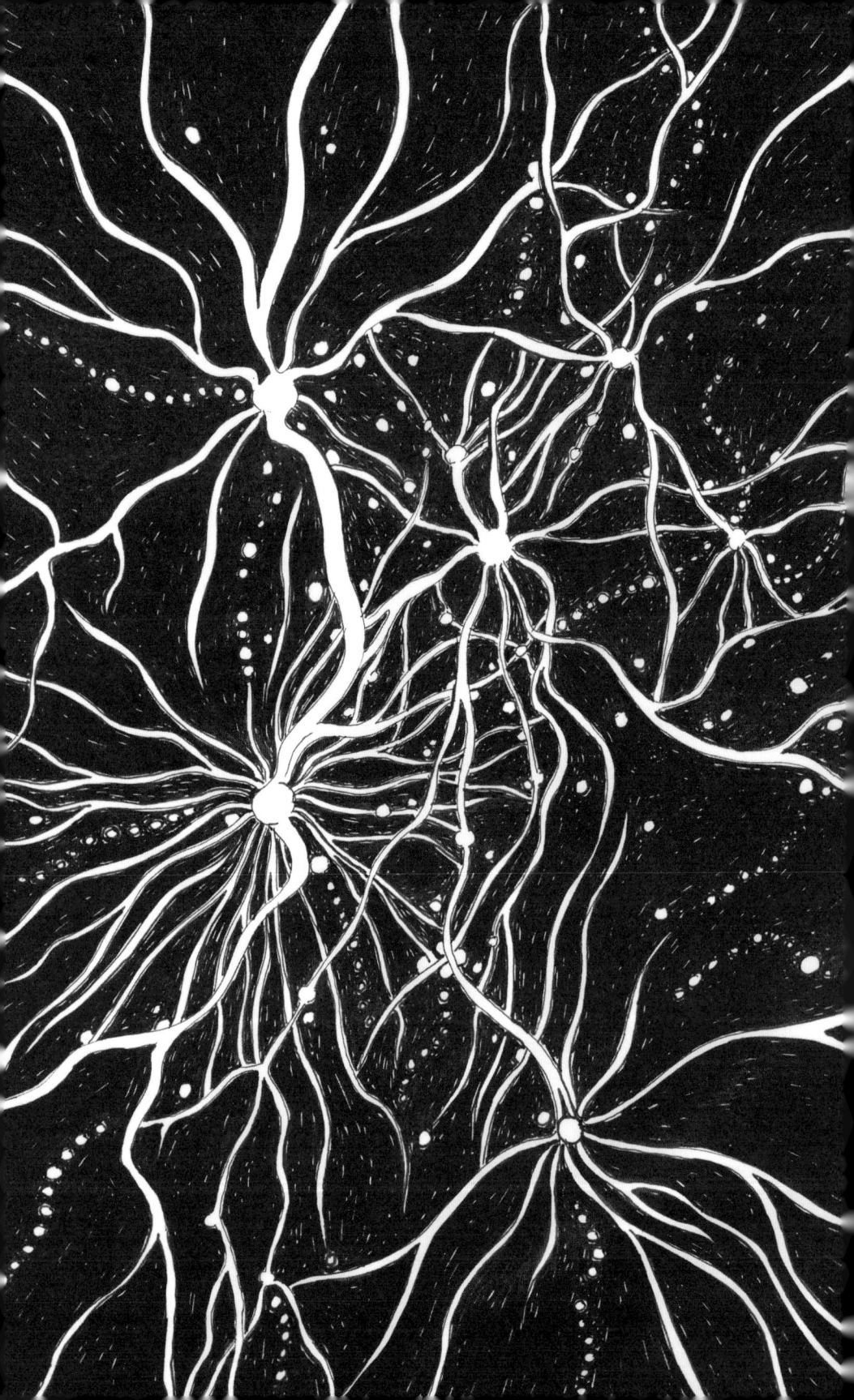

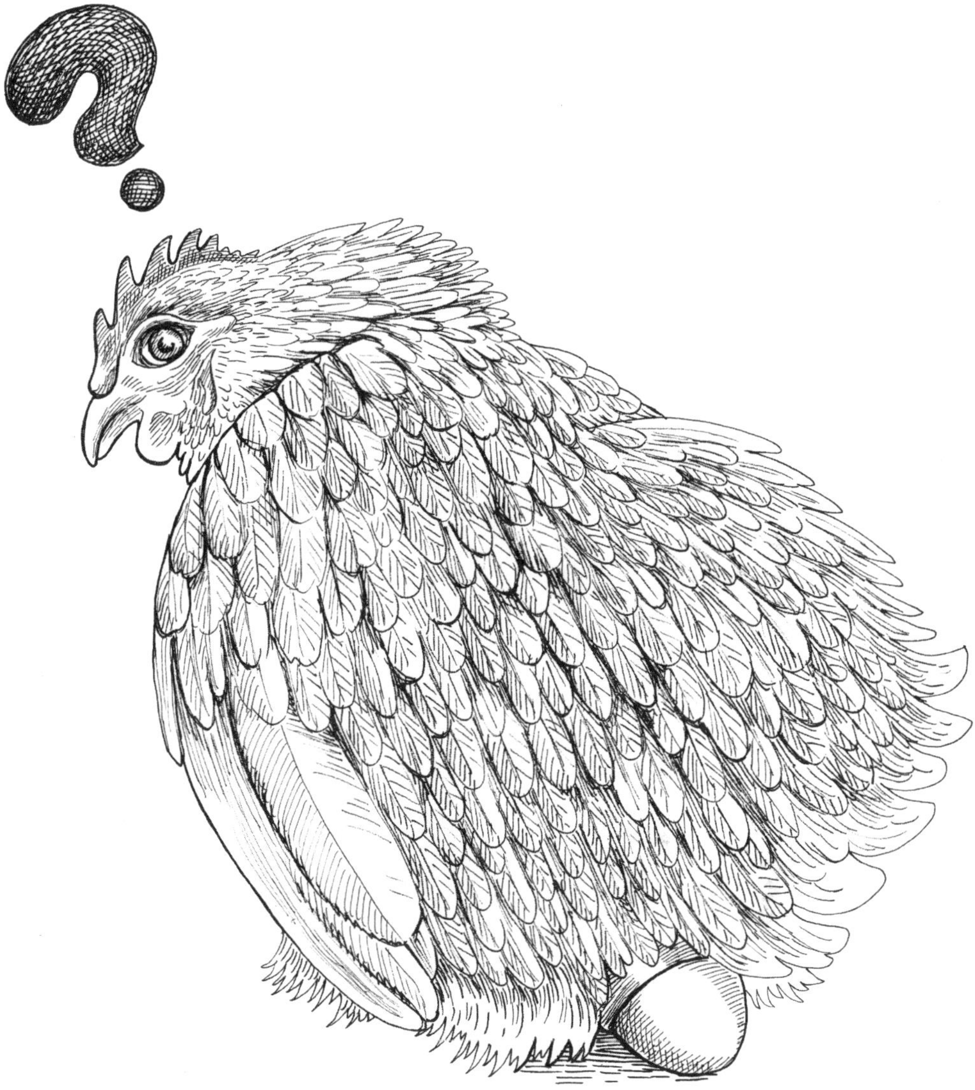

Question: Which came first: the chicken or the egg?

Answer: Neither. They are **one complex system**, best observed together. The egg and its mother are one, observable as generational stages: one inside the other, inseparable.

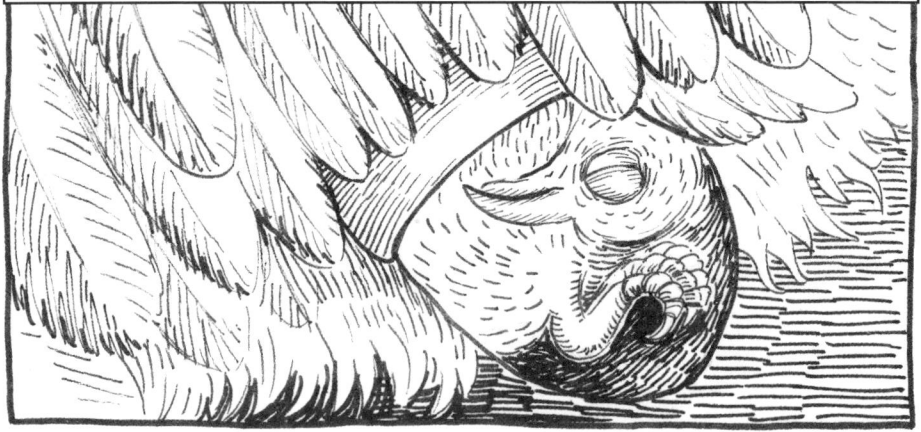

The chicken or the egg, the seed or the plant, night or day...Not one of these can exist without the other. "Or" is best replaced with "and." "Or" is selective, exclusive, and even destructive, as that little word, "OR," stands for "Overly Reductive"!

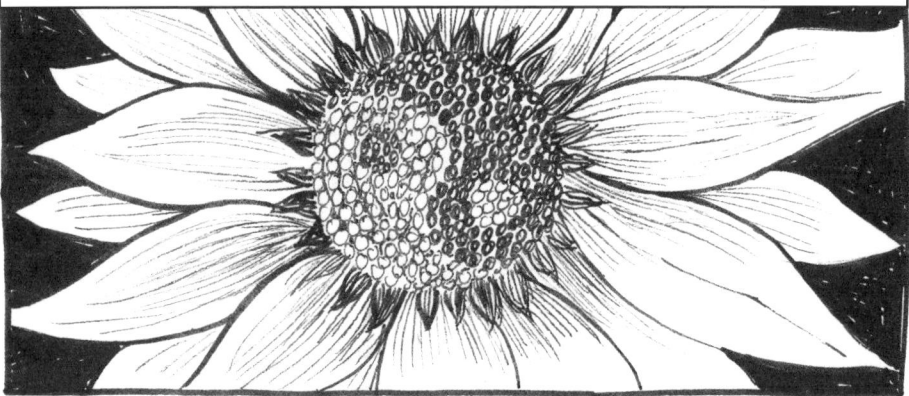

Scandinavian bat researcher and author of *The Darkness Manifesto*, Johan Eklöf, describes the vital and beautiful symbiosis of diurnal and nocturnal rhythms.

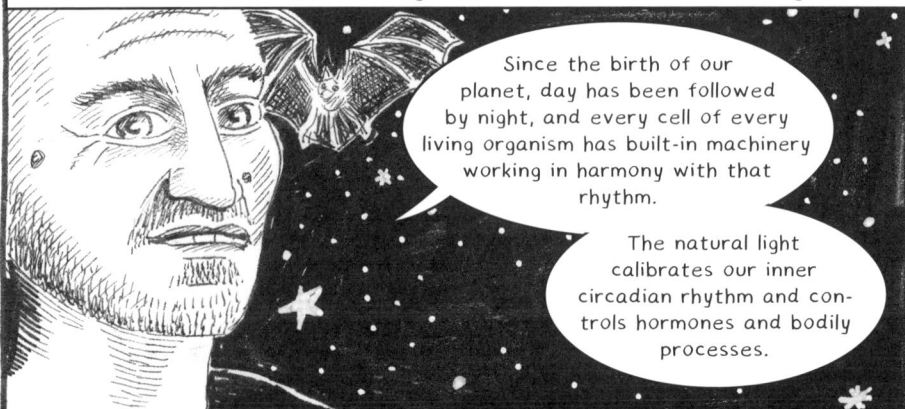

Since the birth of our planet, day has been followed by night, and every cell of every living organism has built-in machinery working in harmony with that rhythm.

The natural light calibrates our inner circadian rhythm and controls hormones and bodily processes.

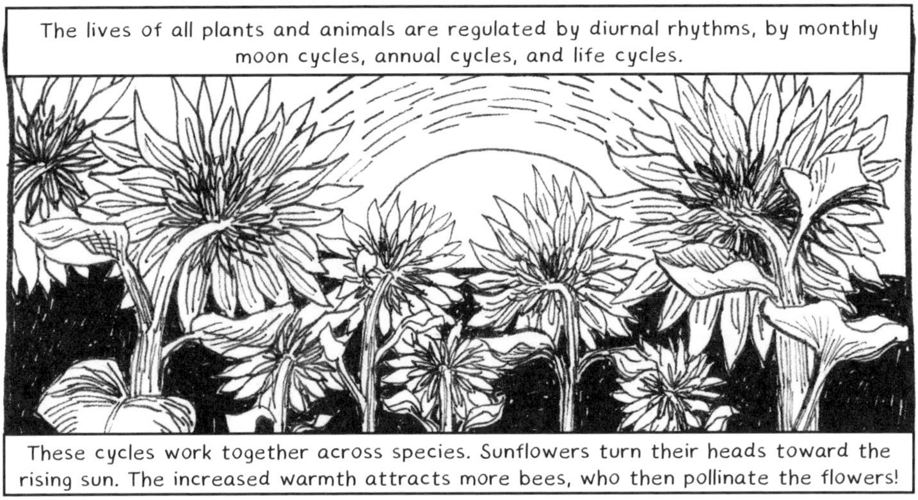
The lives of all plants and animals are regulated by diurnal rhythms, by monthly moon cycles, annual cycles, and life cycles.
These cycles work together across species. Sunflowers turn their heads toward the rising sun. The increased warmth attracts more bees, who then pollinate the flowers!

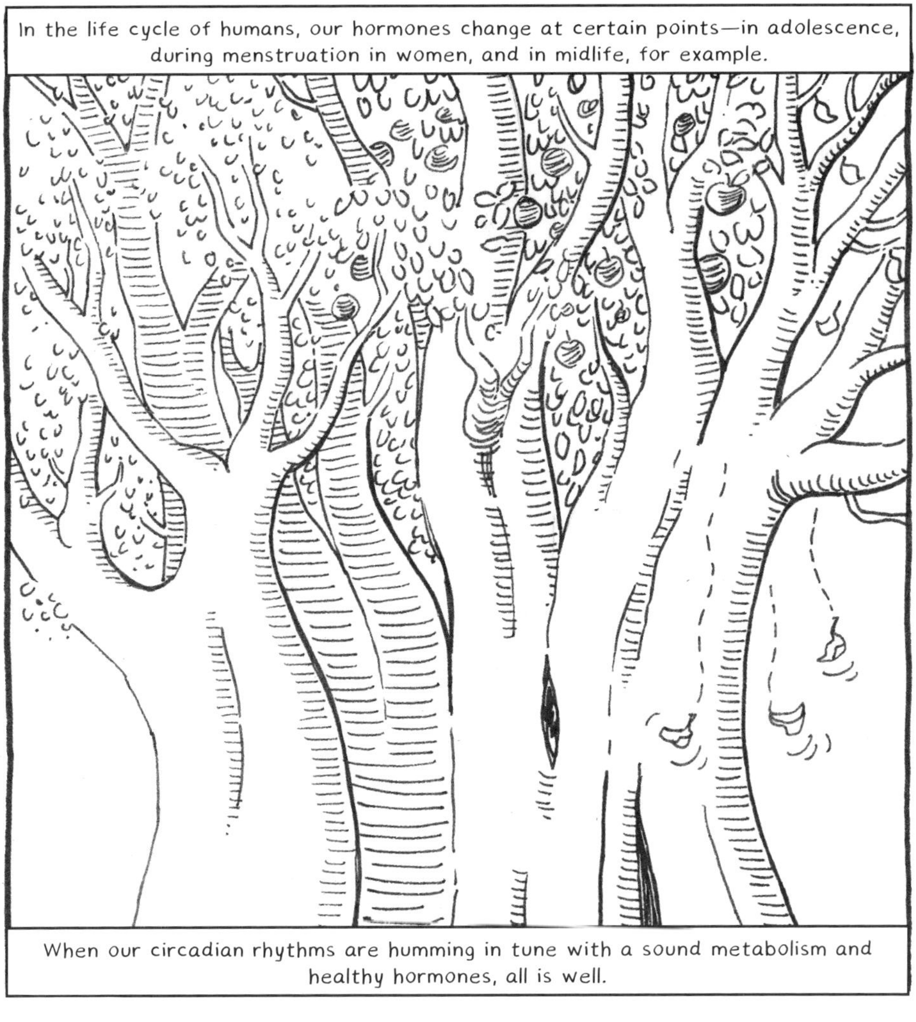
In the life cycle of humans, our hormones change at certain points—in adolescence, during menstruation in women, and in midlife, for example.
When our circadian rhythms are humming in tune with a sound metabolism and healthy hormones, all is well.

If our metabolism, or the process through which we transform food into physical and mental vitality, is the "orchestra" of our embodied manifestation in the world, then you might say that circadian rhythms are our "conductor." In the space-time continuum that is expressed microcosmically in each of us, our circadian rhythms are the master of timing.

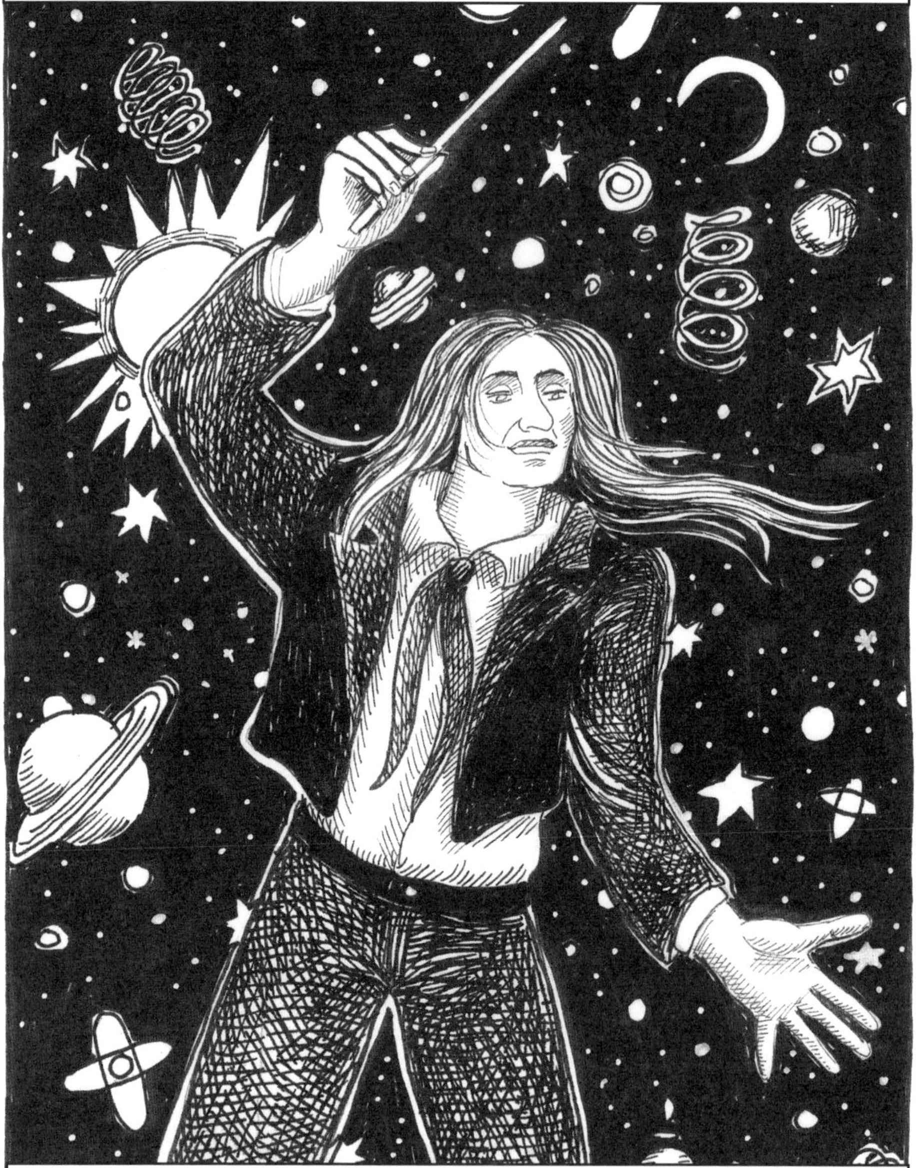

When the metabolic orchestra is out of tune, the circadian conductor has little to work with. Similarly, if the circadian conductor's rhythm is off, the metabolic orchestra is likely to sound just terrible, a veritable cacophony, even if the musicians are talented and each instrument has been well tuned. The two systems aren't separate. Instead, they need to communicate harmoniously and work together to create beautiful music.

This is where good bedtime habits (and regular routines throughout the 24-hour cycle) come in. Overconsumption of inflammatory foods, light, information, and energy is detrimental to our sleep and overall health. Human hyperactivity and hyperproductivity result in a chronic state of hyperarousal, agitation, and inflammation.

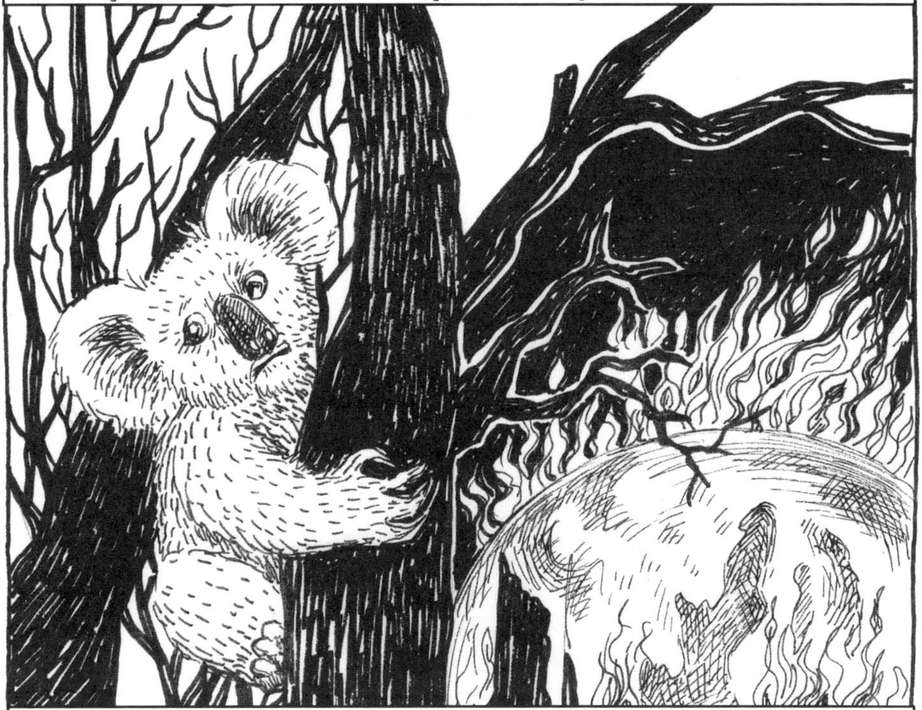

The fire raging within our individual bodies, the global displacement and extinction of other species, and the overheating of the planet are all connected. We tend to overbreathe and overconsume oxygen by inhaling, holding our breath, and forgetting to exhale. We know what oxygen does to fire! Our species and our world are inflamed and out of sync. More than anything else, it's **inflammation** that causes and perpetuates mental and physical illnesses.

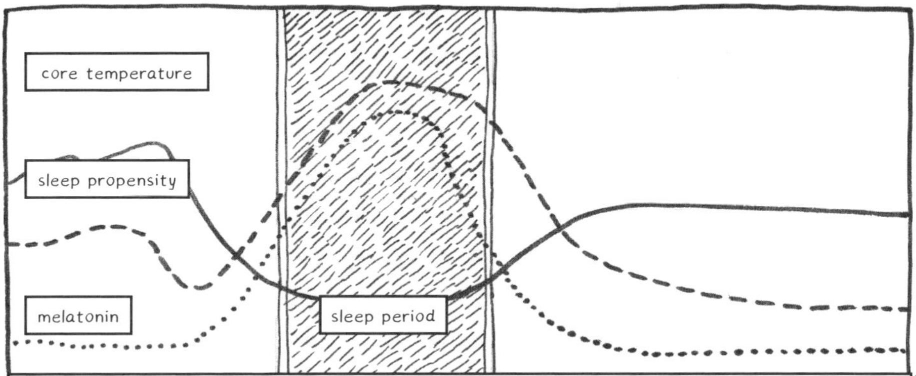
core temperature
sleep propensity
melatonin
sleep period

Especially in the fatter nations, we run hot. We ingest more than we release, work more than we rest. It's no wonder that well over a third of us struggle with sleep problems. People with insomnia often have flattened circadian temperature rhythms and are hotter throughout the circadian cycle. We literally need to chill out!

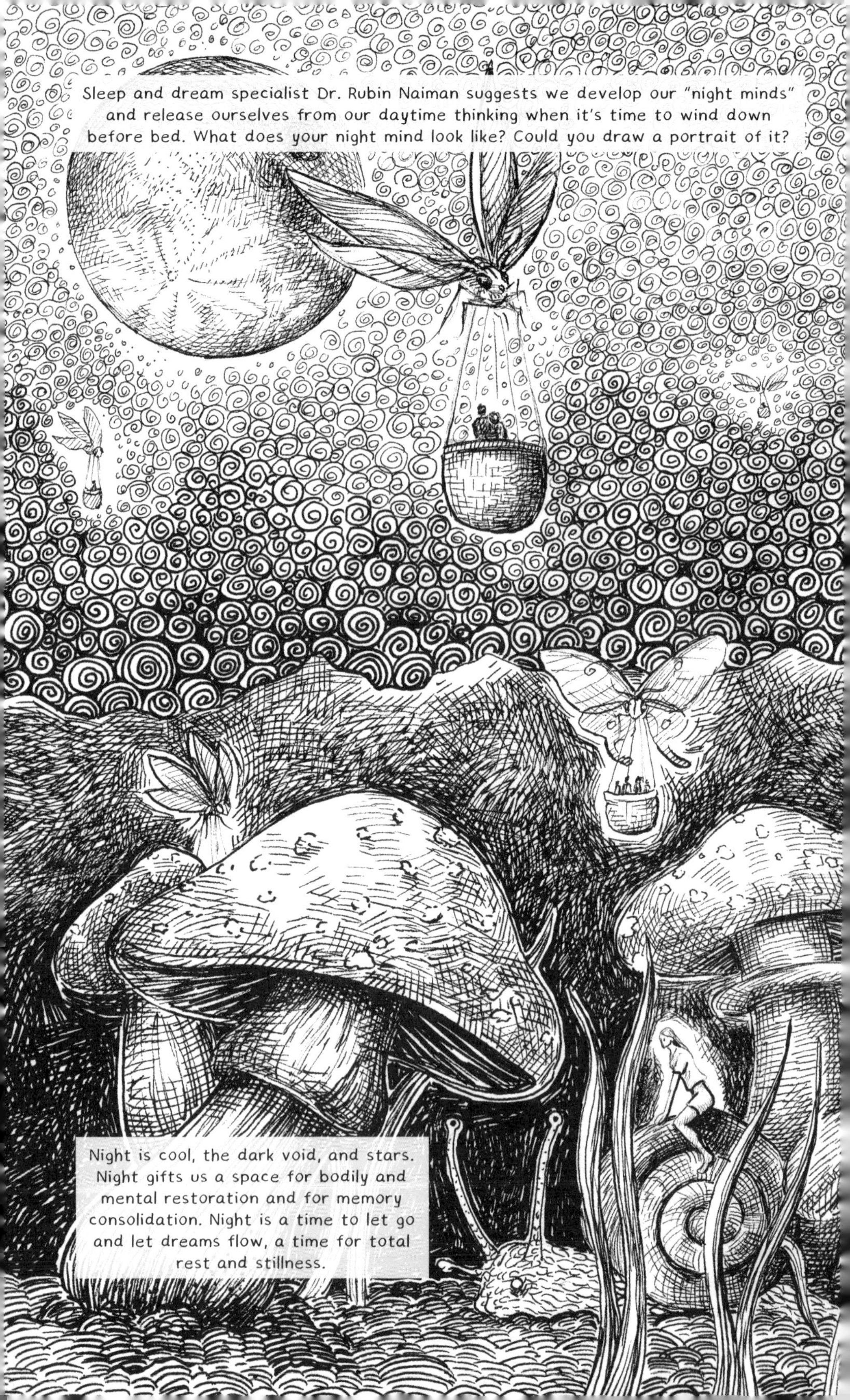
Sleep and dream specialist Dr. Rubin Naiman suggests we develop our "night minds" and release ourselves from our daytime thinking when it's time to wind down before bed. What does your night mind look like? Could you draw a portrait of it?
Night is cool, the dark void, and stars. Night gifts us a space for bodily and mental restoration and for memory consolidation. Night is a time to let go and let dreams flow, a time for total rest and stillness.

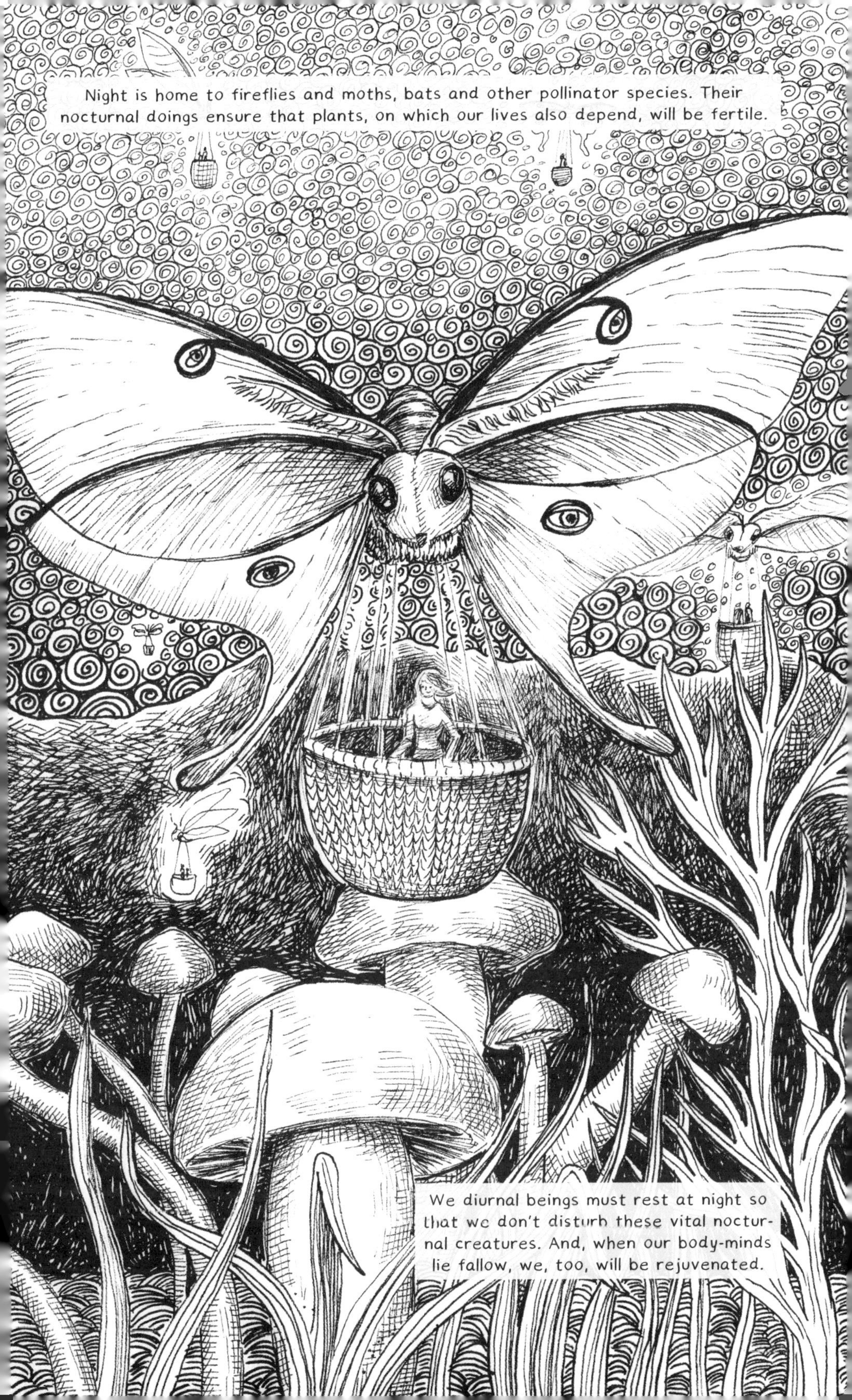
Night is home to fireflies and moths, bats and other pollinator species. Their nocturnal doings ensure that plants, on which our lives also depend, will be fertile.
We diurnal beings must rest at night so that we don't disturb these vital nocturnal creatures. And, when our body-minds lie fallow, we, too, will be rejuvenated.

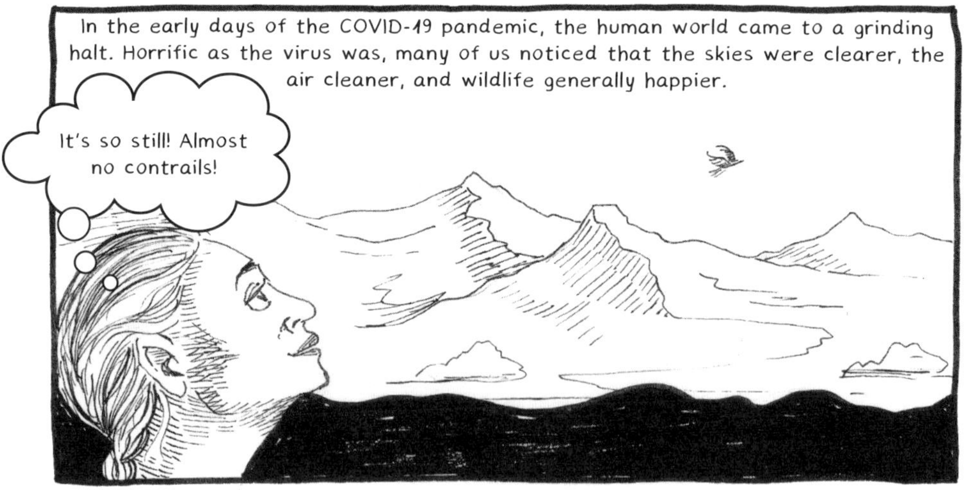
In the early days of the COVID-19 pandemic, the human world came to a grinding halt. Horrific as the virus was, many of us noticed that the skies were clearer, the air cleaner, and wildlife generally happier.
It's so still! Almost no contrails!

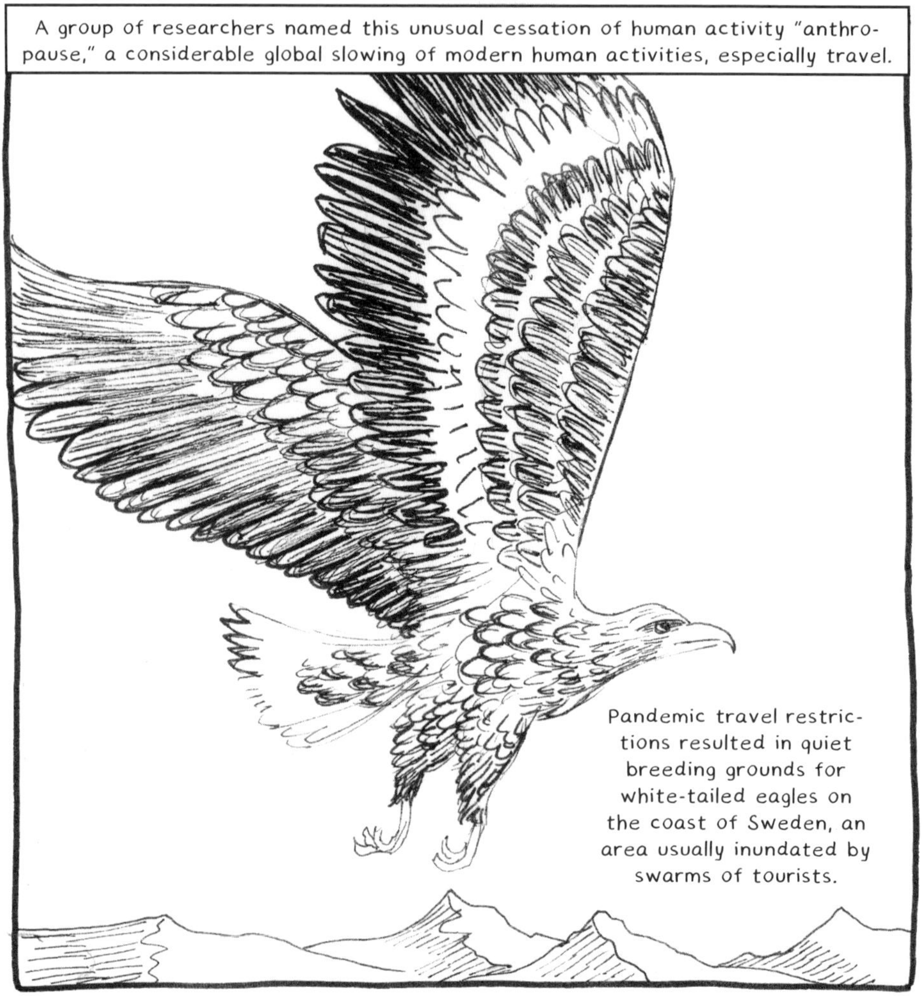
A group of researchers named this unusual cessation of human activity "anthropause," a considerable global slowing of modern human activities, especially travel.
Pandemic travel restrictions resulted in quiet breeding grounds for white-tailed eagles on the coast of Sweden, an area usually inundated by swarms of tourists.

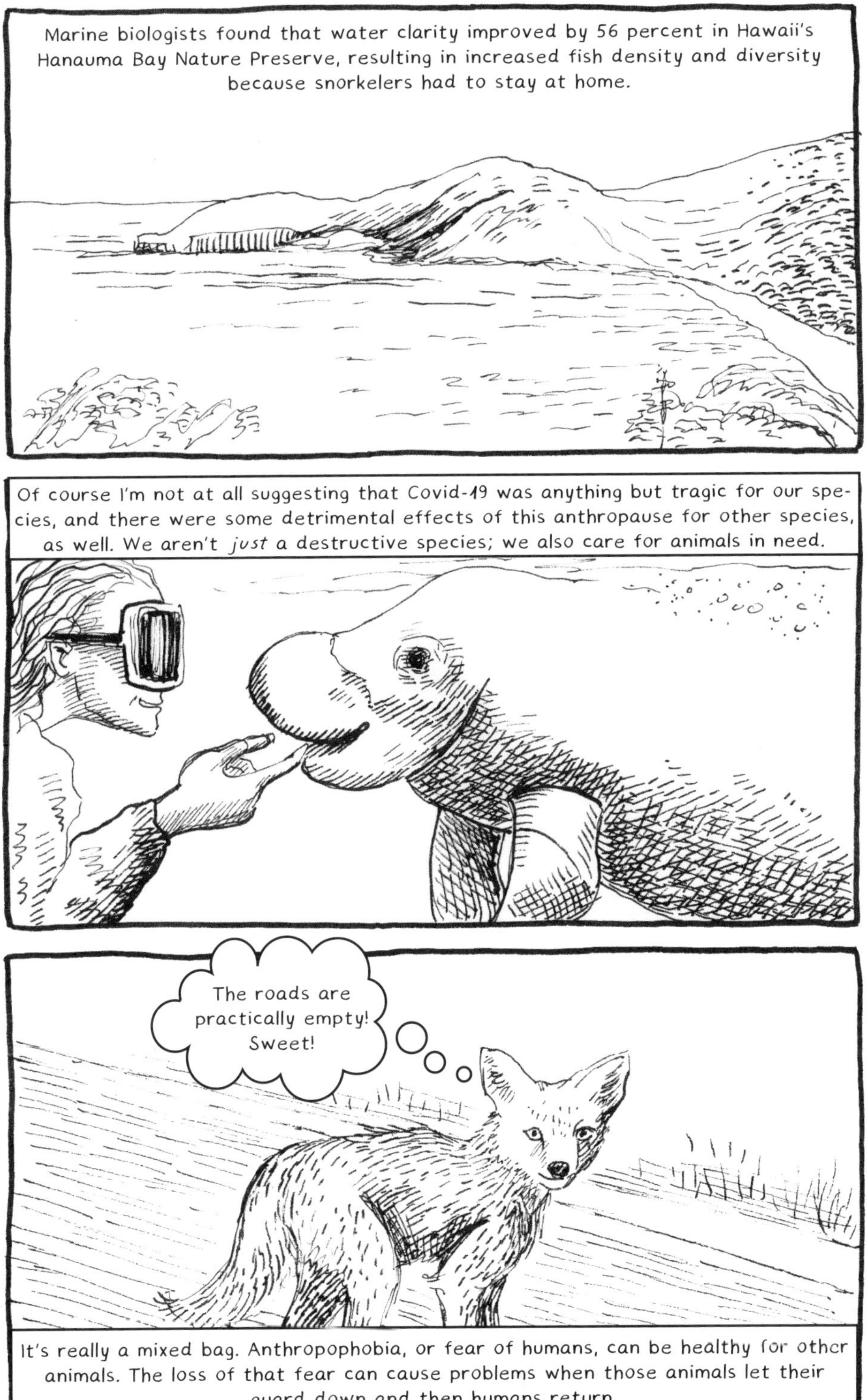
Marine biologists found that water clarity improved by 56 percent in Hawaii's Hanauma Bay Nature Preserve, resulting in increased fish density and diversity because snorkelers had to stay at home.
Of course I'm not at all suggesting that Covid-19 was anything but tragic for our species, and there were some detrimental effects of this anthropause for other species, as well. We aren't *just* a destructive species; we also care for animals in need.
The roads are practically empty! Sweet!
It's really a mixed bag. Anthropophobia, or fear of humans, can be healthy for other animals. The loss of that fear can cause problems when those animals let their guard down and then humans return.

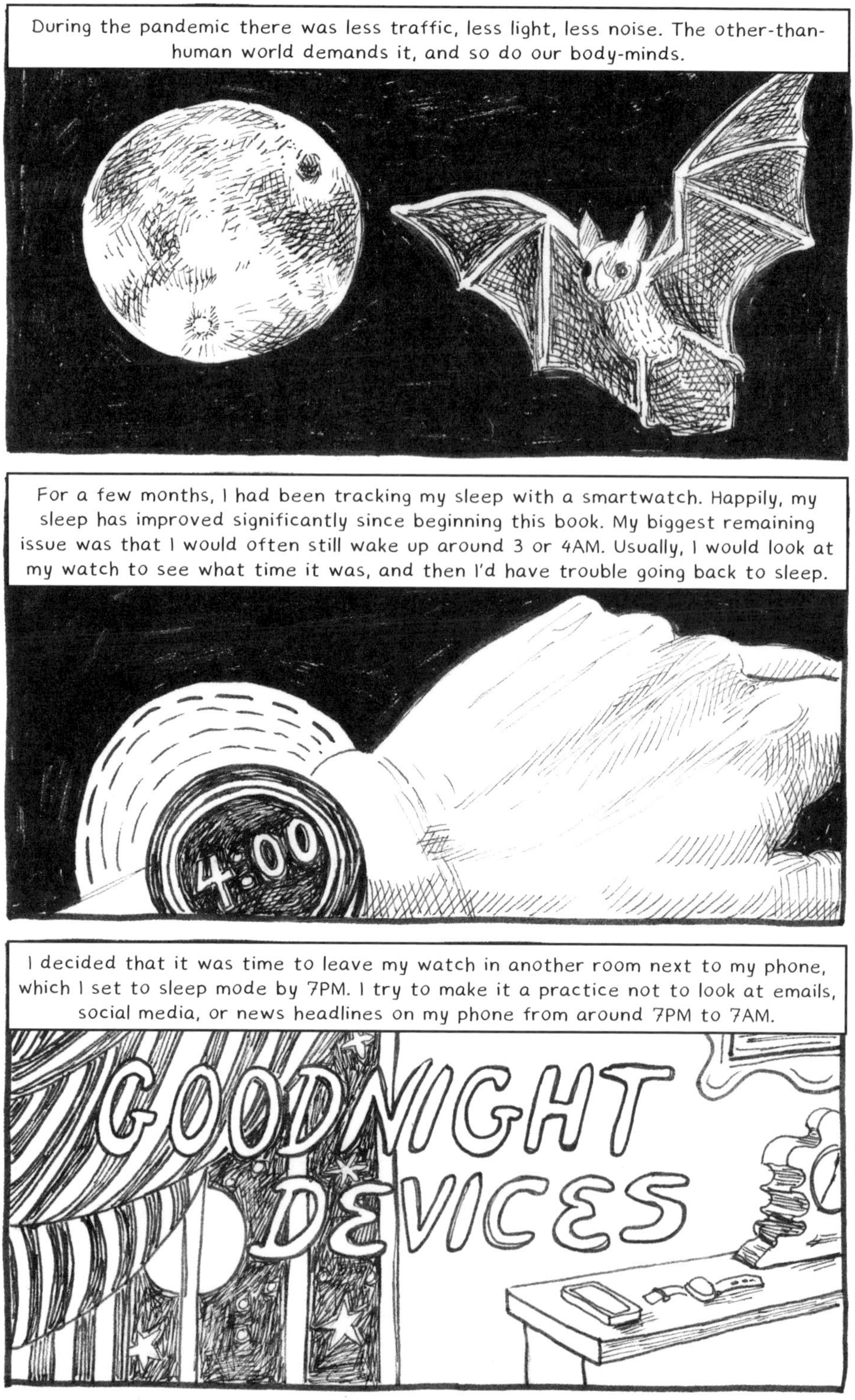
During the pandemic there was less traffic, less light, less noise. The other-than-human world demands it, and so do our body-minds.
For a few months, I had been tracking my sleep with a smartwatch. Happily, my sleep has improved significantly since beginning this book. My biggest remaining issue was that I would often still wake up around 3 or 4AM. Usually, I would look at my watch to see what time it was, and then I'd have trouble going back to sleep.
4:00
I decided that it was time to leave my watch in another room next to my phone, which I set to sleep mode by 7PM. I try to make it a practice not to look at emails, social media, or news headlines on my phone from around 7PM to 7AM.
GOODNIGHT DEVICES

In the interest of silencing our incessantly jabbering thoughts and slipping into night mode, it is as important to do a regular "digital fast" as it is to stop consuming food at night. Without input, our brains can rest and digest information.

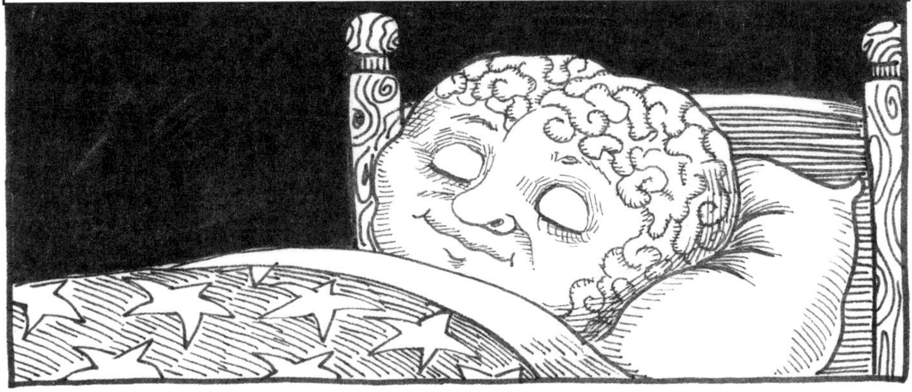

News headlines and emails and social media can wait. Those fun little games on your smartphone that help you wind down? Not worth the blue light they're beaming into your bleary eyeballs! Unless you are an emergency worker of some sort and must be on call, there is no reason to keep devices next to your bed. If you have to set an alarm, find a gentle one and position it so that you can't see the time or light emanating from it.

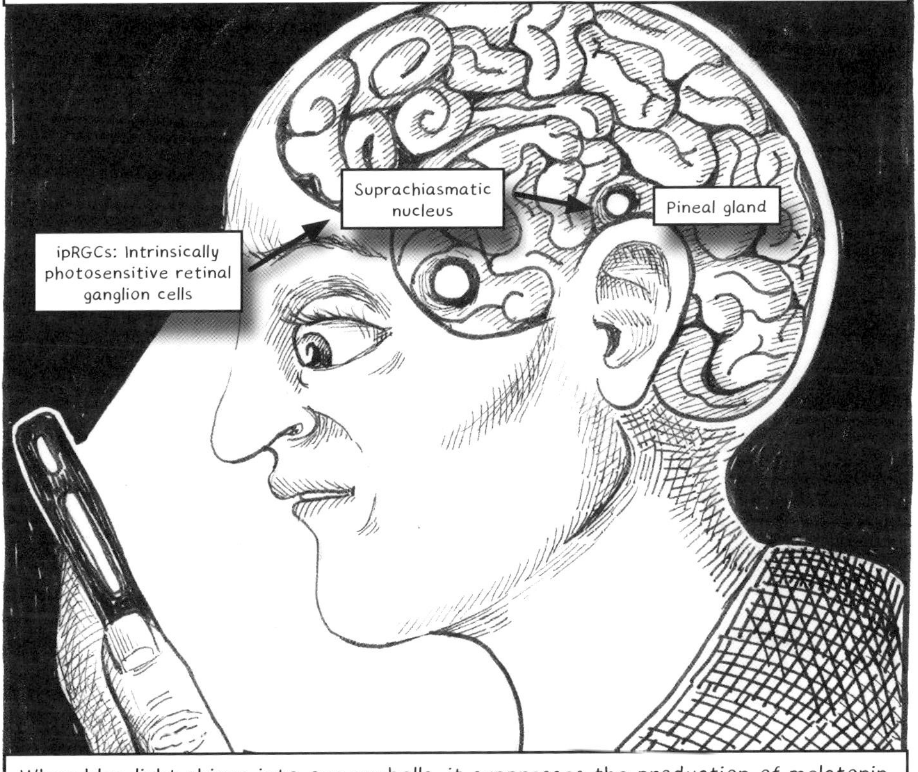
Suprachiasmatic nucleus
Pineal gland
ipRGCs: Intrinsically photosensitive retinal ganglion cells

When blue light shines into our eyeballs, it suppresses the production of melatonin, which is the queen of sleep hormones. Blue-light-blocking glasses can help.

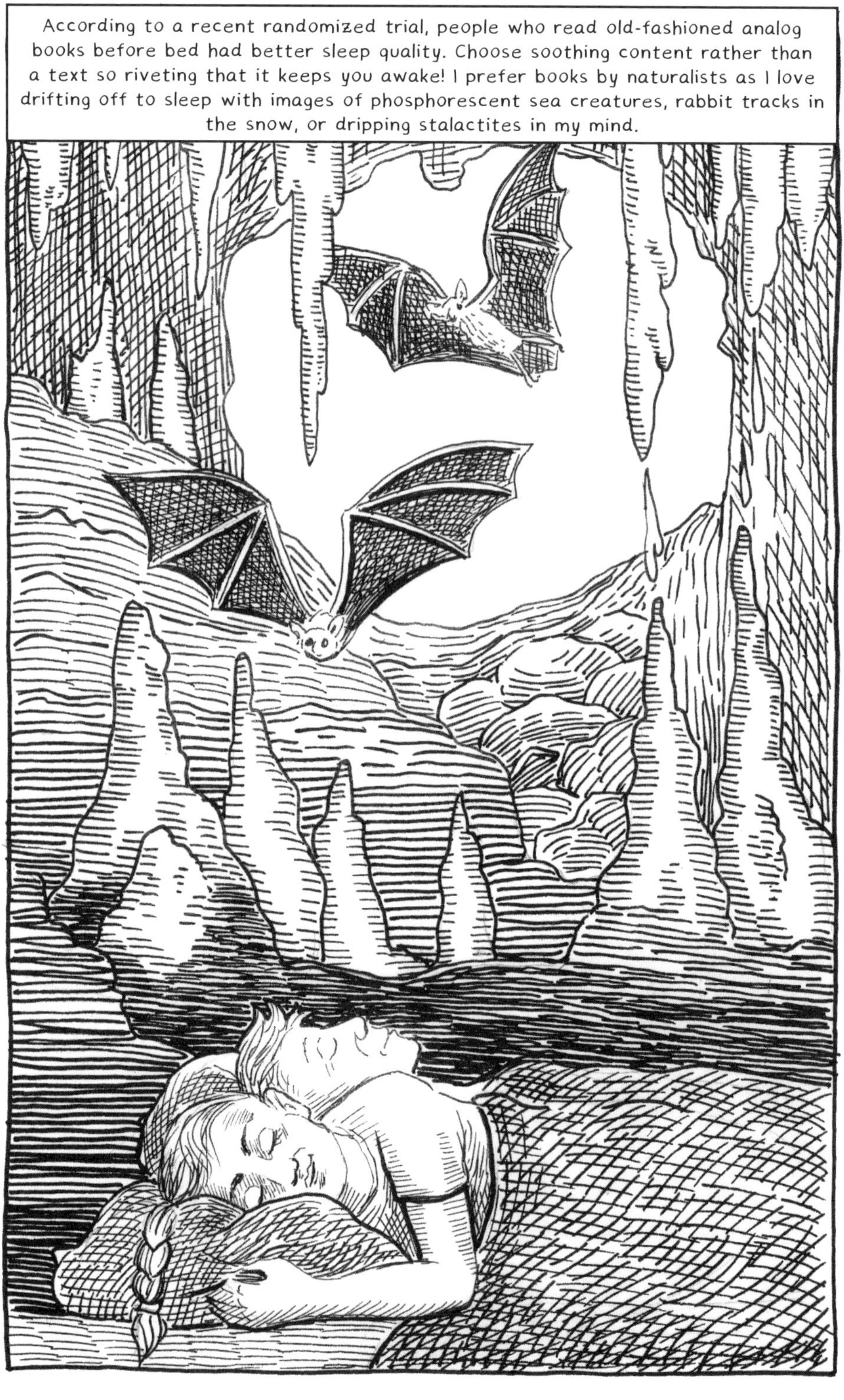
According to a recent randomized trial, people who read old-fashioned analog books before bed had better sleep quality. Choose soothing content rather than a text so riveting that it keeps you awake! I prefer books by naturalists as I love drifting off to sleep with images of phosphorescent sea creatures, rabbit tracks in the snow, or dripping stalactites in my mind.

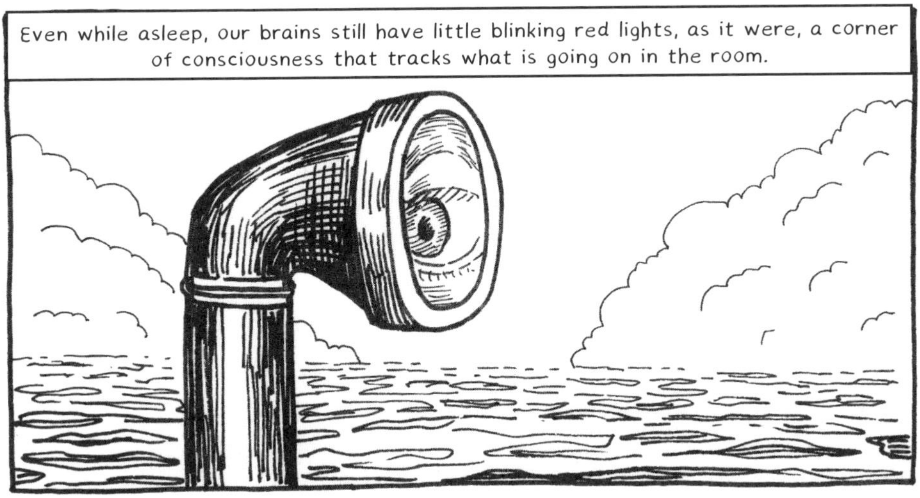
Even while asleep, our brains still have little blinking red lights, as it were, a corner of consciousness that tracks what is going on in the room.

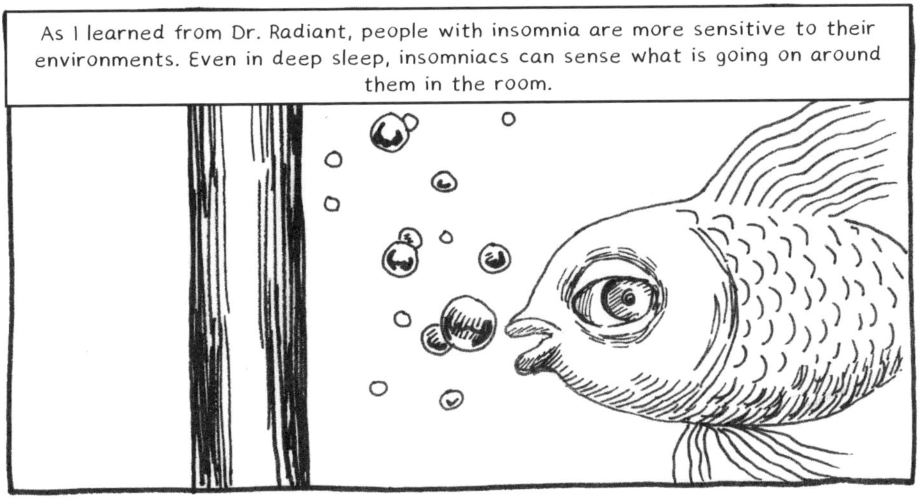
As I learned from Dr. Radiant, people with insomnia are more sensitive to their environments. Even in deep sleep, insomniacs can sense what is going on around them in the room.

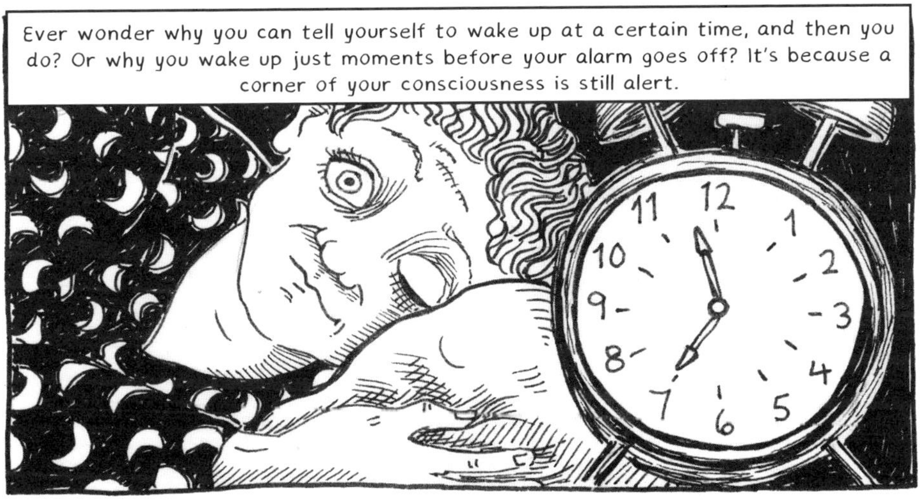
Ever wonder why you can tell yourself to wake up at a certain time, and then you do? Or why you wake up just moments before your alarm goes off? It's because a corner of your consciousness is still alert.

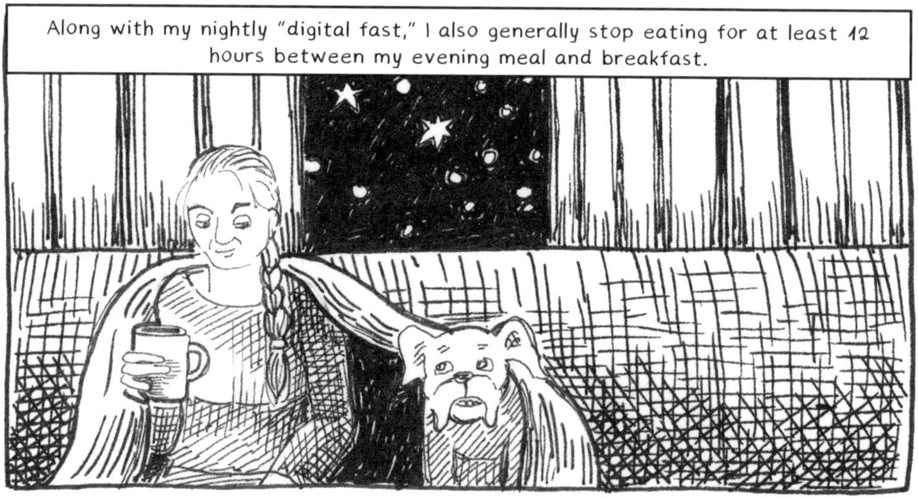
Along with my nightly "digital fast," I also generally stop eating for at least 12 hours between my evening meal and breakfast.

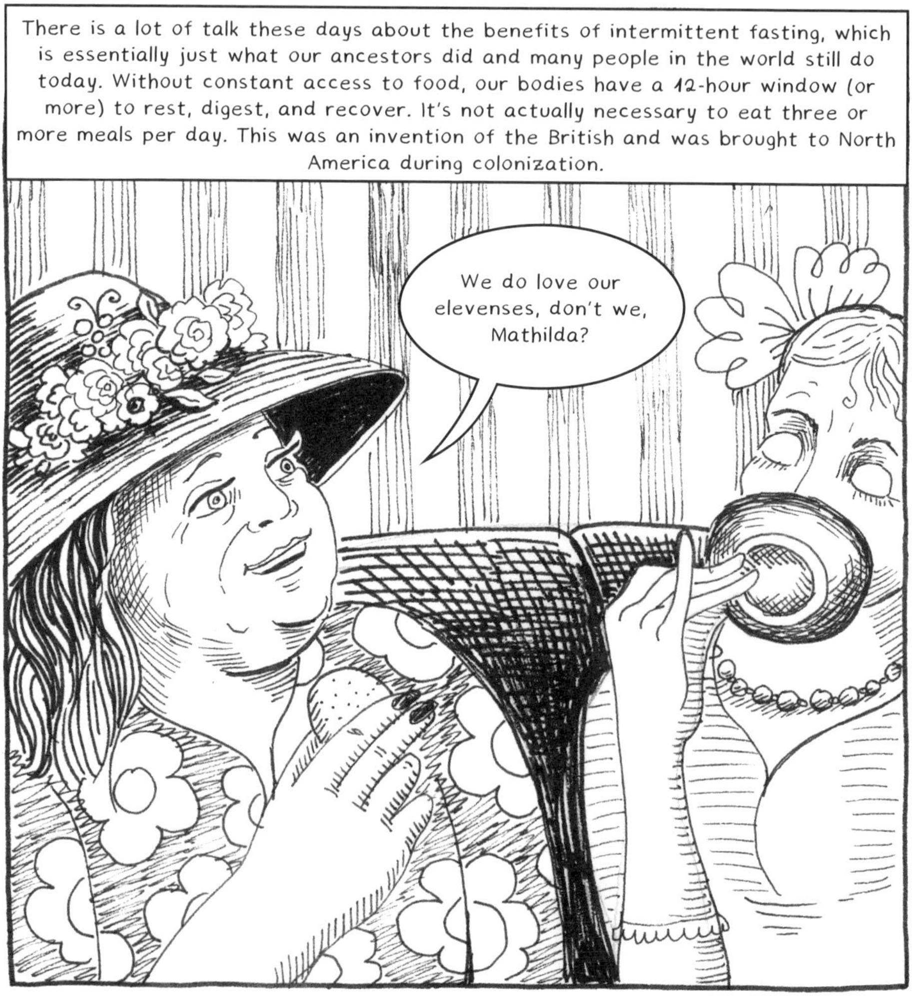
There is a lot of talk these days about the benefits of intermittent fasting, which is essentially just what our ancestors did and many people in the world still do today. Without constant access to food, our bodies have a 12-hour window (or more) to rest, digest, and recover. It's not actually necessary to eat three or more meals per day. This was an invention of the British and was brought to North America during colonization.
We do love our elevenses, don't we, Mathilda?

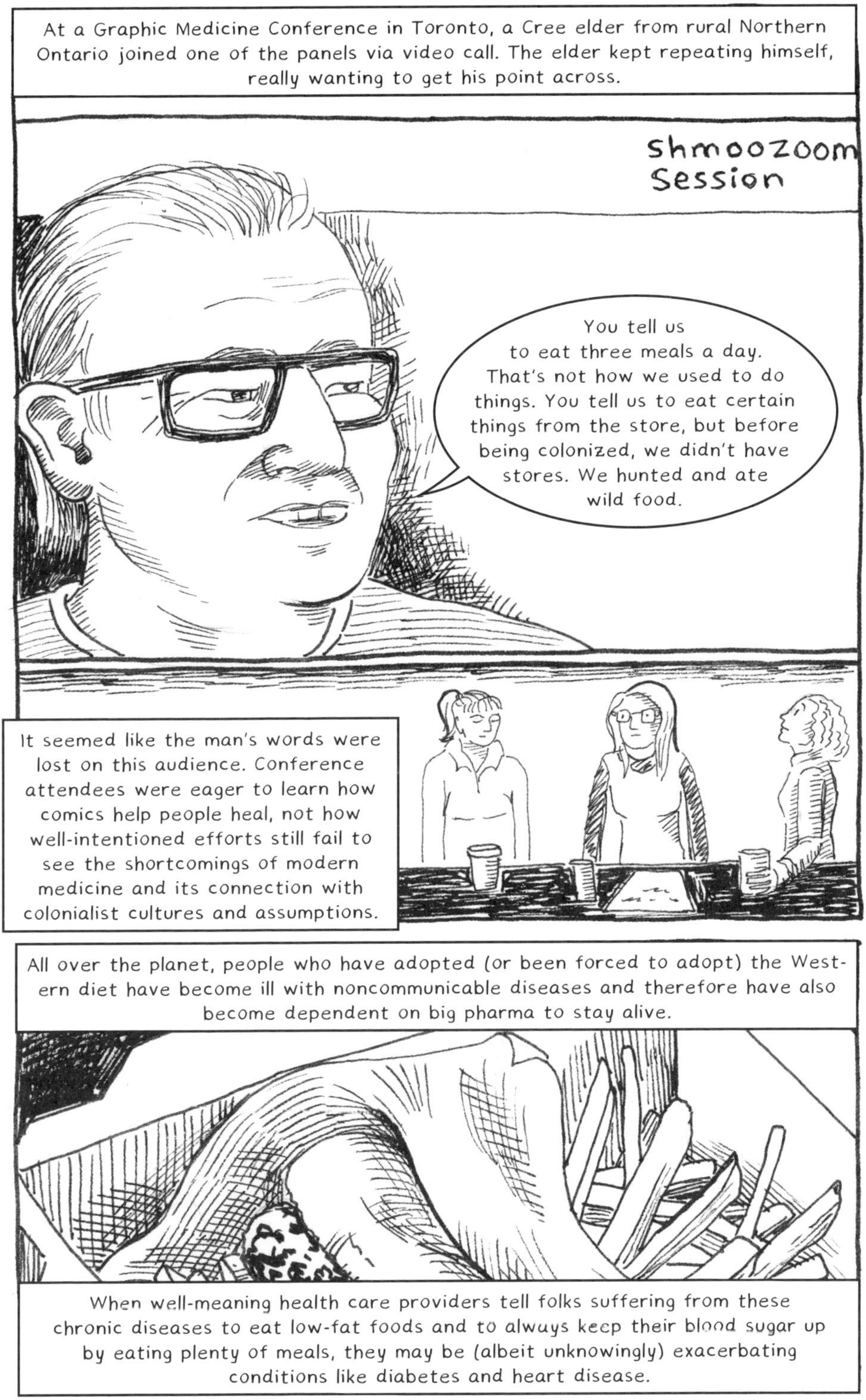

At a Graphic Medicine Conference in Toronto, a Cree elder from rural Northern Ontario joined one of the panels via video call. The elder kept repeating himself, really wanting to get his point across.

Shmoozoom Session

"You tell us to eat three meals a day. That's not how we used to do things. You tell us to eat certain things from the store, but before being colonized, we didn't have stores. We hunted and ate wild food."

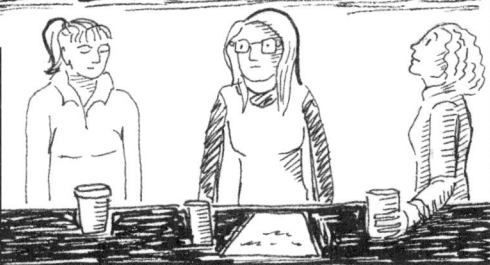

It seemed like the man's words were lost on this audience. Conference attendees were eager to learn how comics help people heal, not how well-intentioned efforts still fail to see the shortcomings of modern medicine and its connection with colonialist cultures and assumptions.

All over the planet, people who have adopted (or been forced to adopt) the Western diet have become ill with noncommunicable diseases and therefore have also become dependent on big pharma to stay alive.

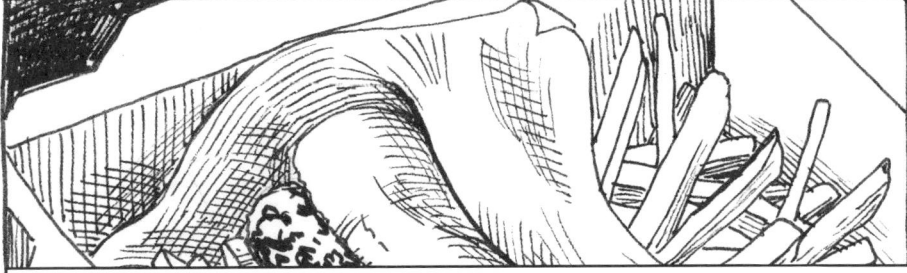

When well-meaning health care providers tell folks suffering from these chronic diseases to eat low-fat foods and to always keep their blood sugar up by eating plenty of meals, they may be (albeit unknowingly) exacerbating conditions like diabetes and heart disease.

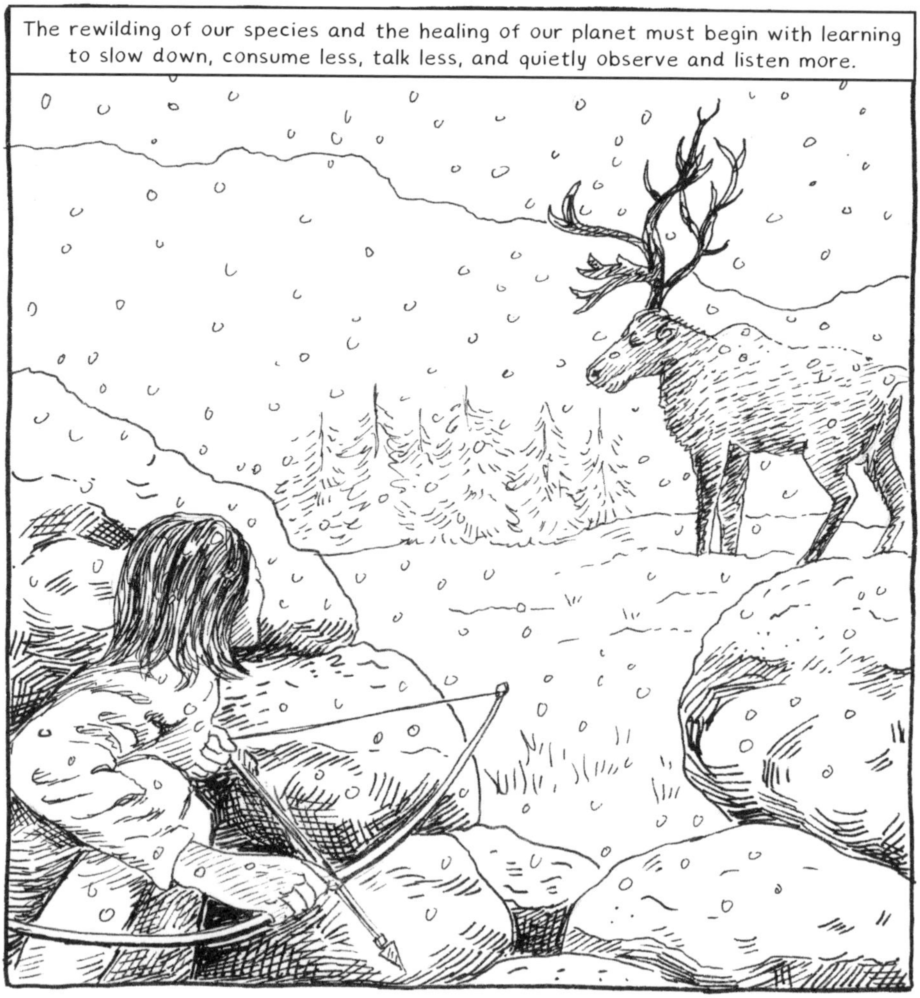
The rewilding of our species and the healing of our planet must begin with learning to slow down, consume less, talk less, and quietly observe and listen more.

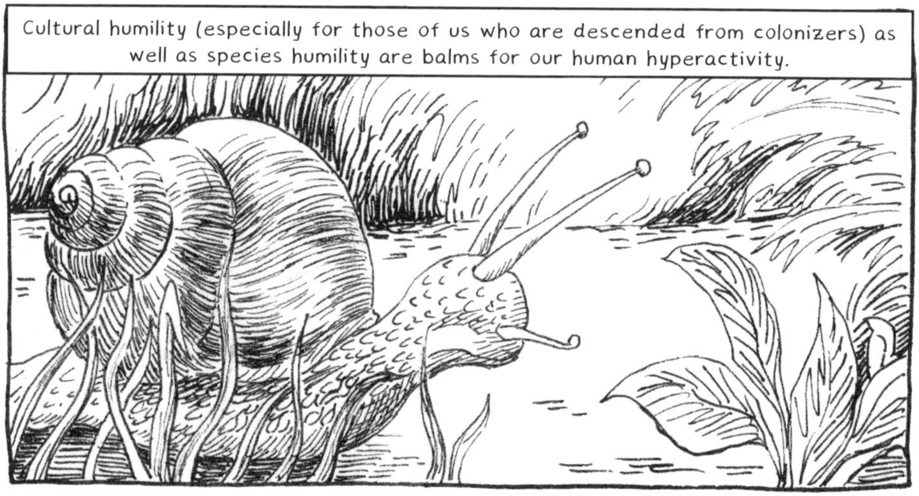
Cultural humility (especially for those of us who are descended from colonizers) as well as species humility are balms for our human hyperactivity.

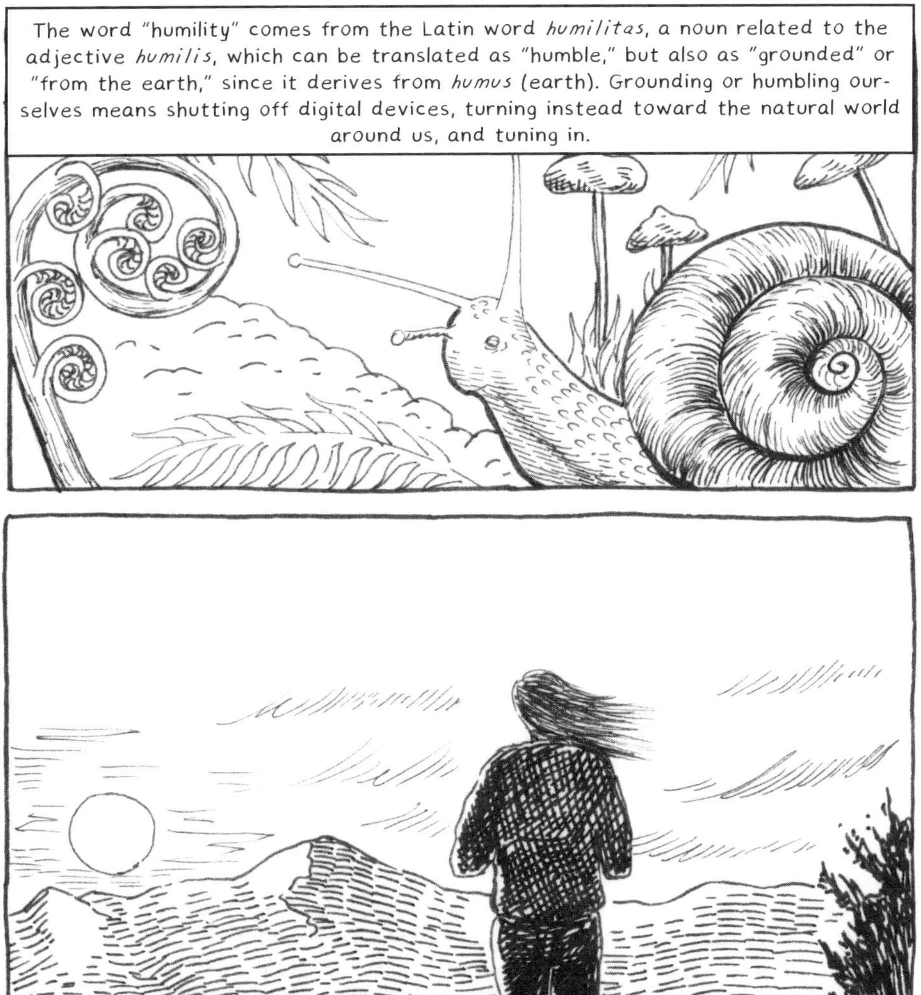
The word "humility" comes from the Latin word *humilitas*, a noun related to the adjective *humilis*, which can be translated as "humble," but also as "grounded" or "from the earth," since it derives from *humus* (earth). Grounding or humbling ourselves means shutting off digital devices, turning instead toward the natural world around us, and tuning in.
Diné, more commonly known as Navajo, tradition includes a daily early morning run toward the East to greet the rising sun, the Creator. *Ha'a'aahjigo dighádídeeshwoł*, I will run to the East. This daily run is a form of prayer, a way to greet the spirits and deities that are most accessible in early morning. And it's a way to show Mother Earth and Father Sky that you're working on being a strong person.

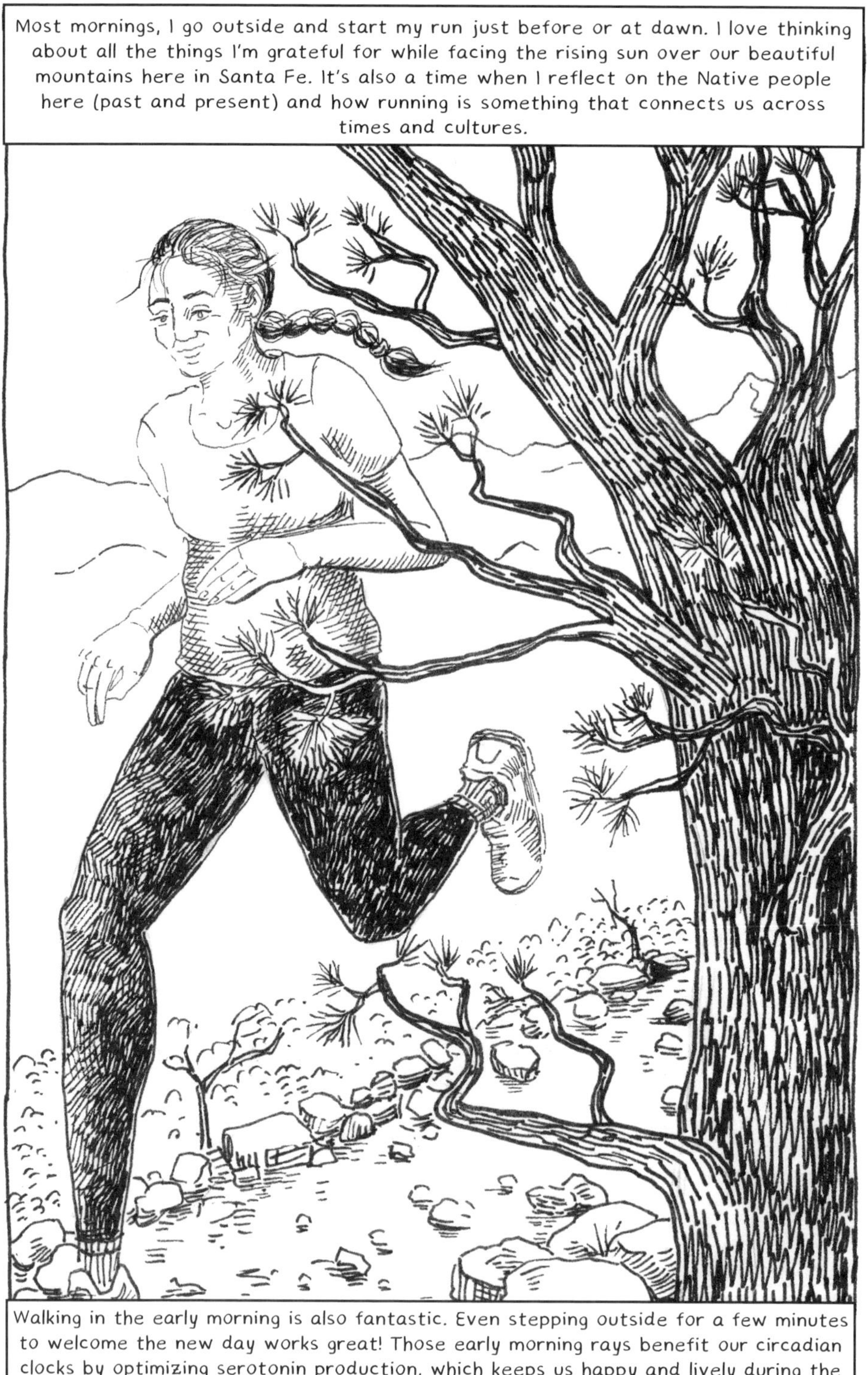
Most mornings, I go outside and start my run just before or at dawn. I love thinking about all the things I'm grateful for while facing the rising sun over our beautiful mountains here in Santa Fe. It's also a time when I reflect on the Native people here (past and present) and how running is something that connects us across times and cultures.
Walking in the early morning is also fantastic. Even stepping outside for a few minutes to welcome the new day works great! Those early morning rays benefit our circadian clocks by optimizing serotonin production, which keeps us happy and lively during the day and ensures adequate melatonin production to make us sleepy at bedtime.

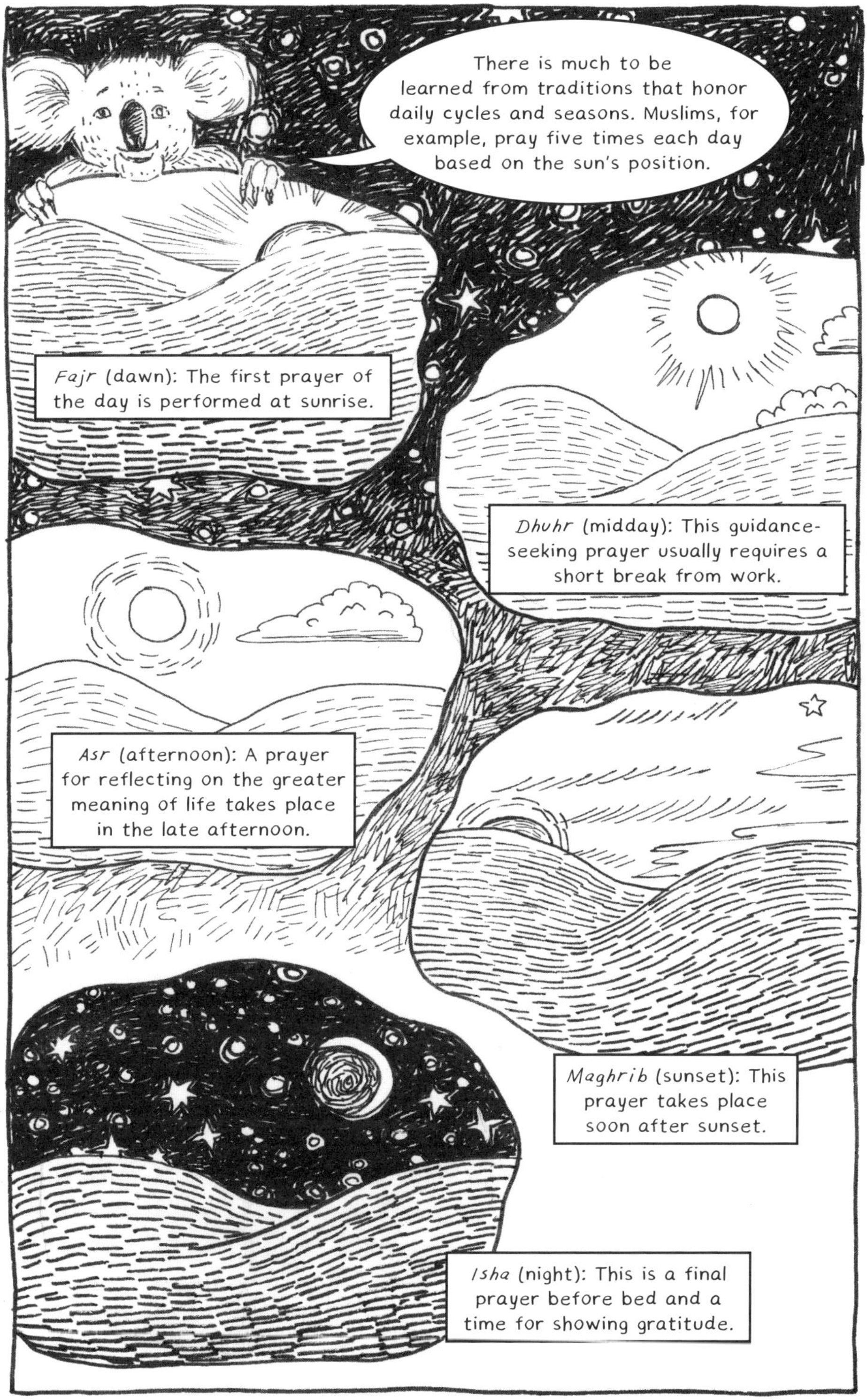
There is much to be learned from traditions that honor daily cycles and seasons. Muslims, for example, pray five times each day based on the sun's position.
Fajr (dawn): The first prayer of the day is performed at sunrise.
Dhuhr (midday): This guidance-seeking prayer usually requires a short break from work.
Asr (afternoon): A prayer for reflecting on the greater meaning of life takes place in the late afternoon.
Maghrib (sunset): This prayer takes place soon after sunset.
Isha (night): This is a final prayer before bed and a time for showing gratitude.

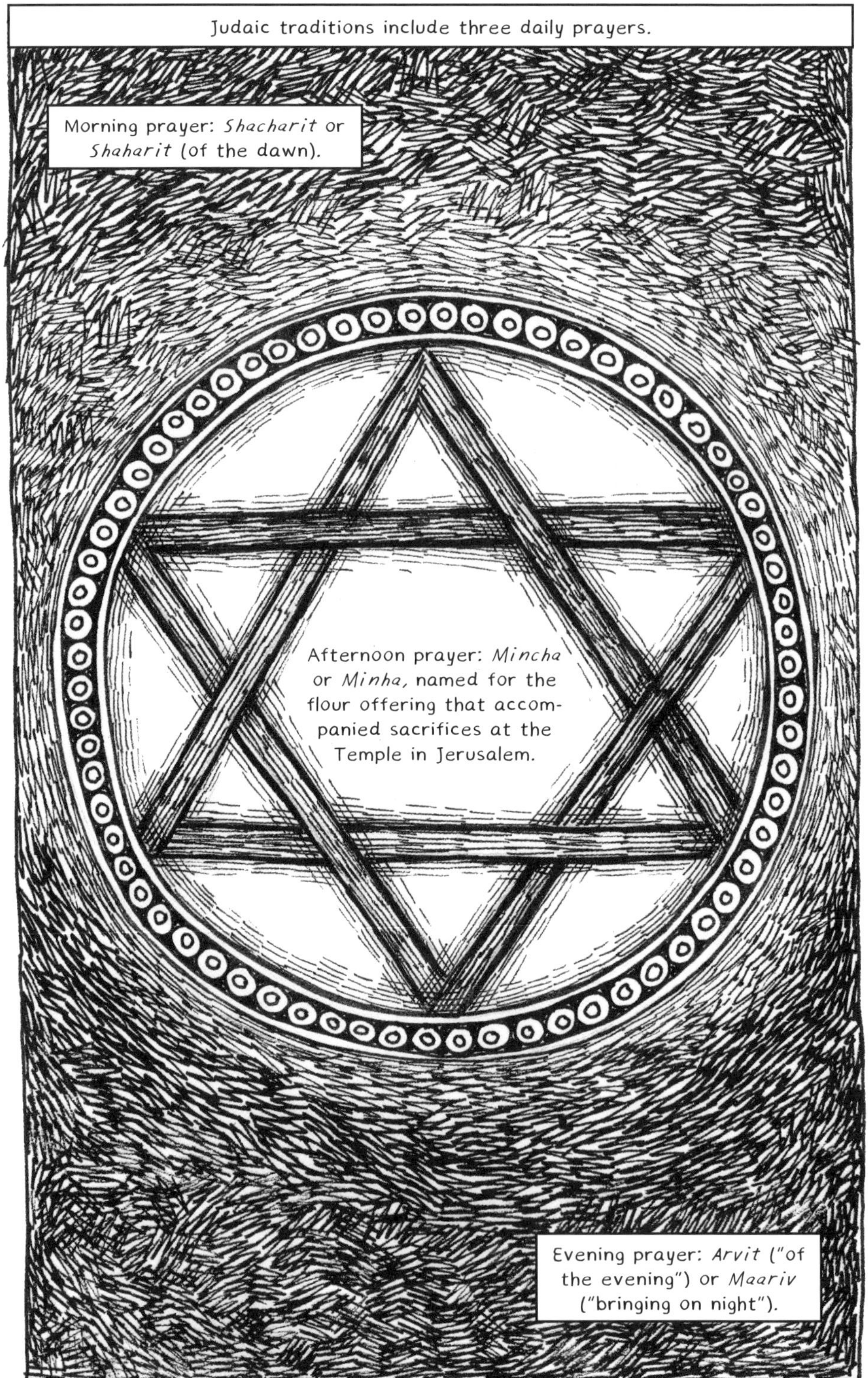
Judaic traditions include three daily prayers.
Morning prayer: *Shacharit* or *Shaharit* (of the dawn).
Afternoon prayer: *Mincha* or *Minha,* named for the flour offering that accompanied sacrifices at the Temple in Jerusalem.
Evening prayer: *Arvit* ("of the evening") or *Maariv* ("bringing on night").

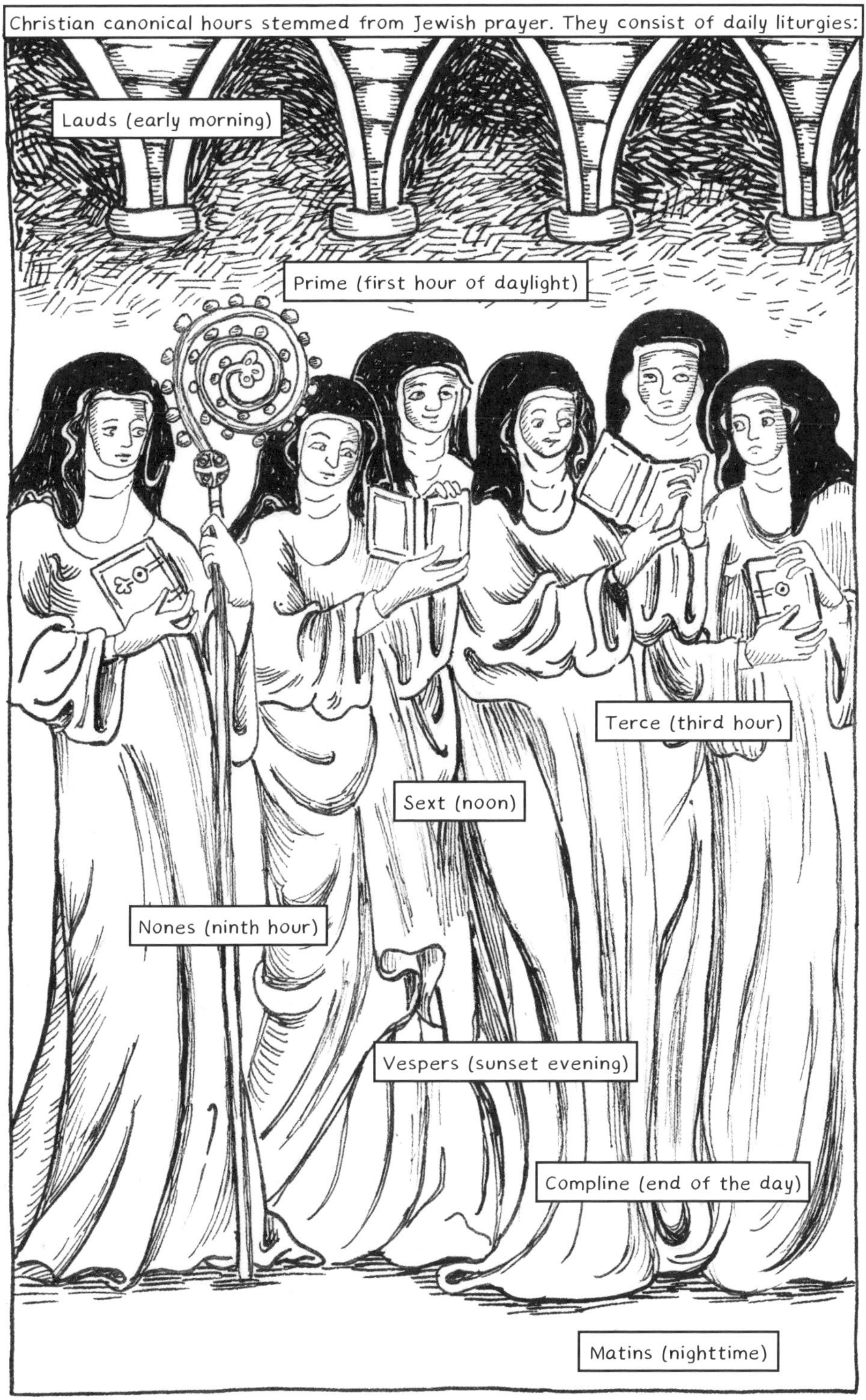
Christian canonical hours stemmed from Jewish prayer. They consist of daily liturgies:
Lauds (early morning)
Prime (first hour of daylight)
Terce (third hour)
Sext (noon)
Nones (ninth hour)
Vespers (sunset evening)
Compline (end of the day)
Matins (nighttime)

None of these traditions feel like home to me. In my early twenties, I turned to Wicca/Paganism to help me observe my own daily and seasonal rhythms. The philosophy of being in tune with diurnal, lunar, and seasonal cycles has always resonated with me.

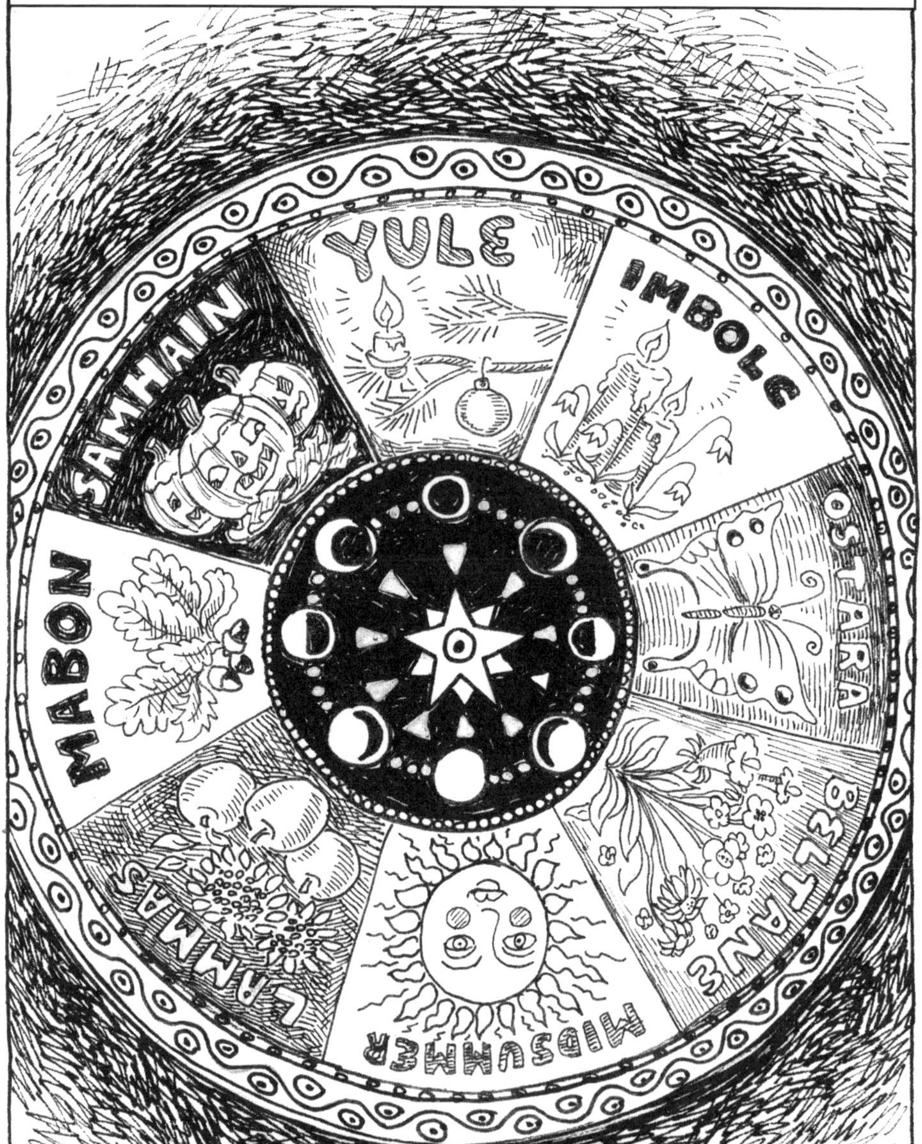
YULE
IMBOLC
OSTARA
BELTANE
MIDSUMMER
LAMMAS
MABON
SAMHAIN

In significant ways, these ideas are similar to Ayurvedic principles (*Ayur* = life and *veda* = knowledge or science). Ayurveda originated in India and is probably the most ancient system of medicine. Some sources indicate Ayurveda is at least 5,000 years old.

A key principle of Ayurvedic philosophy is *Dinacharya*, or daily routine. *Dinacharya* is the concept that improved mental and physical health must begin with a good daily routine.

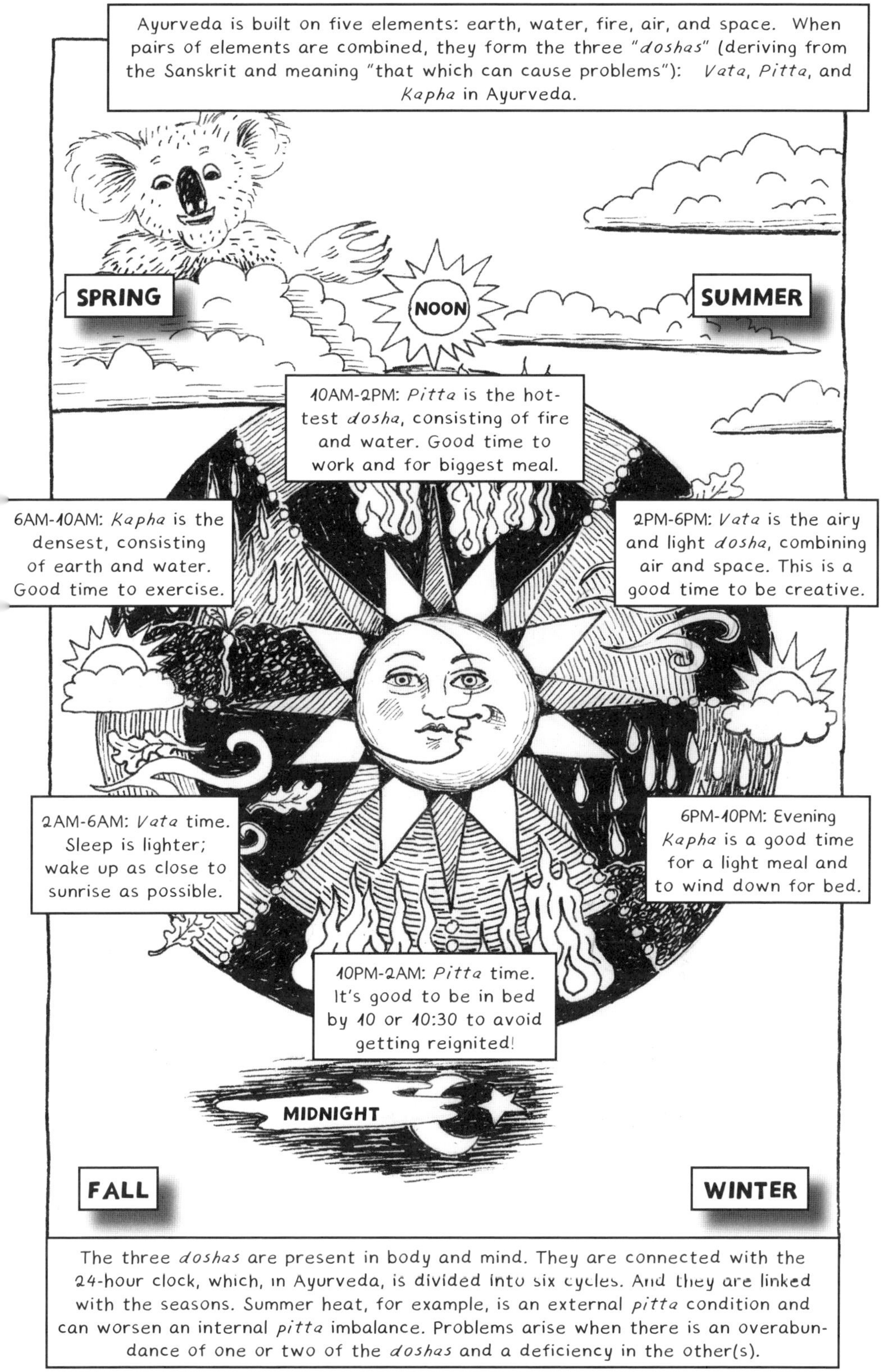

Ayurveda is built on five elements: earth, water, fire, air, and space. When pairs of elements are combined, they form the three "*doshas*" (deriving from the Sanskrit and meaning "that which can cause problems"): *Vata*, *Pitta*, and *Kapha* in Ayurveda.
SPRING
NOON
SUMMER
10AM-2PM: *Pitta* is the hottest *dosha*, consisting of fire and water. Good time to work and for biggest meal.
6AM-10AM: *Kapha* is the densest, consisting of earth and water. Good time to exercise.
2PM-6PM: *Vata* is the airy and light *dosha*, combining air and space. This is a good time to be creative.
2AM-6AM: *Vata* time. Sleep is lighter; wake up as close to sunrise as possible.
6PM-10PM: Evening *Kapha* is a good time for a light meal and to wind down for bed.
10PM-2AM: *Pitta* time. It's good to be in bed by 10 or 10:30 to avoid getting reignited!
MIDNIGHT
FALL
WINTER
The three *doshas* are present in body and mind. They are connected with the 24-hour clock, which, in Ayurveda, is divided into six cycles. And they are linked with the seasons. Summer heat, for example, is an external *pitta* condition and can worsen an internal *pitta* imbalance. Problems arise when there is an overabundance of one or two of the *doshas* and a deficiency in the other(s).

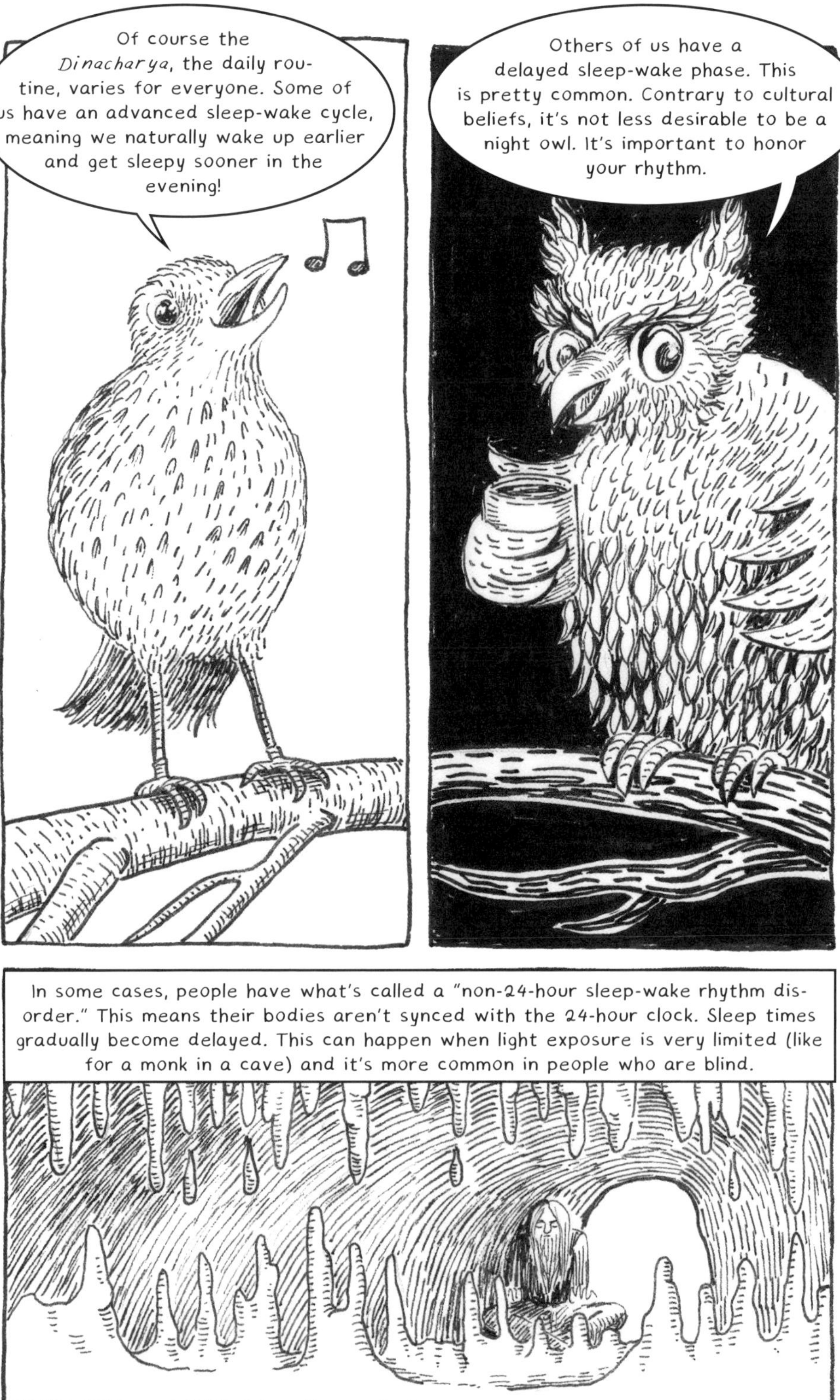
Of course the *Dinacharya*, the daily routine, varies for everyone. Some of us have an advanced sleep-wake cycle, meaning we naturally wake up earlier and get sleepy sooner in the evening!
Others of us have a delayed sleep-wake phase. This is pretty common. Contrary to cultural beliefs, it's not less desirable to be a night owl. It's important to honor your rhythm.
In some cases, people have what's called a "non-24-hour sleep-wake rhythm disorder." This means their bodies aren't synced with the 24-hour clock. Sleep times gradually become delayed. This can happen when light exposure is very limited (like for a monk in a cave) and it's more common in people who are blind.

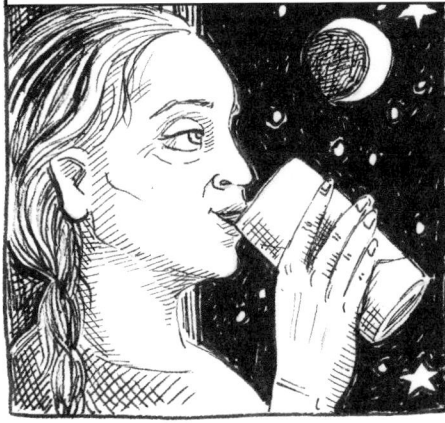

I'm an early bird and typically rise before the sun. I drink a glass of water.

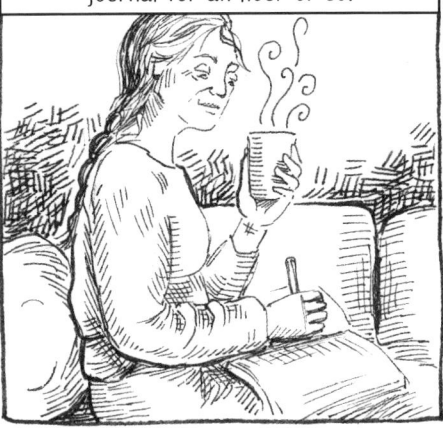

Then I have a coffee and write in my journal for an hour or so.

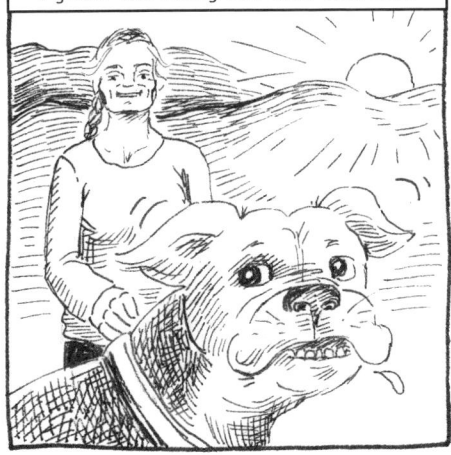

I greet the rising sun with exercise.

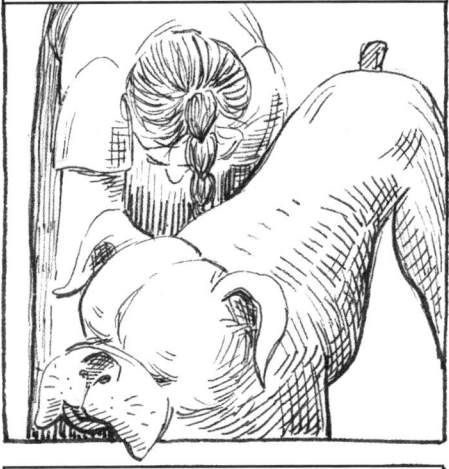

Often, I do a little yoga.

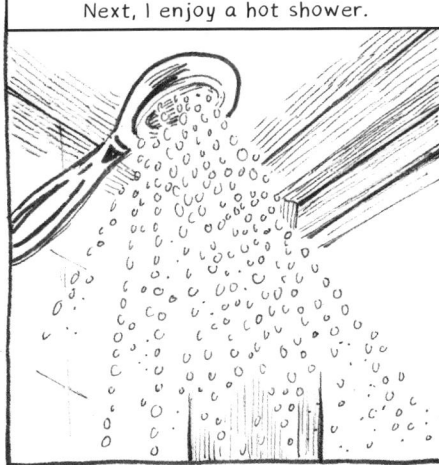

Next, I enjoy a hot shower.

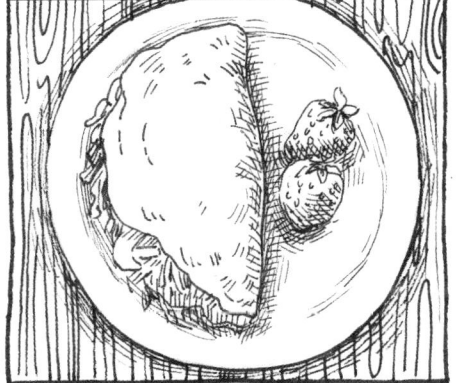

I like to eat a big breakfast before getting to work. Hearty omelets or soup are favorites!

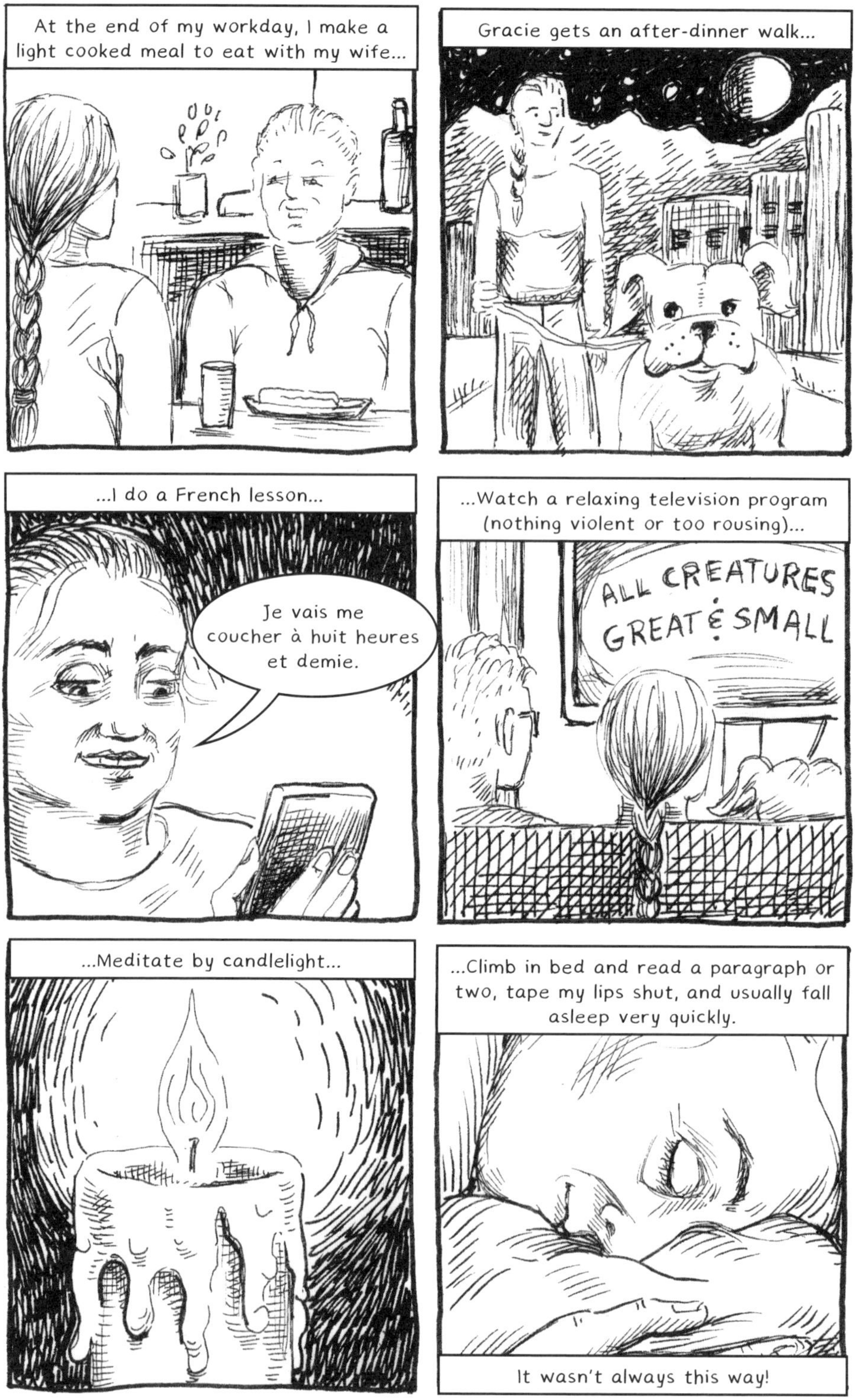
At the end of my workday, I make a light cooked meal to eat with my wife...
Gracie gets an after-dinner walk...
...I do a French lesson...
Je vais me coucher à huit heures et demie.
...Watch a relaxing television program (nothing violent or too rousing)...
ALL CREATURES GREAT & SMALL
...Meditate by candlelight...
...Climb in bed and read a paragraph or two, tape my lips shut, and usually fall asleep very quickly.
It wasn't always this way!

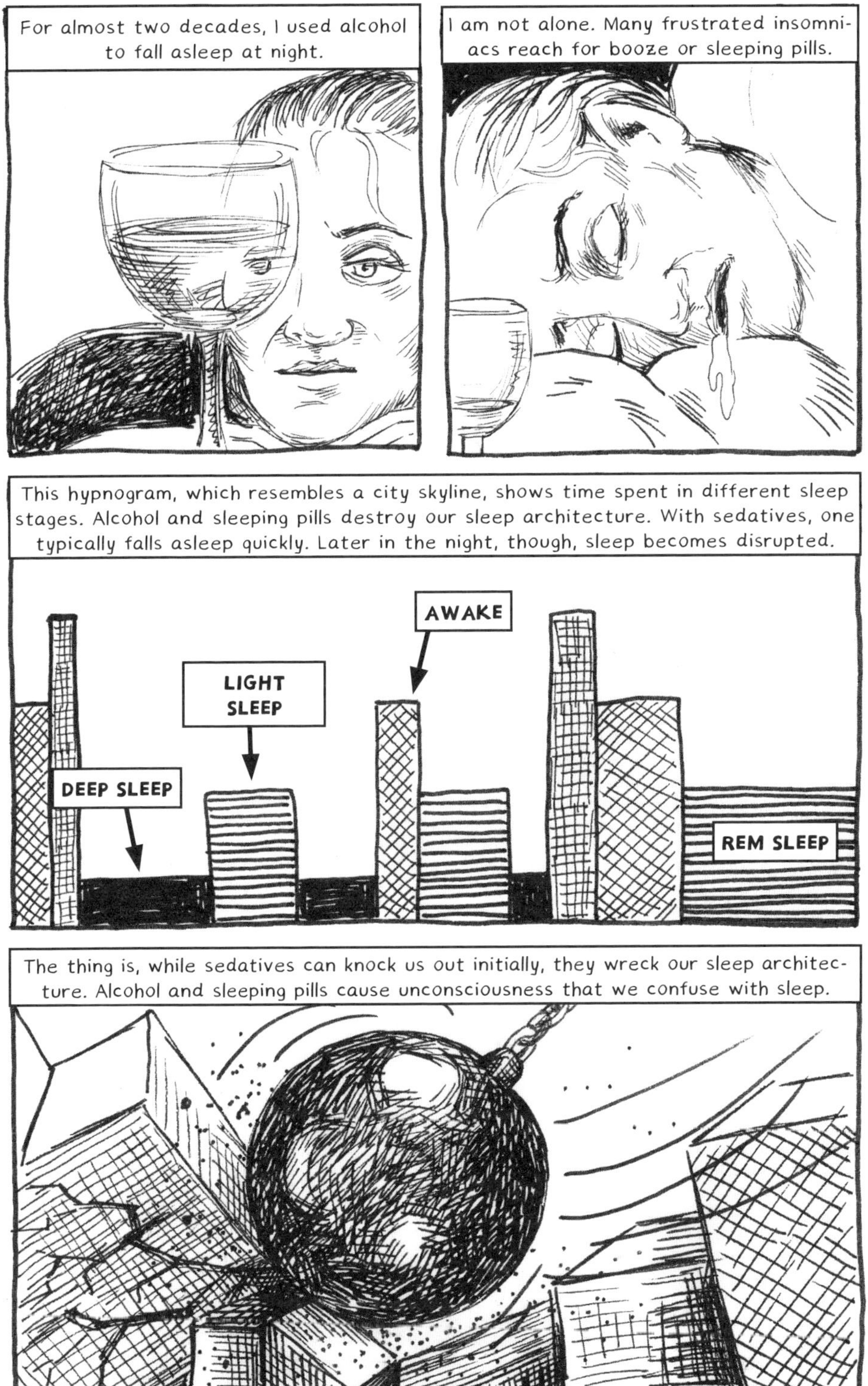
For almost two decades, I used alcohol to fall asleep at night.
I am not alone. Many frustrated insomniacs reach for booze or sleeping pills.
This hypnogram, which resembles a city skyline, shows time spent in different sleep stages. Alcohol and sleeping pills destroy our sleep architecture. With sedatives, one typically falls asleep quickly. Later in the night, though, sleep becomes disrupted.
AWAKE
LIGHT SLEEP
DEEP SLEEP
REM SLEEP
The thing is, while sedatives can knock us out initially, they wreck our sleep architecture. Alcohol and sleeping pills cause unconsciousness that we confuse with sleep.

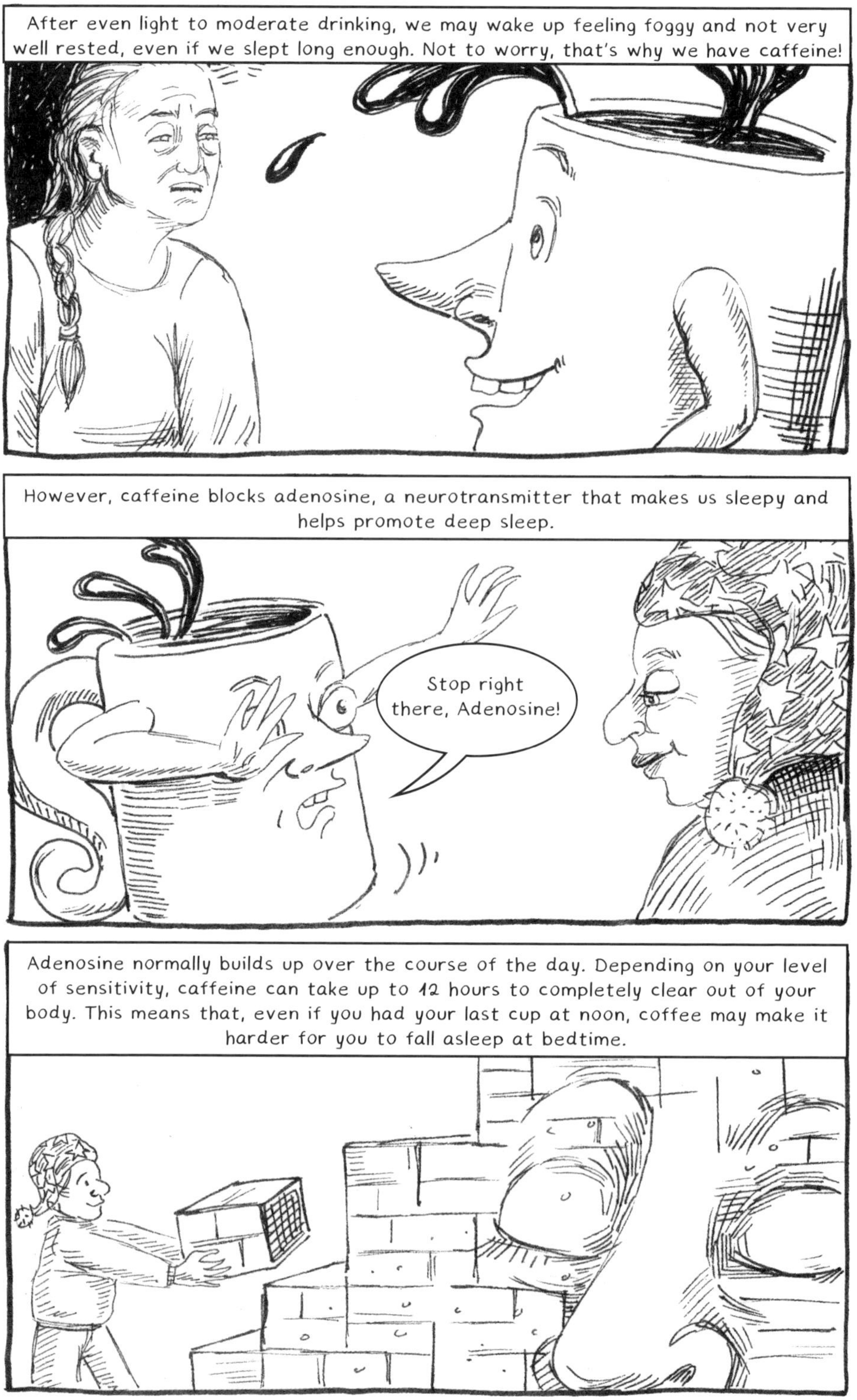
After even light to moderate drinking, we may wake up feeling foggy and not very well rested, even if we slept long enough. Not to worry, that's why we have caffeine!
However, caffeine blocks adenosine, a neurotransmitter that makes us sleepy and helps promote deep sleep.
Stop right there, Adenosine!
Adenosine normally builds up over the course of the day. Depending on your level of sensitivity, caffeine can take up to 12 hours to completely clear out of your body. This means that, even if you had your last cup at noon, coffee may make it harder for you to fall asleep at bedtime.

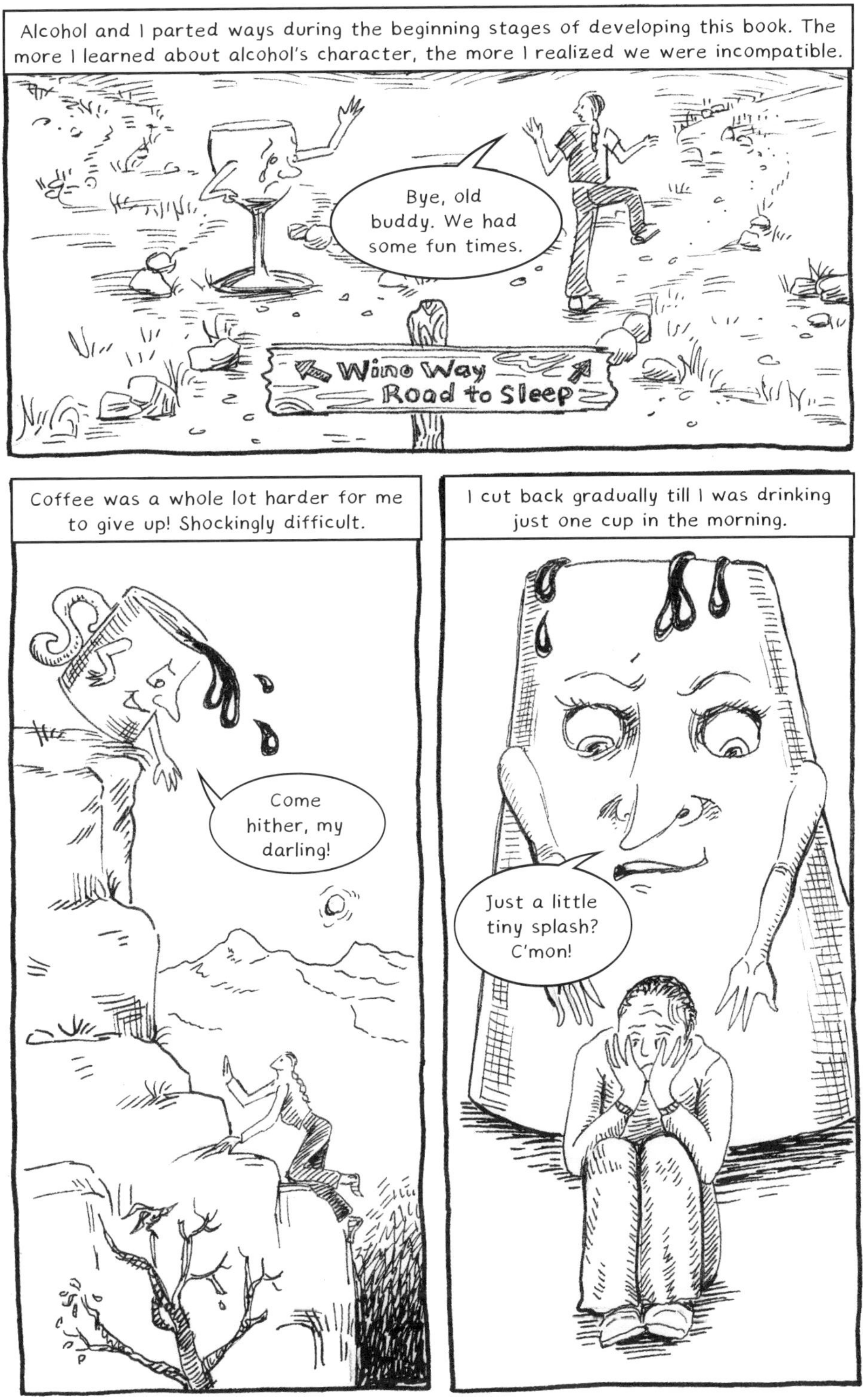
Alcohol and I parted ways during the beginning stages of developing this book. The more I learned about alcohol's character, the more I realized we were incompatible.
Bye, old buddy. We had some fun times.
Wino Way
Road to Sleep
Coffee was a whole lot harder for me to give up! Shockingly difficult.
Come hither, my darling!
I cut back gradually till I was drinking just one cup in the morning.
Just a little tiny splash? C'mon!

Everyone has to experiment with how much, if any, caffeine works for them. Someone with tired adrenal glands, for example, might want to avoid it altogether.

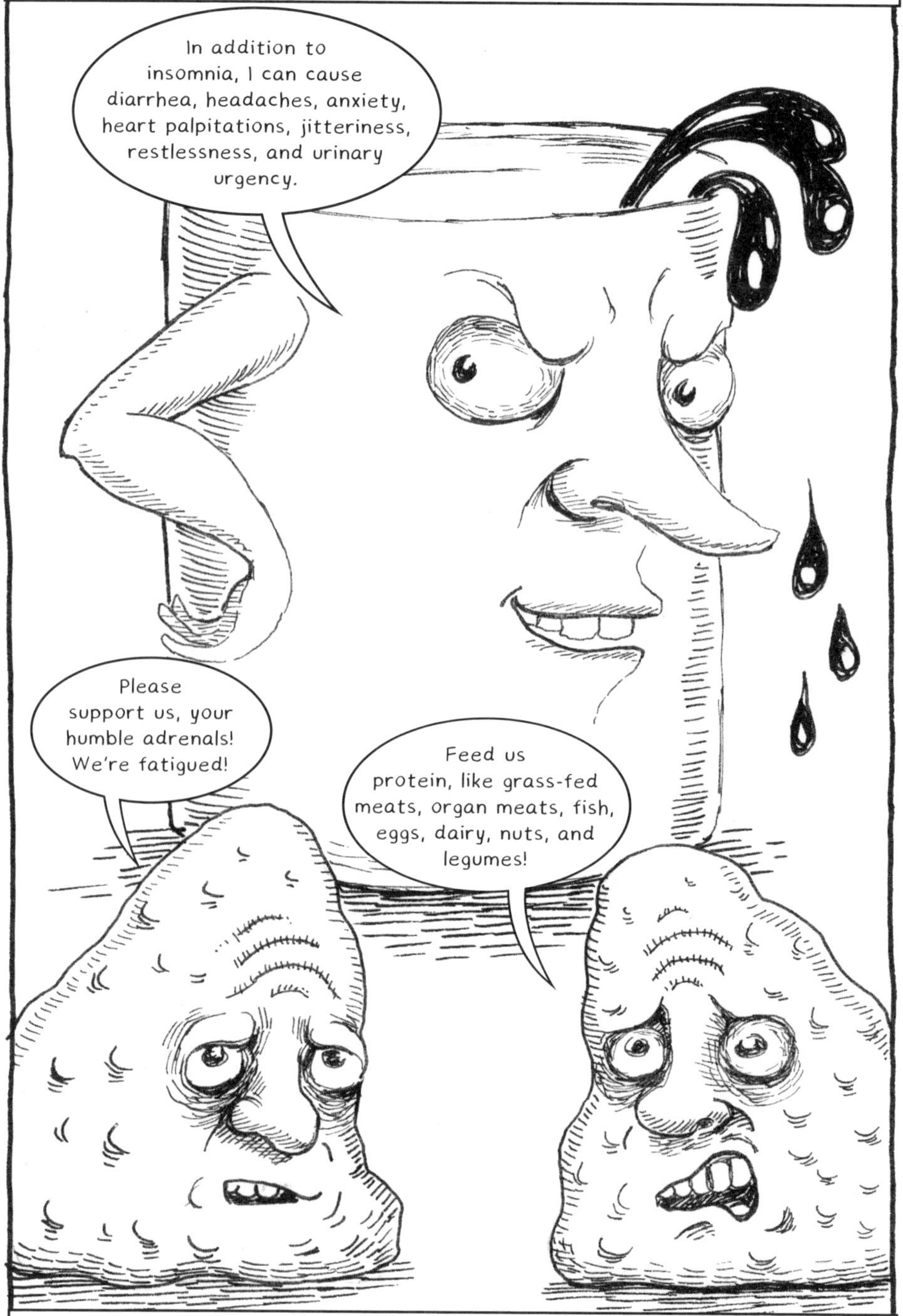
In addition to insomnia, I can cause diarrhea, headaches, anxiety, heart palpitations, jitteriness, restlessness, and urinary urgency.
Please support us, your humble adrenals! We're fatigued!
Feed us protein, like grass-fed meats, organ meats, fish, eggs, dairy, nuts, and legumes!

When we have tired, burned-out adrenals, we often crave caffeine just to function. But caffeine doesn't help those adrenals one bit, so it might be a good idea to support our tired glands with wholesome foods and adequate rest while cutting back on caffeine.

Those of us who suffer from chronic insomnia often develop a real fear of bedtime. Bed, instead of being a safe nest for rest, becomes a site of plight.

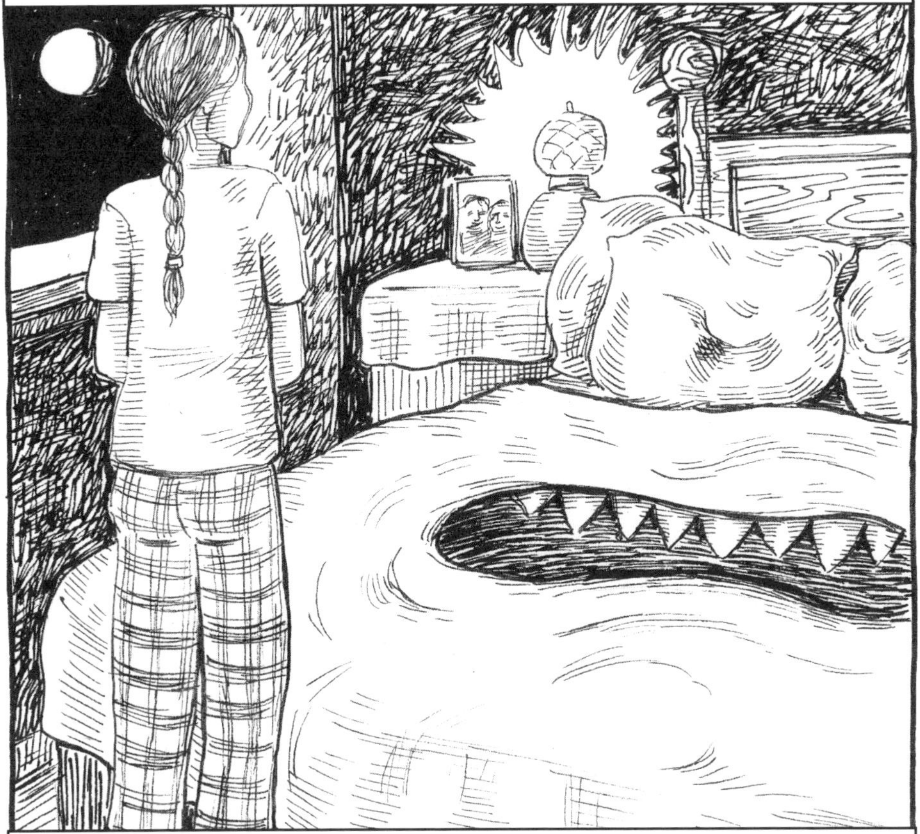

It's not actually the bed we're afraid of, of course. It's essentially a broken sense of trust in the body-mind and its ability to rest and recover. Bed becomes symbolic of failure, of chronic dysfunction and misery.

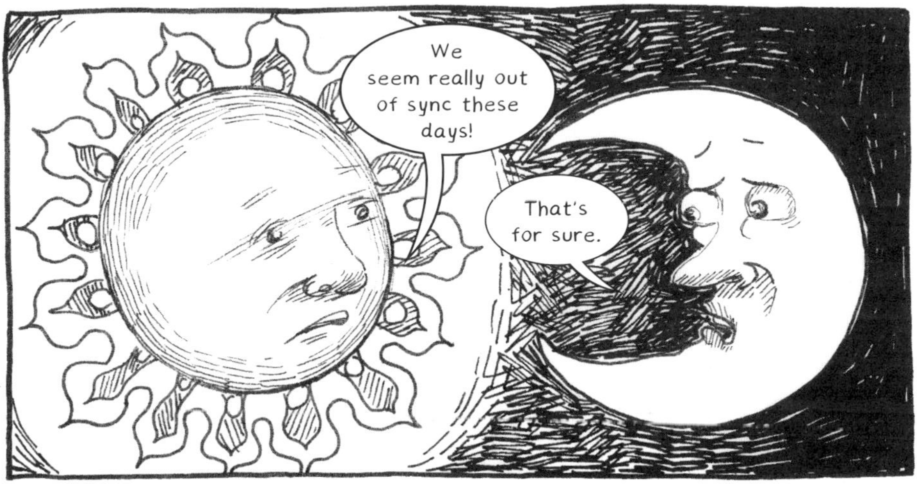
We seem really out of sync these days!
That's for sure.

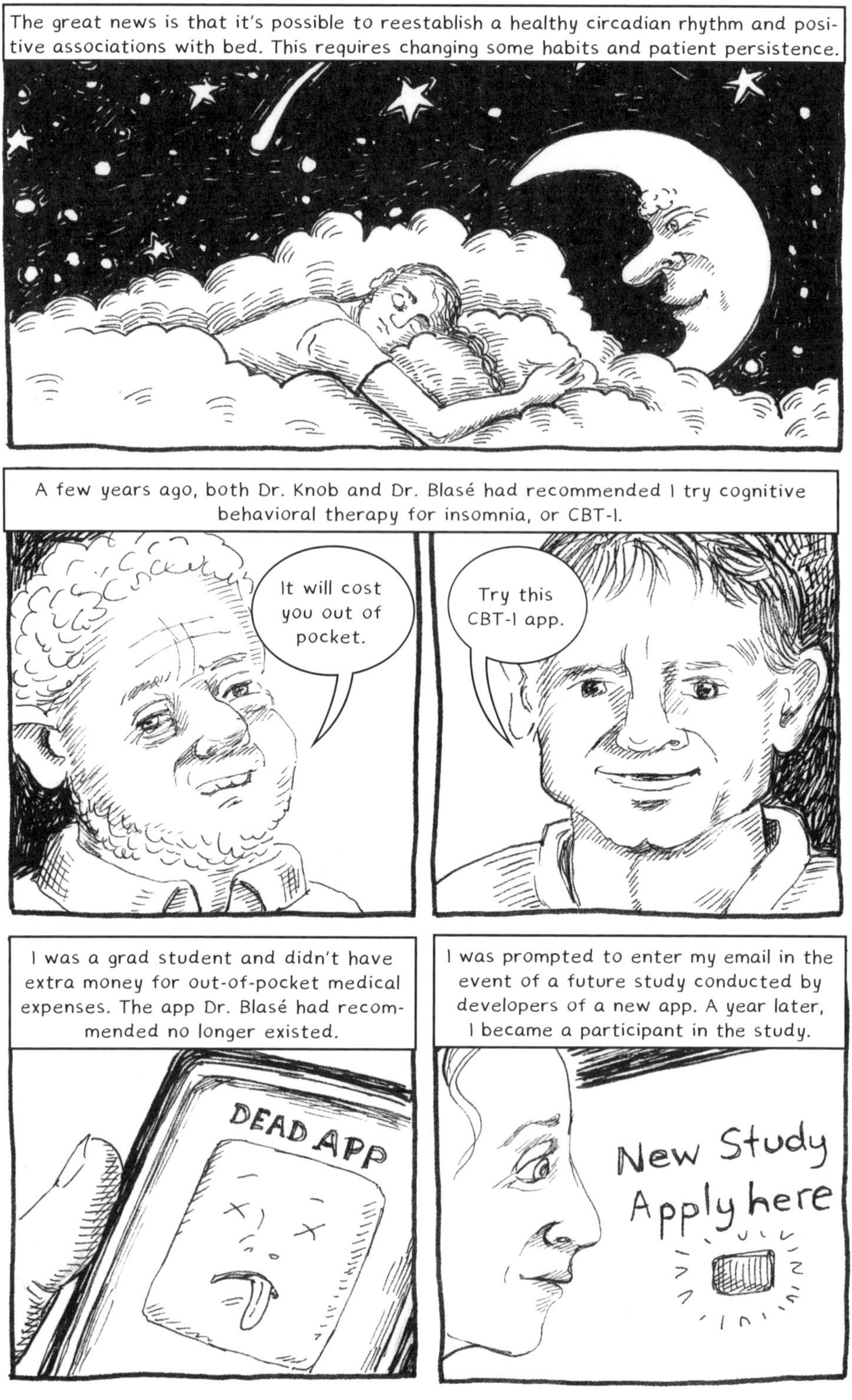
The great news is that it's possible to reestablish a healthy circadian rhythm and positive associations with bed. This requires changing some habits and patient persistence.
A few years ago, both Dr. Knob and Dr. Blasé had recommended I try cognitive behavioral therapy for insomnia, or CBT-I.
It will cost you out of pocket.
Try this CBT-I app.
I was a grad student and didn't have extra money for out-of-pocket medical expenses. The app Dr. Blasé had recommended no longer existed.
DEAD APP
I was prompted to enter my email in the event of a future study conducted by developers of a new app. A year later, I became a participant in the study.
New Study
Apply here

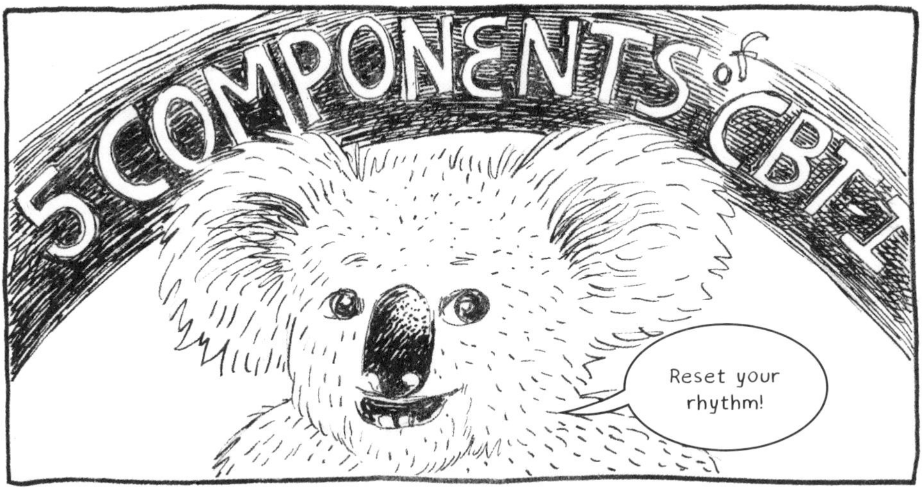
5 COMPONENTS of CBT-I
Reset your rhythm!

CBT-I ELEMENT 1: SLEEP RESTRICTION

This is tough in the beginning, but very well worth it! The principle: People with insomnia spend a lot of time lying in bed awake. They have poor sleep EFFICIENCY. To improve this, the first step is sleep restriction therapy, which prompts you to spend less time in bed at first. As sleep efficiency improves, the amount of time spent in bed asleep increases.

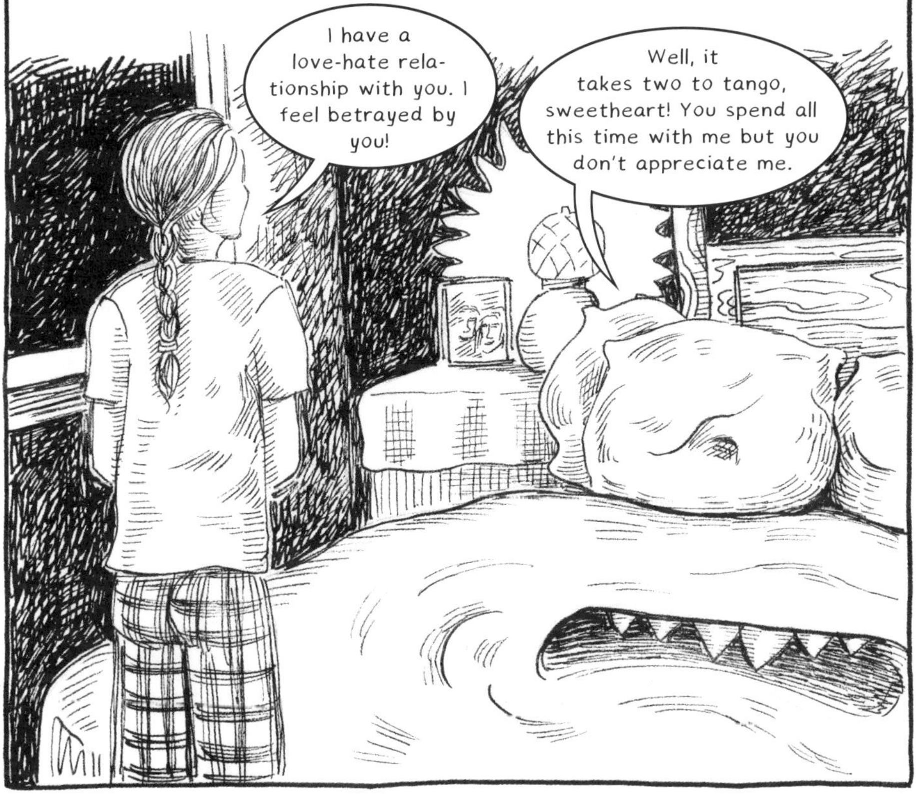
I have a love-hate relationship with you. I feel betrayed by you!
Well, it takes two to tango, sweetheart! You spend all this time with me but you don't appreciate me.

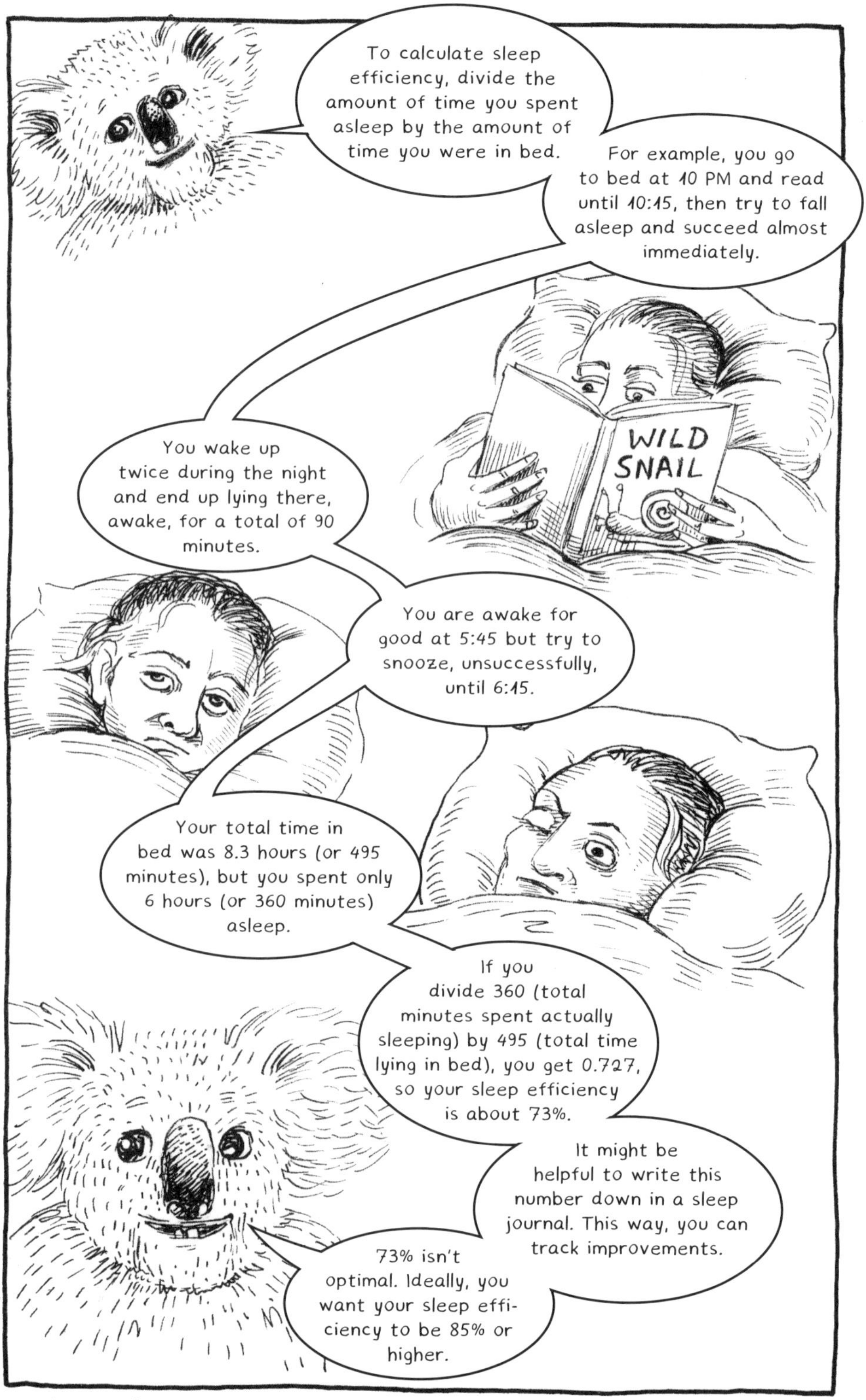
To calculate sleep efficiency, divide the amount of time you spent asleep by the amount of time you were in bed.
For example, you go to bed at 10 PM and read until 10:15, then try to fall asleep and succeed almost immediately.
WILD SNAIL
You wake up twice during the night and end up lying there, awake, for a total of 90 minutes.
You are awake for good at 5:45 but try to snooze, unsuccessfully, until 6:15.
Your total time in bed was 8.3 hours (or 495 minutes), but you spent only 6 hours (or 360 minutes) asleep.
If you divide 360 (total minutes spent actually sleeping) by 495 (total time lying in bed), you get 0.727, so your sleep efficiency is about 73%.
It might be helpful to write this number down in a sleep journal. This way, you can track improvements.
73% isn't optimal. Ideally, you want your sleep efficiency to be 85% or higher.

To bypass all this math, oogle "sleep efficiency calculator" and plug in your numbers!

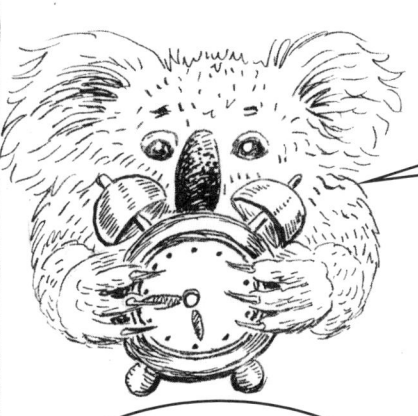

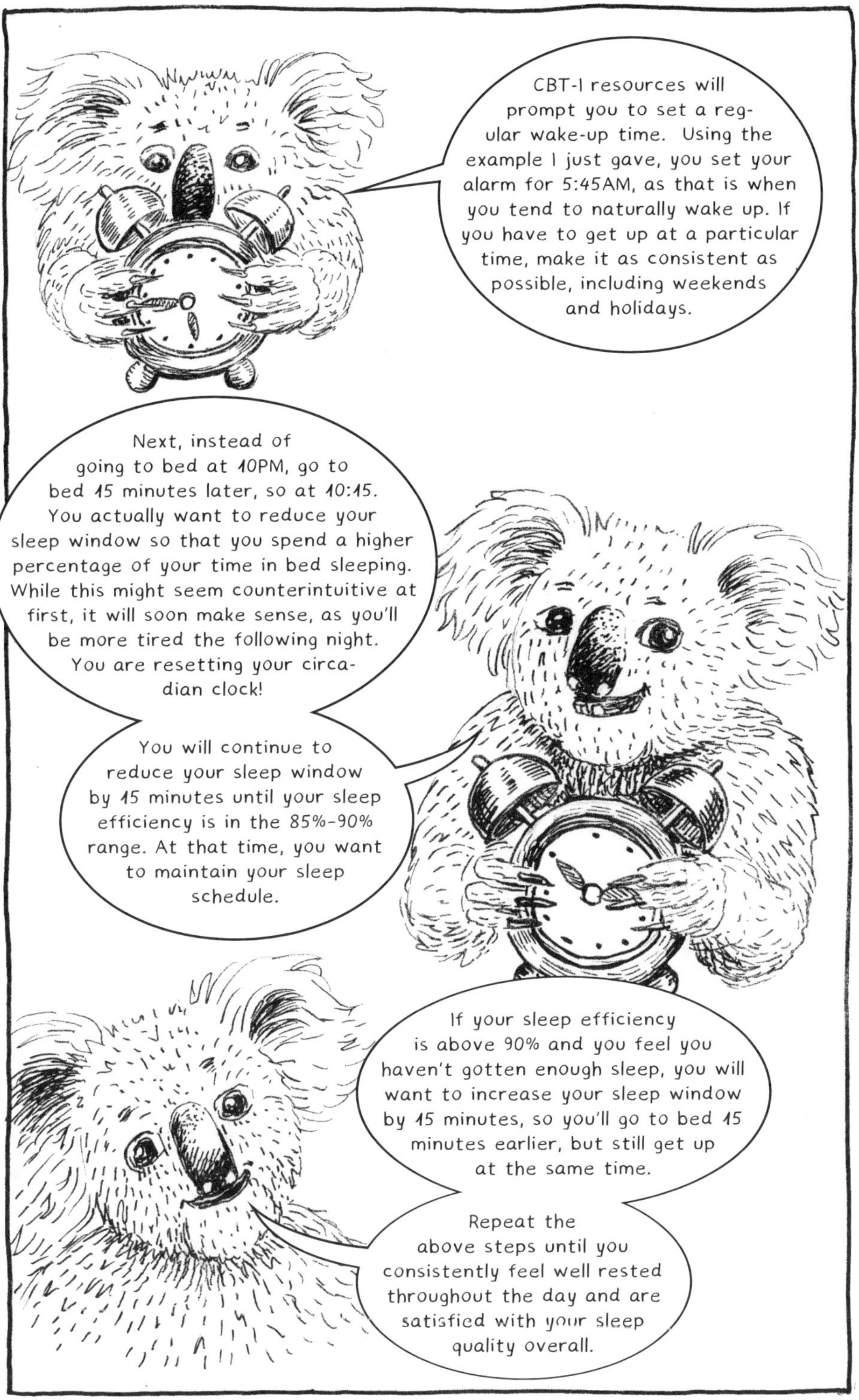

CBT-I resources will prompt you to set a regular wake-up time. Using the example I just gave, you set your alarm for 5:45AM, as that is when you tend to naturally wake up. If you have to get up at a particular time, make it as consistent as possible, including weekends and holidays.

Next, instead of going to bed at 10PM, go to bed 15 minutes later, so at 10:15. You actually want to reduce your sleep window so that you spend a higher percentage of your time in bed sleeping. While this might seem counterintuitive at first, it will soon make sense, as you'll be more tired the following night. You are resetting your circadian clock!

You will continue to reduce your sleep window by 15 minutes until your sleep efficiency is in the 85%-90% range. At that time, you want to maintain your sleep schedule.

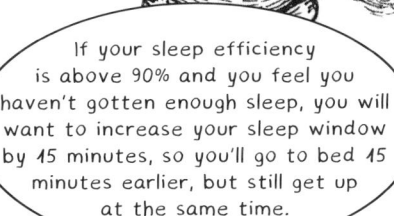

If your sleep efficiency is above 90% and you feel you haven't gotten enough sleep, you will want to increase your sleep window by 15 minutes, so you'll go to bed 15 minutes earlier, but still get up at the same time.

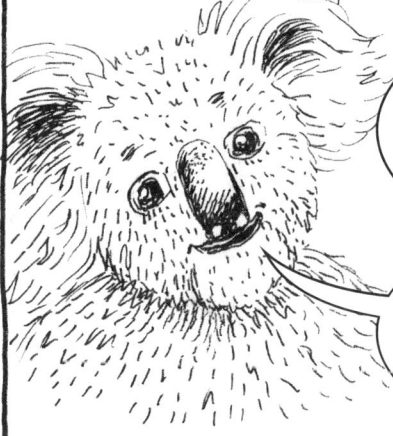

Repeat the above steps until you consistently feel well rested throughout the day and are satisfied with your sleep quality overall.

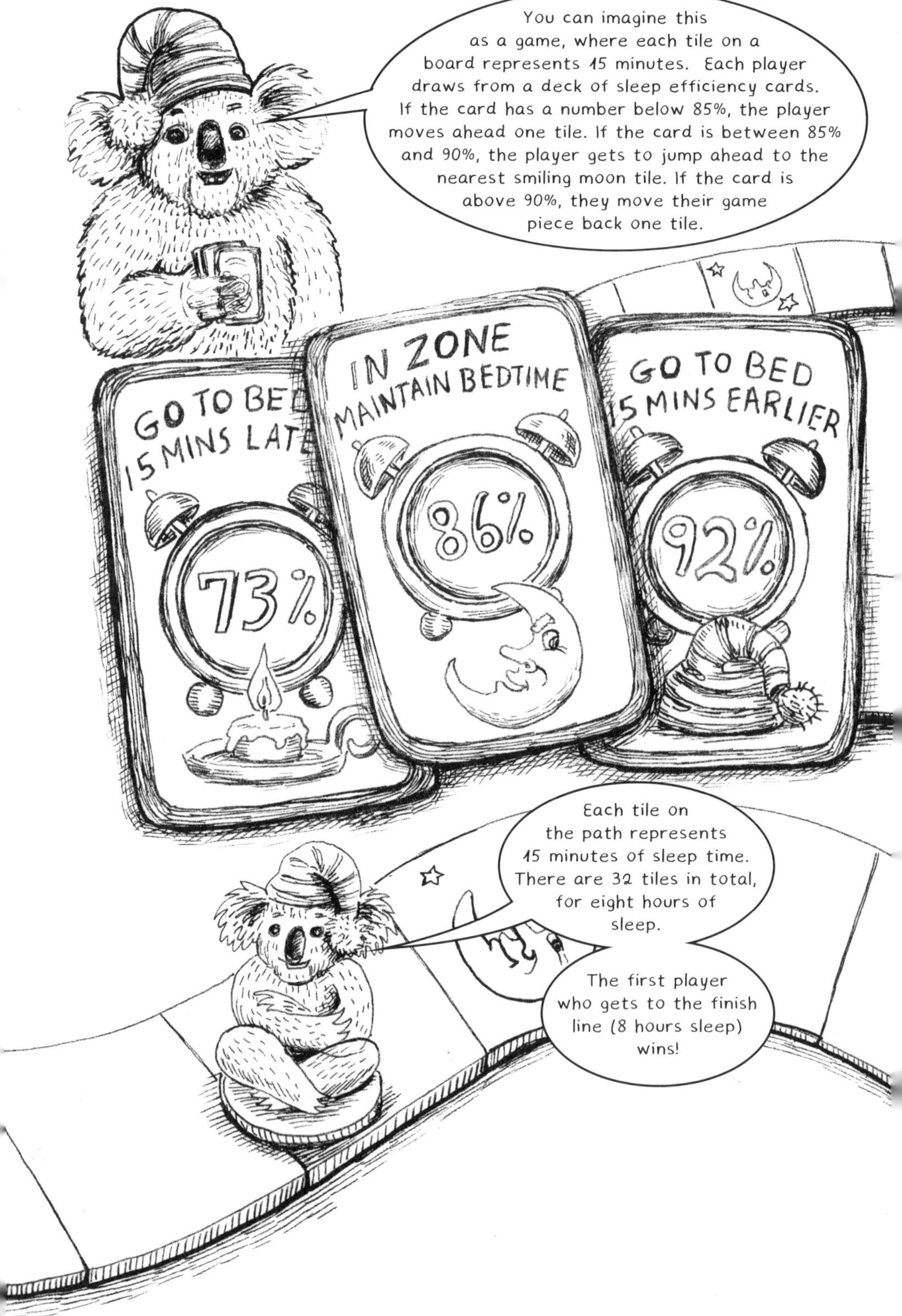
You can imagine this as a game, where each tile on a board represents 15 minutes. Each player draws from a deck of sleep efficiency cards. If the card has a number below 85%, the player moves ahead one tile. If the card is between 85% and 90%, the player gets to jump ahead to the nearest smiling moon tile. If the card is above 90%, they move their game piece back one tile.
GO TO BE
15 MINS LAT
73%
IN ZONE
MAINTAIN BEDTIME
86%
GO TO BED
15 MINS EARLIER
92%
Each tile on the path represents 15 minutes of sleep time. There are 32 tiles in total, for eight hours of sleep.
The first player who gets to the finish line (8 hours sleep) wins!

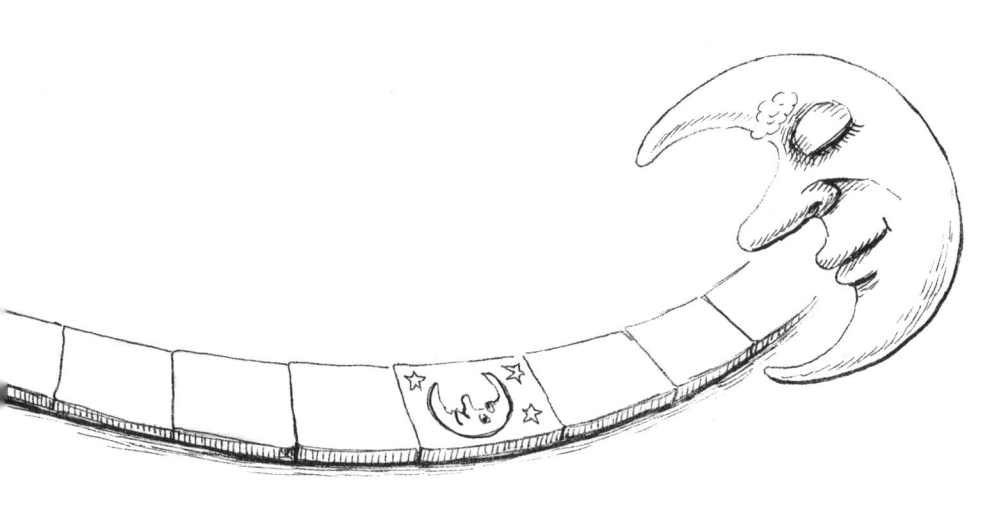

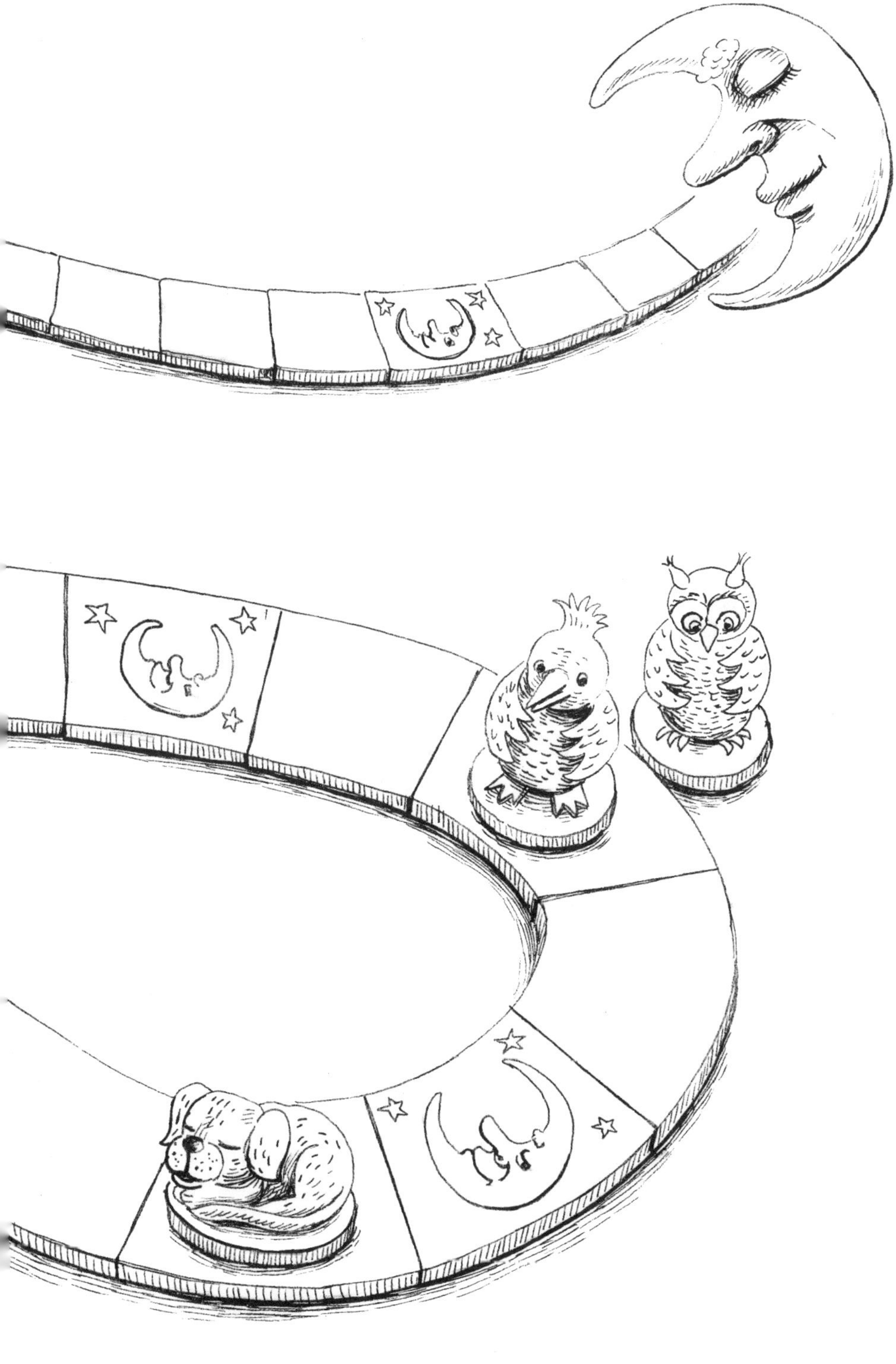

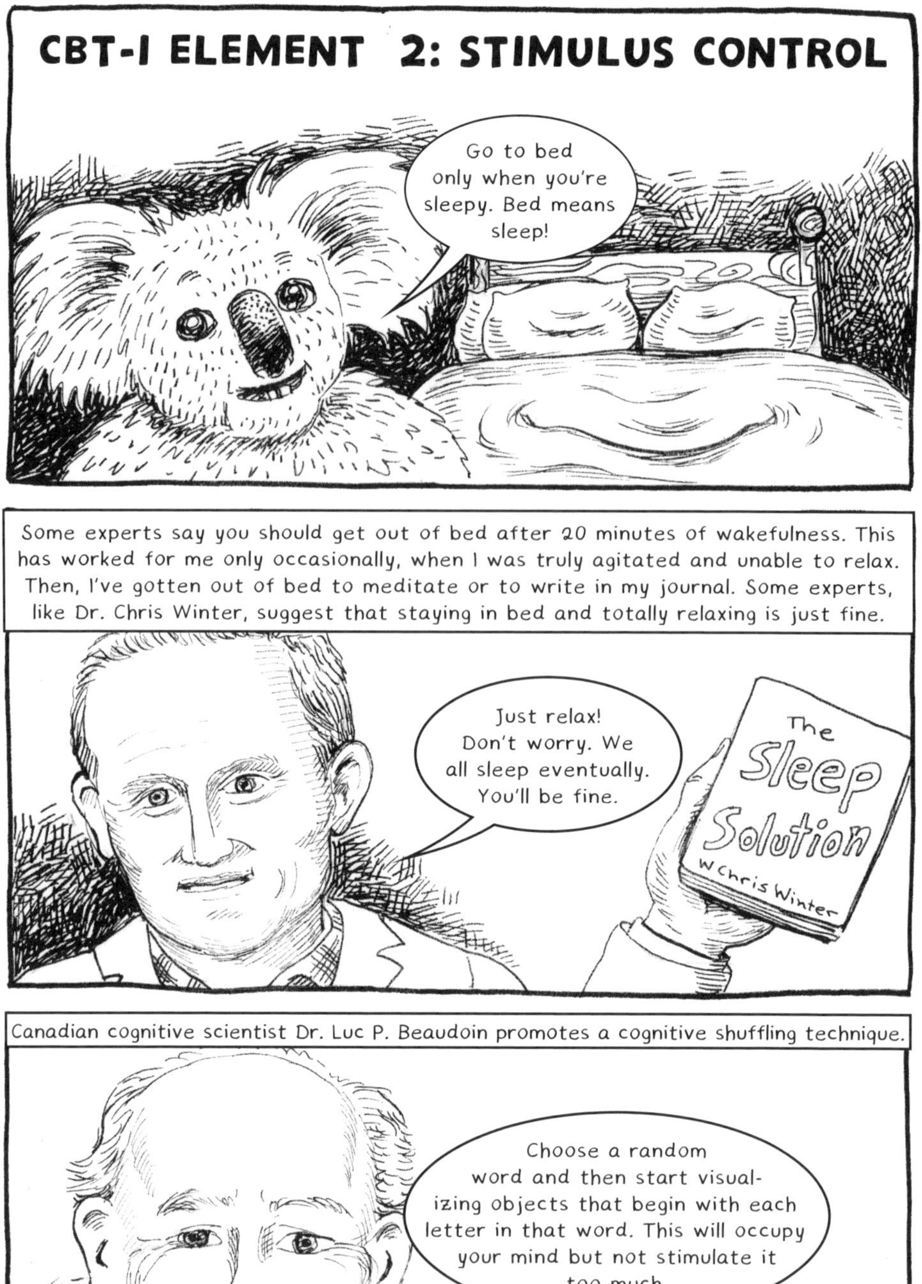
CBT-I ELEMENT 2: STIMULUS CONTROL
Go to bed only when you're sleepy. Bed means sleep!
Some experts say you should get out of bed after 20 minutes of wakefulness. This has worked for me only occasionally, when I was truly agitated and unable to relax. Then, I've gotten out of bed to meditate or to write in my journal. Some experts, like Dr. Chris Winter, suggest that staying in bed and totally relaxing is just fine.
Just relax! Don't worry. We all sleep eventually. You'll be fine.
The Sleep Solution
W Chris Winter
Canadian cognitive scientist Dr. Luc P. Beaudoin promotes a cognitive shuffling technique.
Choose a random word and then start visualizing objects that begin with each letter in that word. This will occupy your mind but not stimulate it too much.
If you have trouble coming up with words on your own, you can use the app I created. It's called mySleepButton.

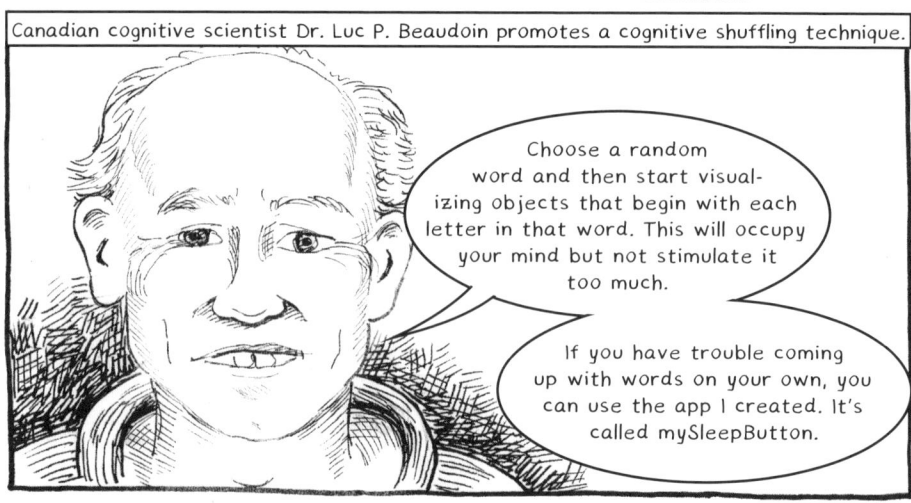

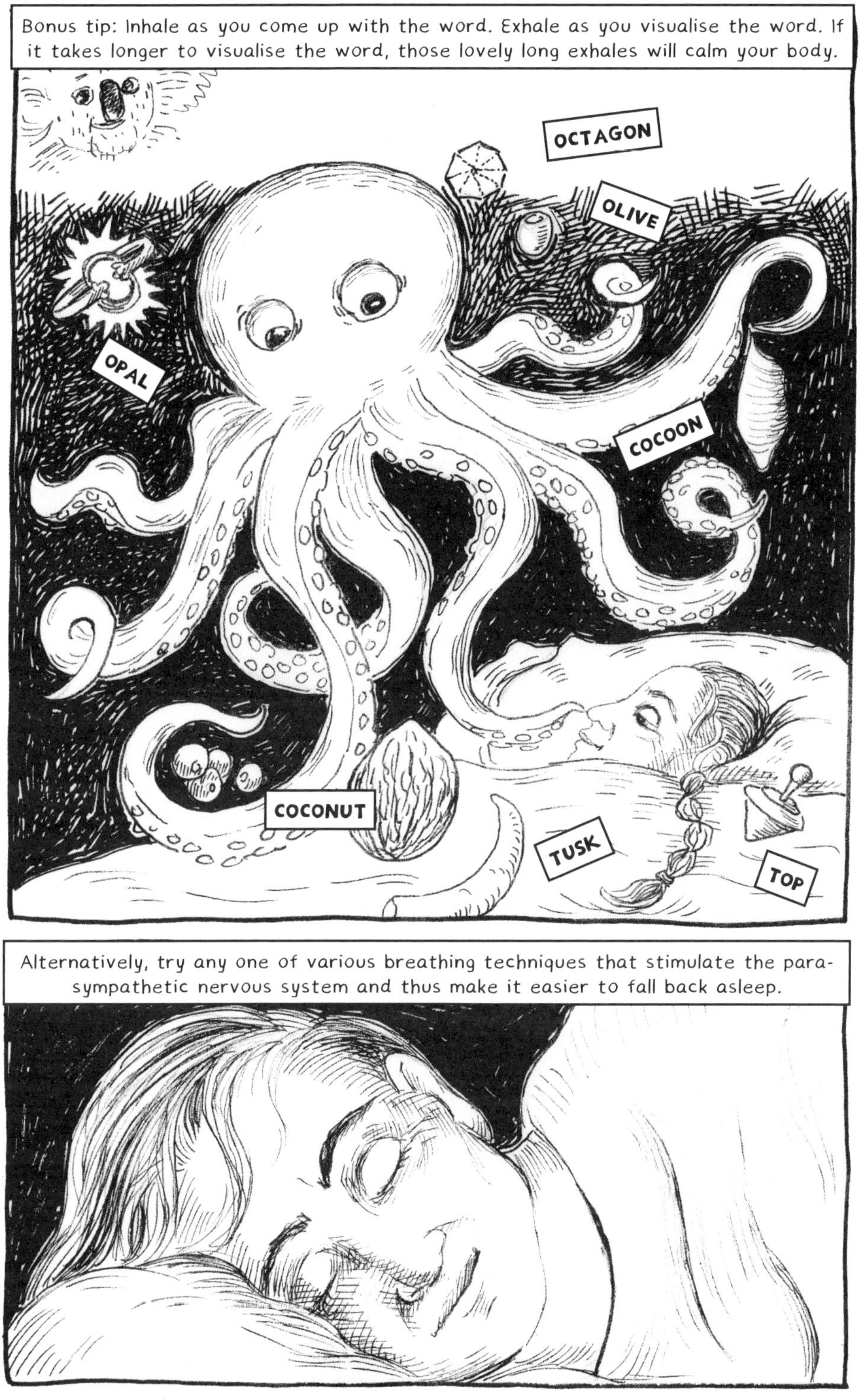
Bonus tip: Inhale as you come up with the word. Exhale as you visualise the word. If it takes longer to visualise the word, those lovely long exhales will calm your body.
OCTAGON
OLIVE
OPAL
COCOON
COCONUT
TUSK
TOP
Alternatively, try any one of various breathing techniques that stimulate the para-sympathetic nervous system and thus make it easier to fall back asleep.

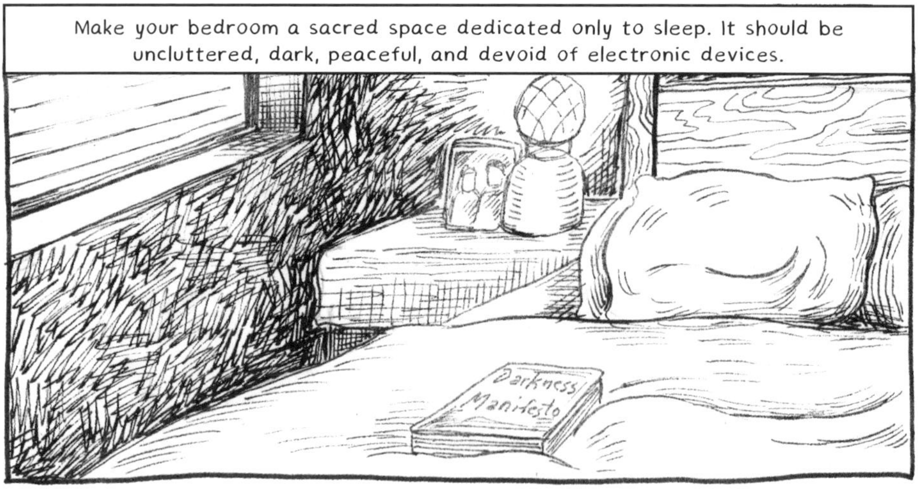
Make your bedroom a sacred space dedicated only to sleep. It should be uncluttered, dark, peaceful, and devoid of electronic devices.
Darkness Manifesto

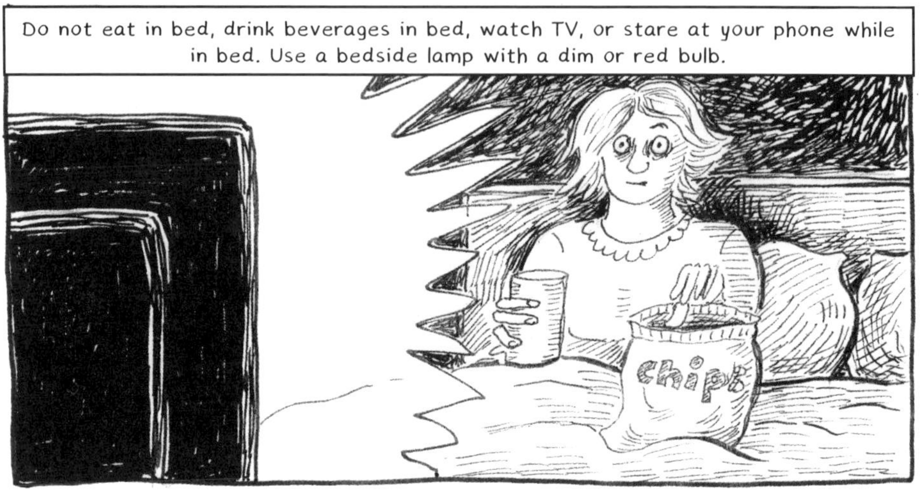
Do not eat in bed, drink beverages in bed, watch TV, or stare at your phone while in bed. Use a bedside lamp with a dim or red bulb.
chips

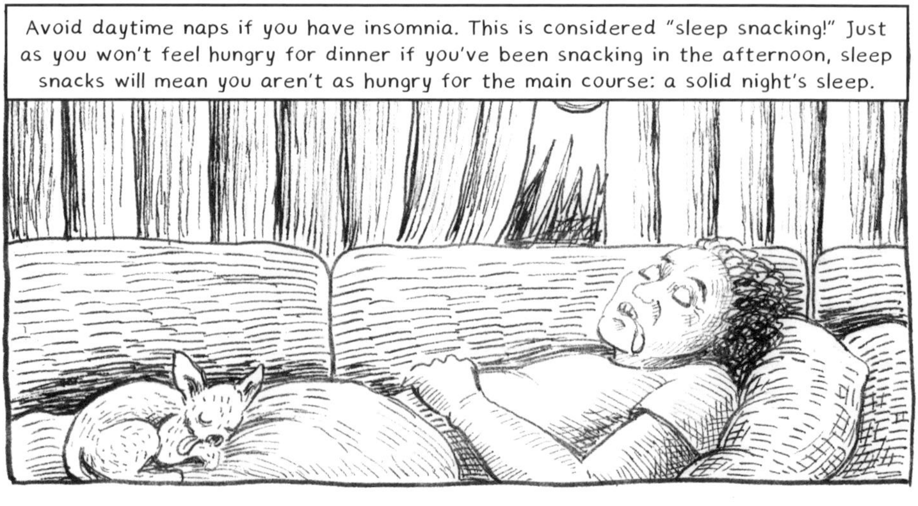
Avoid daytime naps if you have insomnia. This is considered "sleep snacking!" Just as you won't feel hungry for dinner if you've been snacking in the afternoon, sleep snacks will mean you aren't as hungry for the main course: a solid night's sleep.

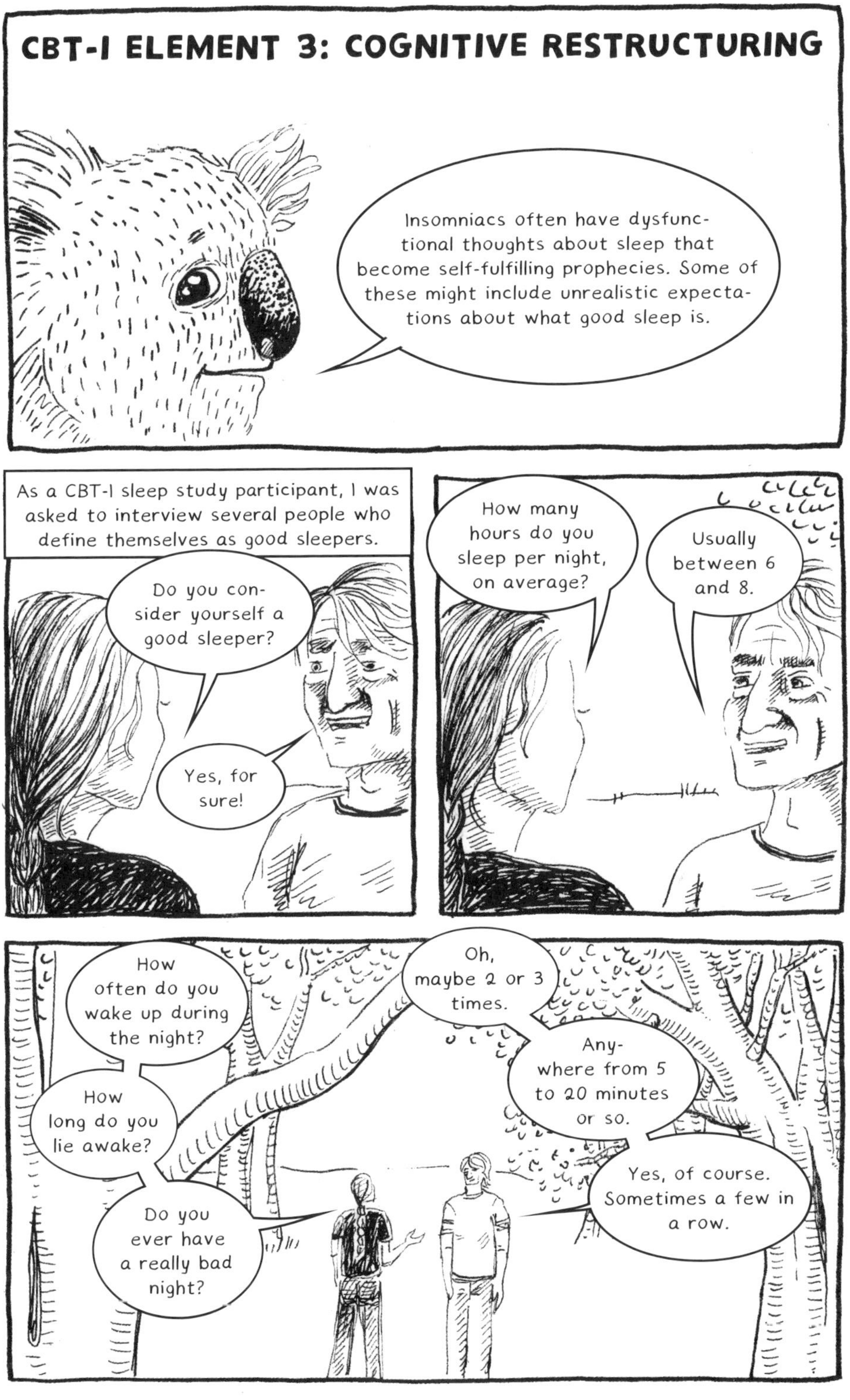
CBT-I ELEMENT 3: COGNITIVE RESTRUCTURING
Insomniacs often have dysfunctional thoughts about sleep that become self-fulfilling prophecies. Some of these might include unrealistic expectations about what good sleep is.
As a CBT-I sleep study participant, I was asked to interview several people who define themselves as good sleepers.
Do you consider yourself a good sleeper?
Yes, for sure!
How many hours do you sleep per night, on average?
Usually between 6 and 8.
How often do you wake up during the night?
Oh, maybe 2 or 3 times.
How long do you lie awake?
Anywhere from 5 to 20 minutes or so.
Do you ever have a really bad night?
Yes, of course. Sometimes a few in a row.

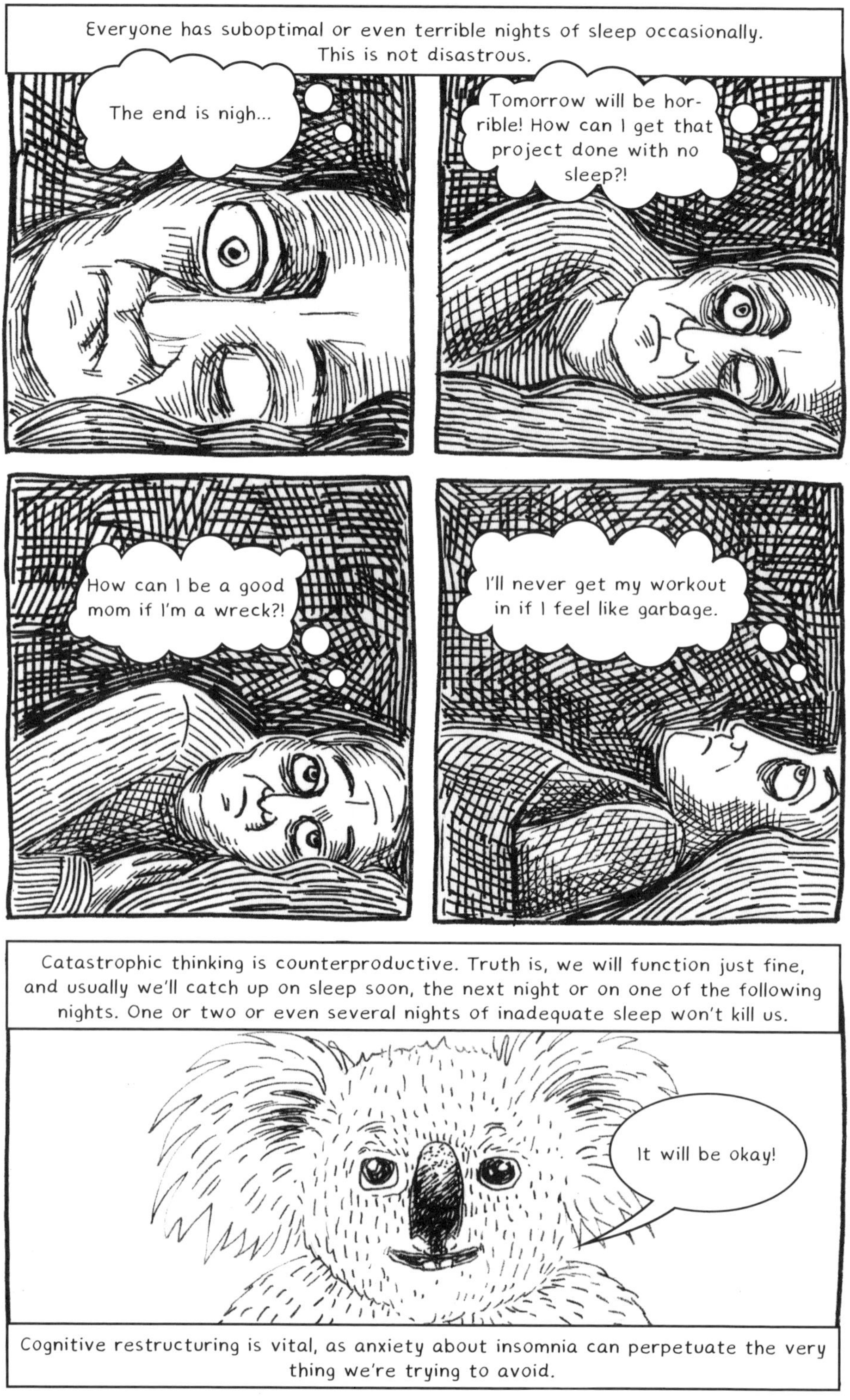
Everyone has suboptimal or even terrible nights of sleep occasionally. This is not disastrous.
The end is nigh...
Tomorrow will be horrible! How can I get that project done with no sleep?!
How can I be a good mom if I'm a wreck?!
I'll never get my workout in if I feel like garbage.
Catastrophic thinking is counterproductive. Truth is, we will function just fine, and usually we'll catch up on sleep soon, the next night or on one of the following nights. One or two or even several nights of inadequate sleep won't kill us.
It will be okay!
Cognitive restructuring is vital, as anxiety about insomnia can perpetuate the very thing we're trying to avoid.

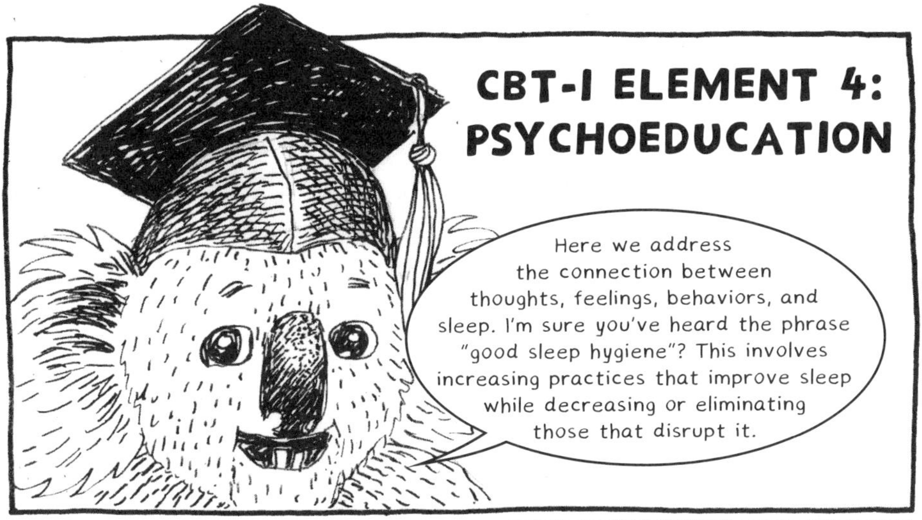
CBT-I ELEMENT 4: PSYCHOEDUCATION
Here we address the connection between thoughts, feelings, behaviors, and sleep. I'm sure you've heard the phrase "good sleep hygiene"? This involves increasing practices that improve sleep while decreasing or eliminating those that disrupt it.

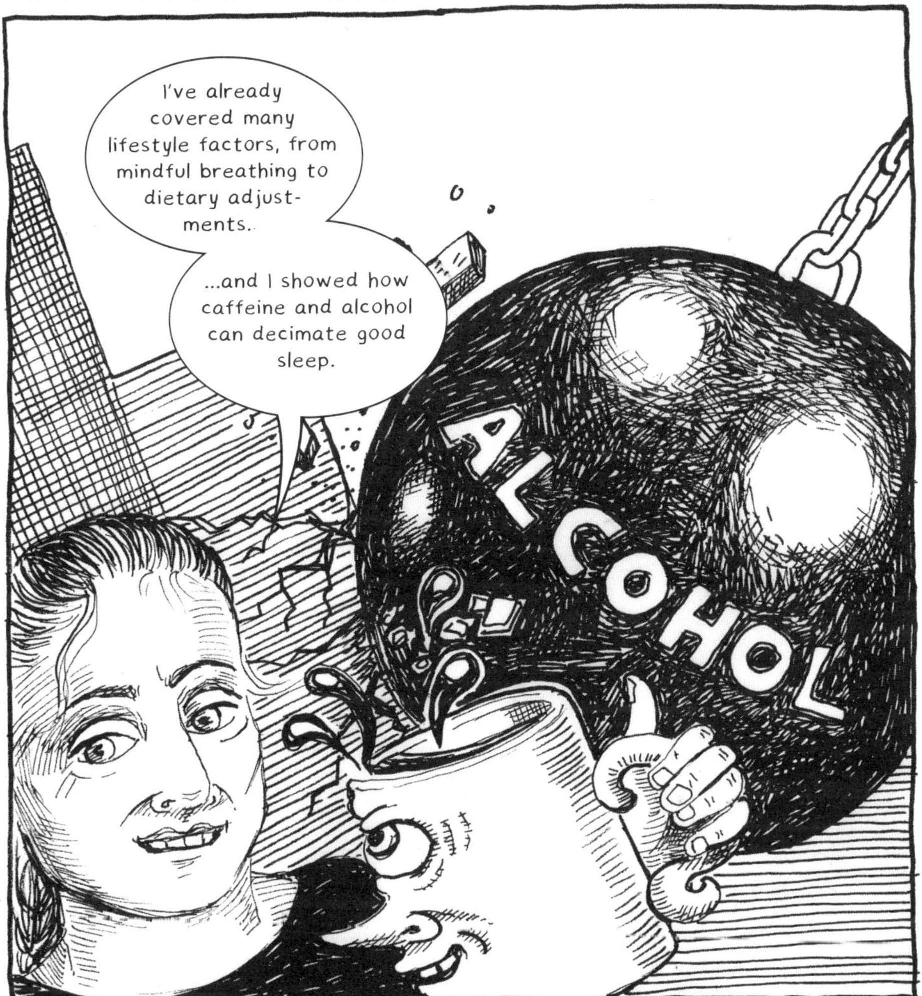
I've already covered many lifestyle factors, from mindful breathing to dietary adjust-ments.
...and I showed how caffeine and alcohol can decimate good sleep.
ALCOHOL

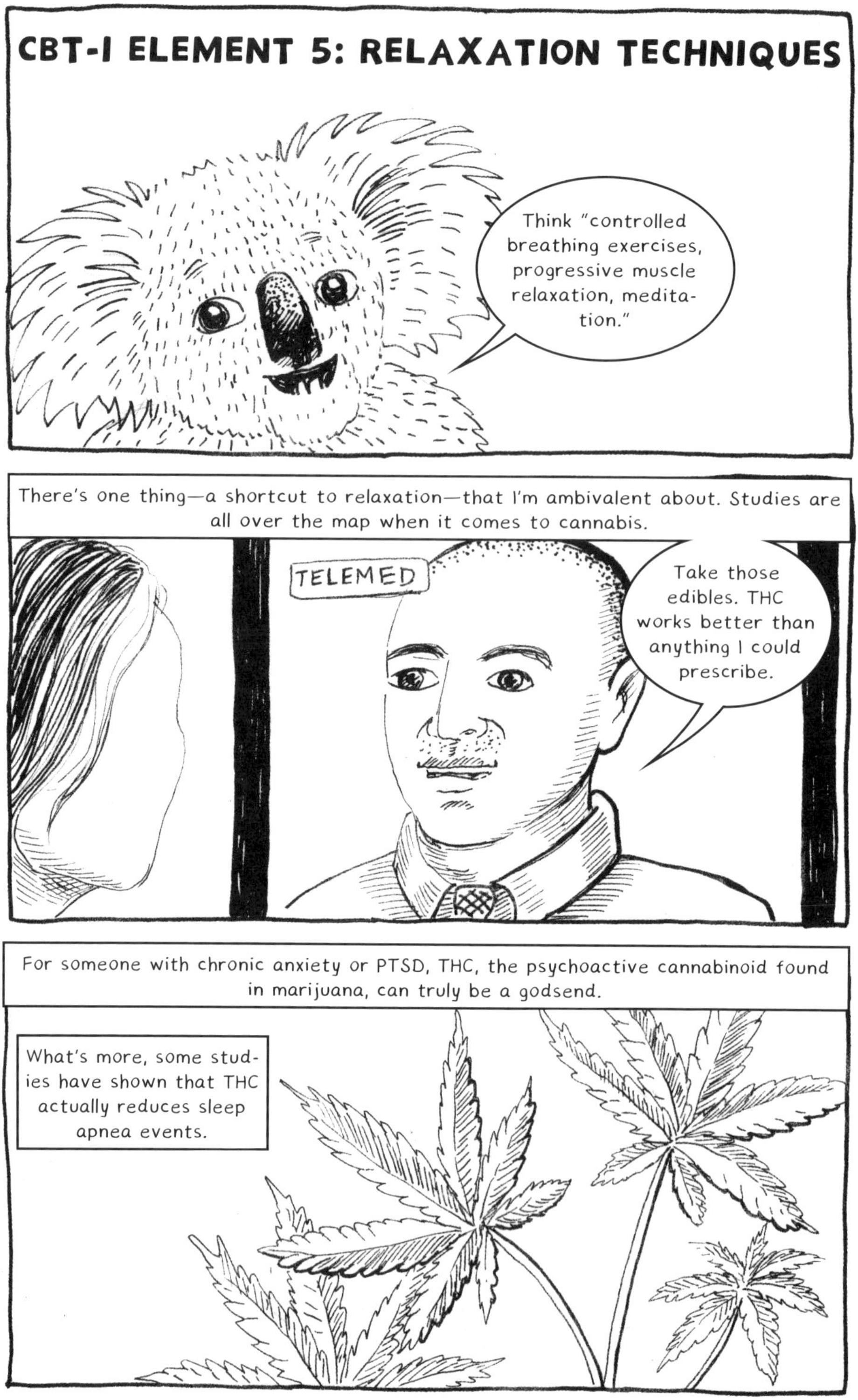
CBT-I ELEMENT 5: RELAXATION TECHNIQUES
Think "controlled breathing exercises, progressive muscle relaxation, medita-tion."
There's one thing—a shortcut to relaxation—that I'm ambivalent about. Studies are all over the map when it comes to cannabis.
TELEMED
Take those edibles. THC works better than anything I could prescribe.
For someone with chronic anxiety or PTSD, THC, the psychoactive cannabinoid found in marijuana, can truly be a godsend.
What's more, some stud-ies have shown that THC actually reduces sleep apnea events.

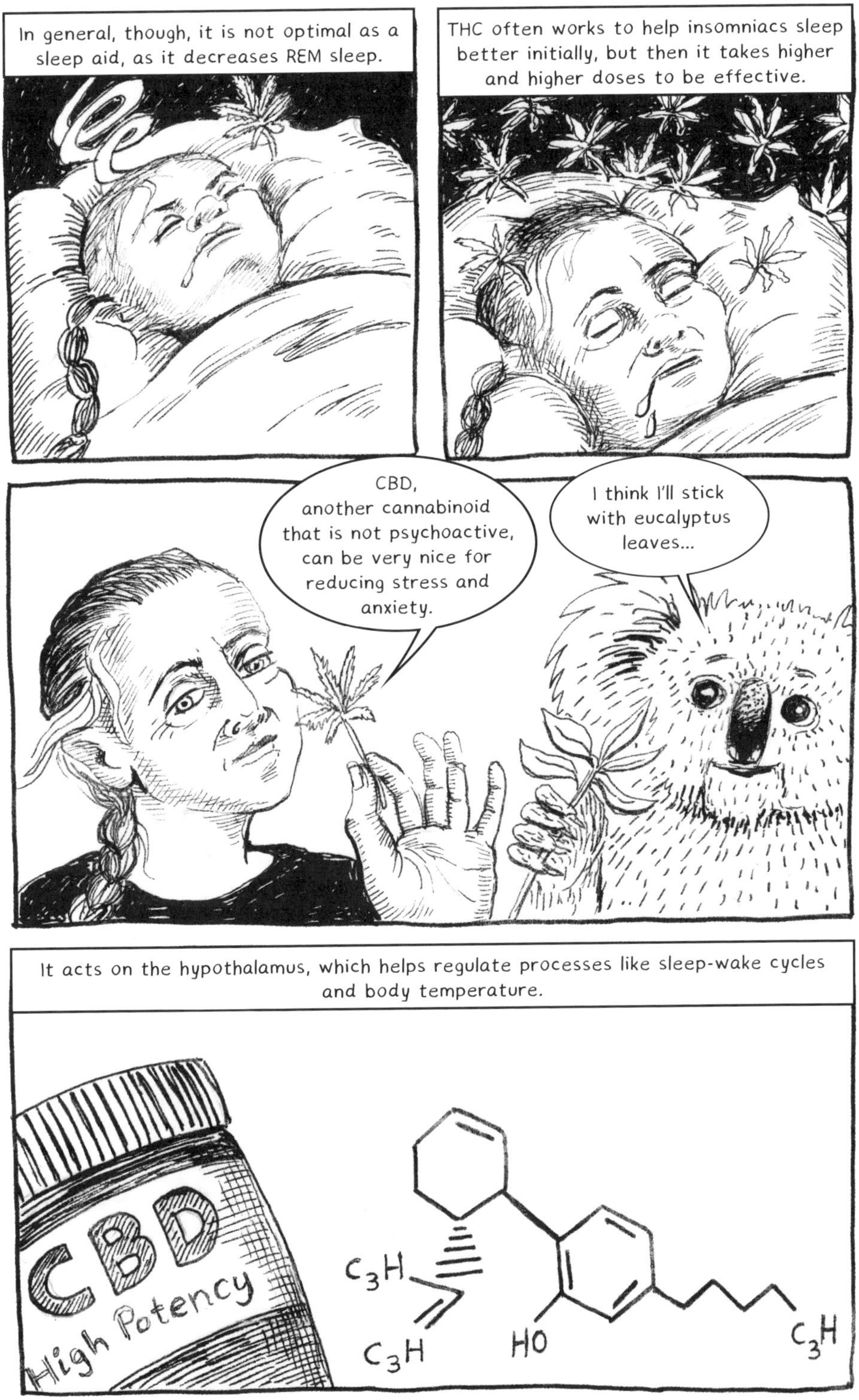
In general, though, it is not optimal as a sleep aid, as it decreases REM sleep.
THC often works to help insomniacs sleep better initially, but then it takes higher and higher doses to be effective.
CBD, another cannabinoid that is not psychoactive, can be very nice for reducing stress and anxiety.
I think I'll stick with eucalyptus leaves...
It acts on the hypothalamus, which helps regulate processes like sleep-wake cycles and body temperature.
CBD
High Potency
C3H
C3H
HO
C3H

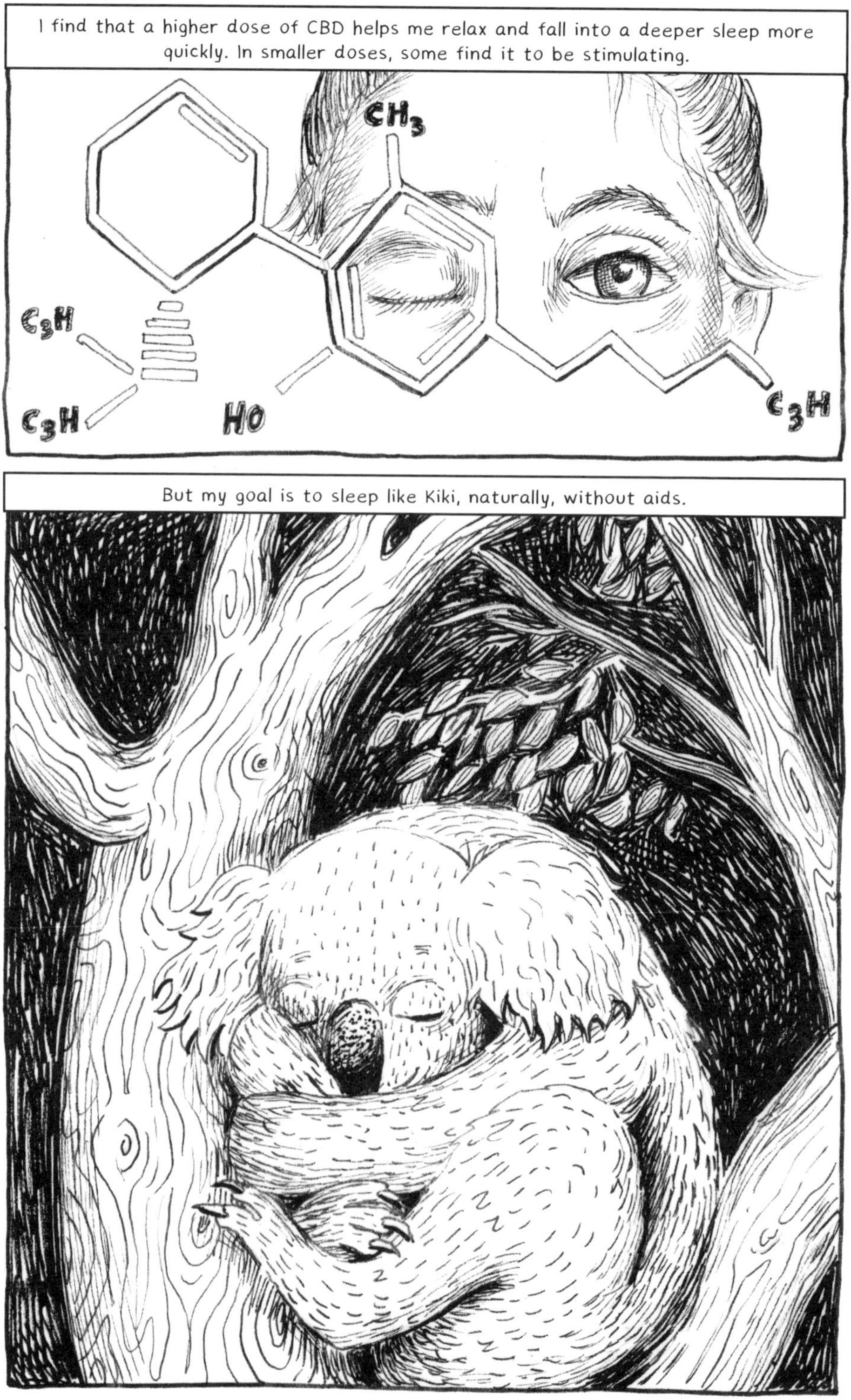

I find that a higher dose of CBD helps me relax and fall into a deeper sleep more quickly. In smaller doses, some find it to be stimulating.

But my goal is to sleep like Kiki, naturally, without aids.

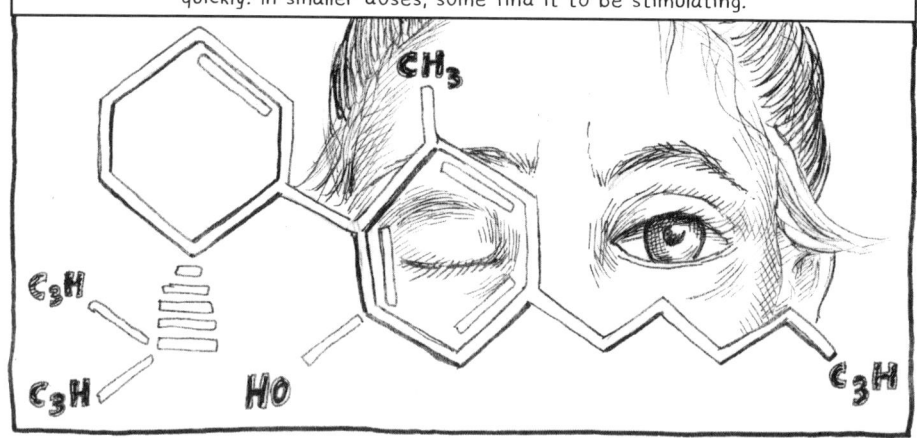

Typically, I now fall asleep very easily and enjoy seven to eight hours of sleep per night with good sleep efficiency. I almost never wake for more than a few minutes. I'm no longer roused by pesky vasomotor symptoms. I wake up organically, feeling rested and ready for the day.

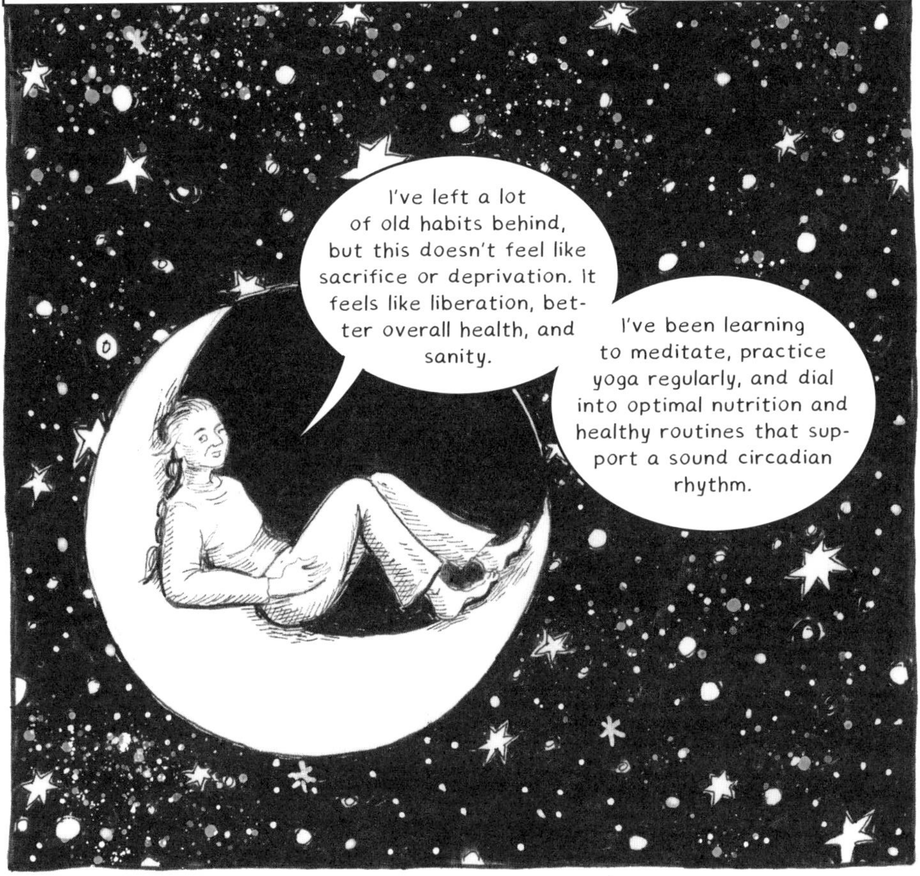
I've left a lot of old habits behind, but this doesn't feel like sacrifice or deprivation. It feels like liberation, better overall health, and sanity.
I've been learning to meditate, practice yoga regularly, and dial into optimal nutrition and healthy routines that support a sound circadian rhythm.

Despite these gains, Dr. Radiant's words still resonate with me, that due to a life deeply affected by childhood and young adulthood trauma, I may find that I need a crutch now and again.

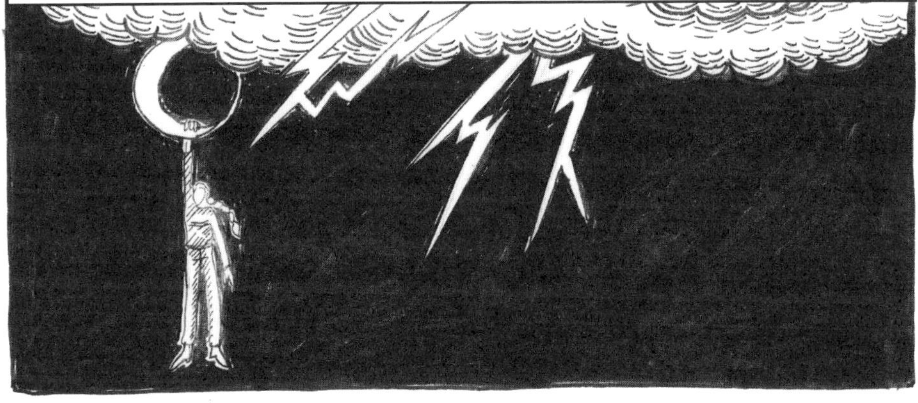

We live in an anxious world. Postindustrial cultures push us to reach for stimulants that cause us to ignore or circumvent difficult thoughts and feelings. Instead of grounding ourselves, we attempt to deal with anxiety by going higher or moving faster. Remember learning to "stop, drop, and roll" during those fire drills in grade school? Stop, drop (or ground), and breathe is a good mantra anytime past traumas or current anxieties catch up with us.

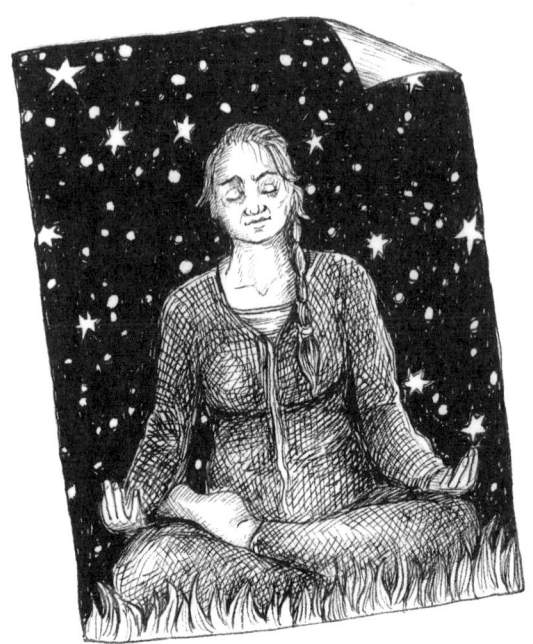

Is it possible to deepen my meditation, yoga, and breathwork practices so that I never need to reach for CBD capsules or THC again? I'm hopeful.

PART FOUR: WATER

THE RIVER TEACHER

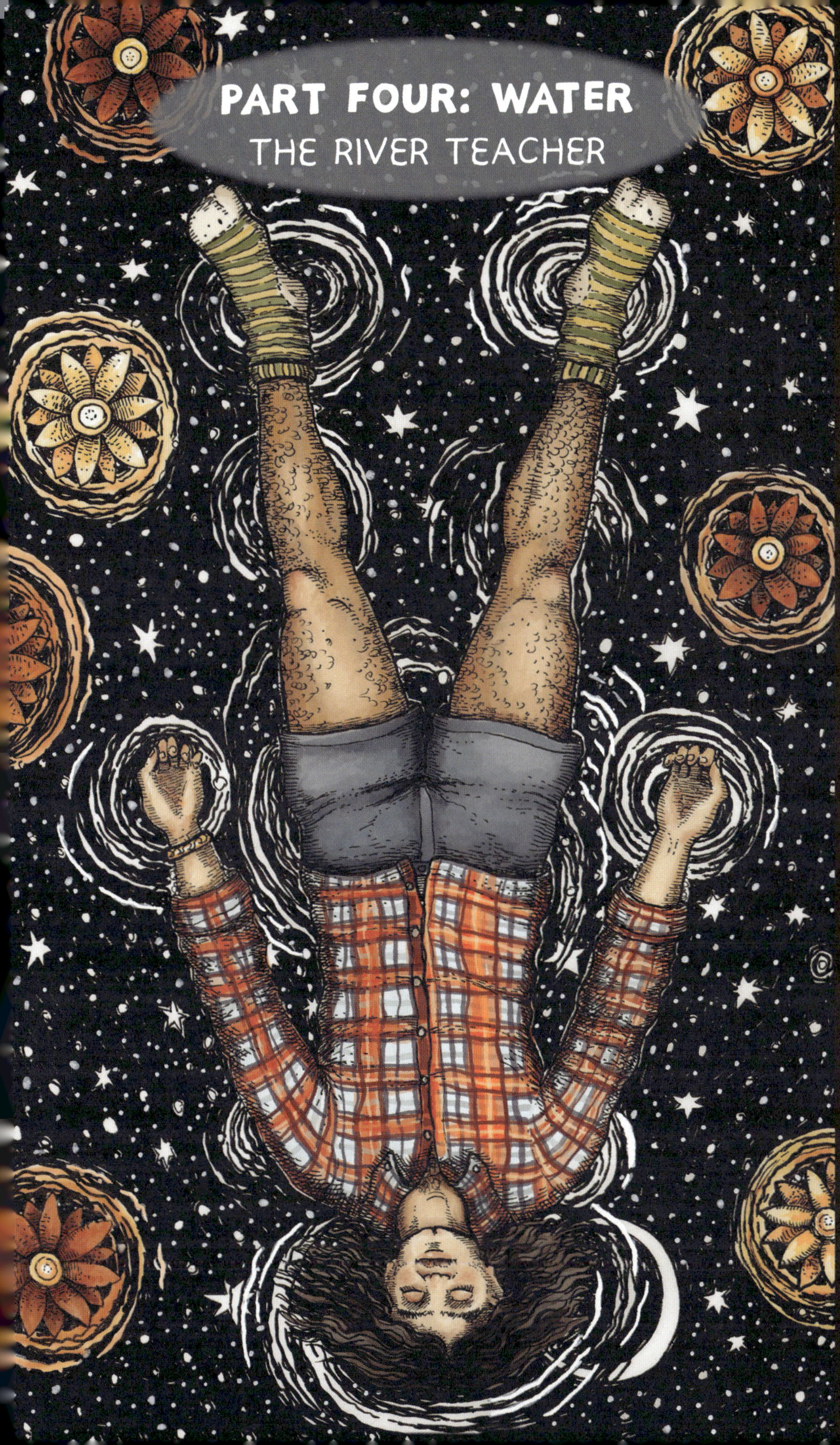

"Be like water making its way through cracks. Do not be assertive, but adjust to the object, and you shall find a way around or through it. If nothing within you stays rigid, outward things will disclose themselves.

Empty your mind, be formless. Shapeless, like water. If you put water into a cup, it becomes the cup. You put water into a bottle and it becomes the bottle. You put it in a teapot, it becomes the teapot. Now, water can flow or it can crash. Be water, my friend."

—Bruce Lee

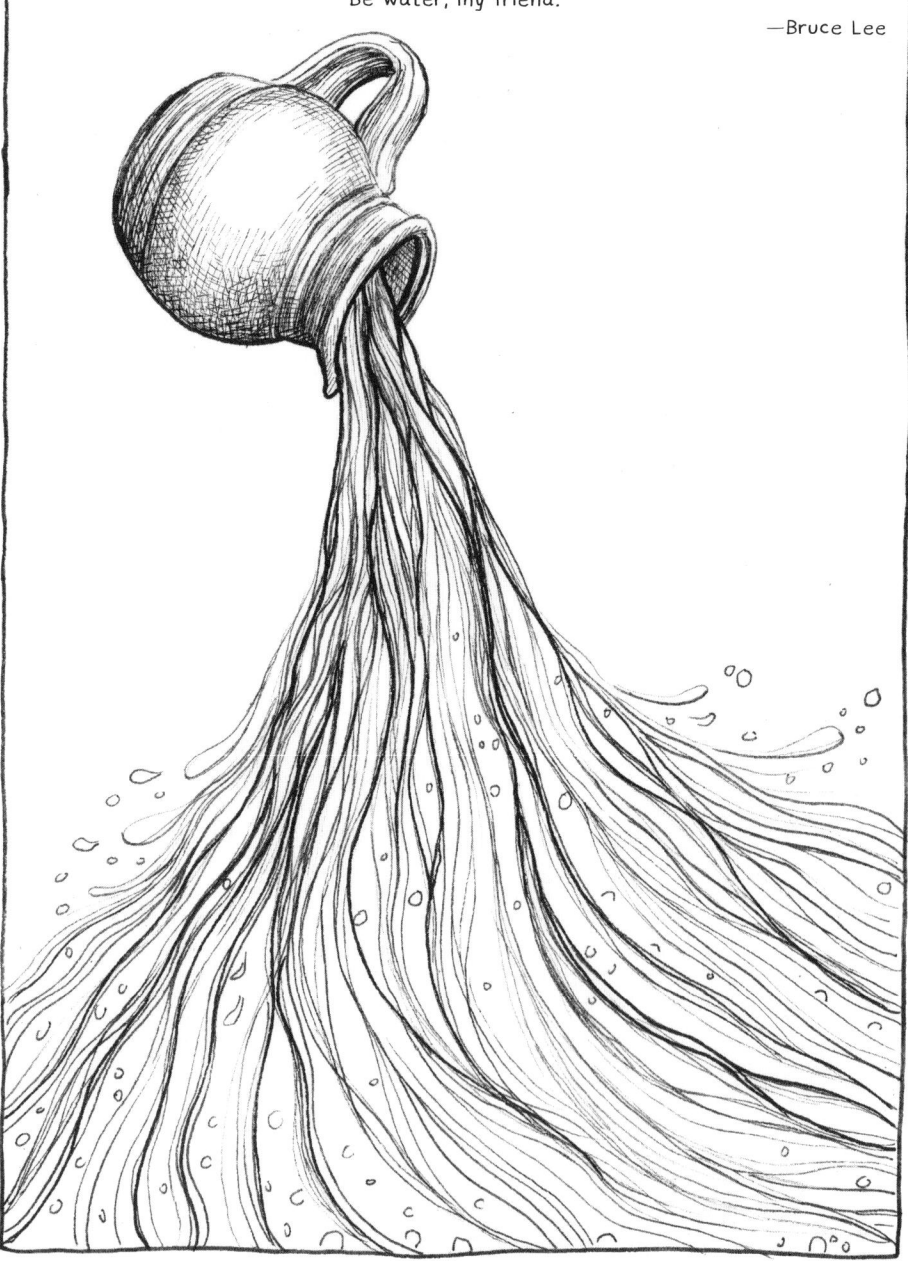

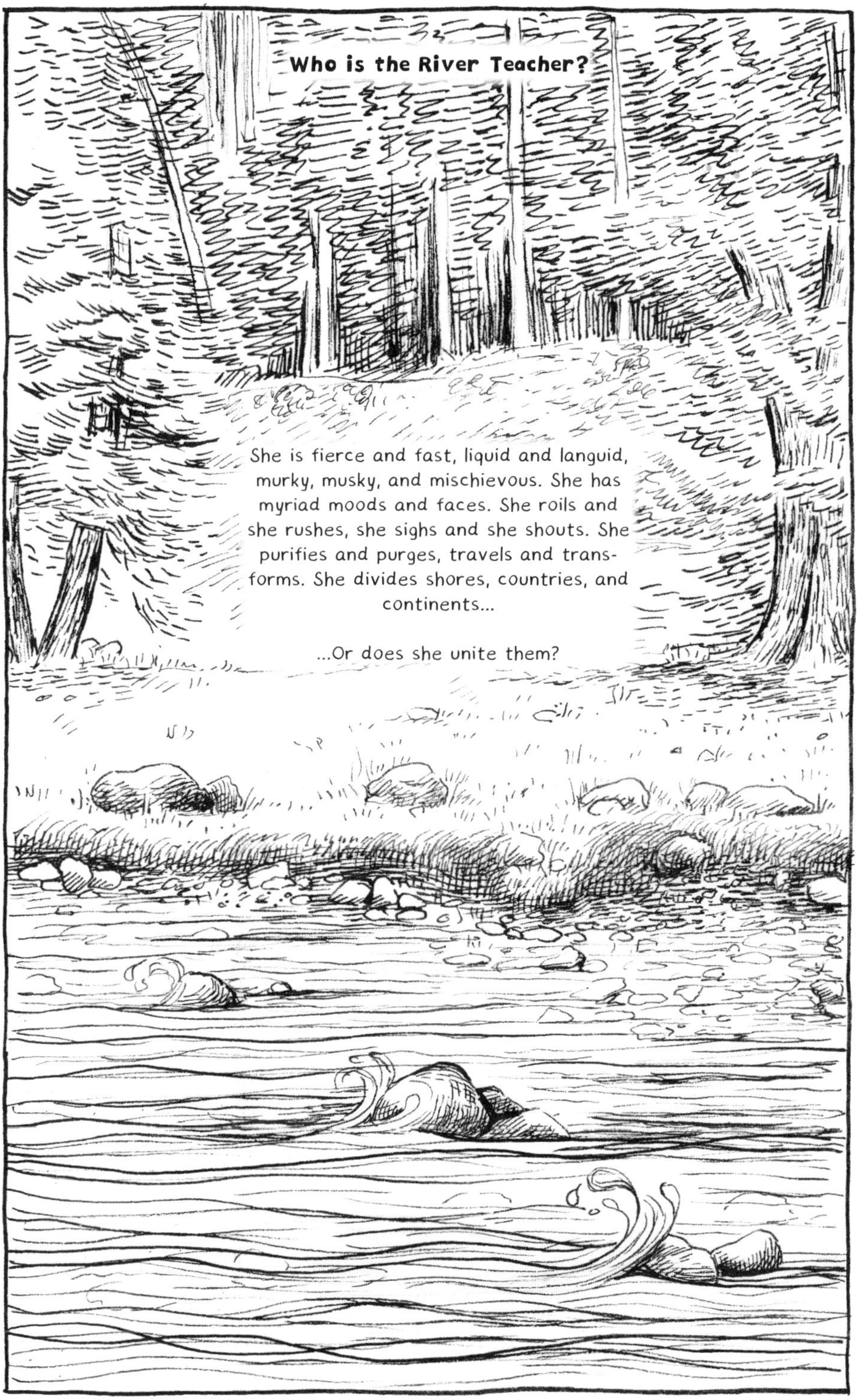
Who is the River Teacher?
She is fierce and fast, liquid and languid, murky, musky, and mischievous. She has myriad moods and faces. She roils and she rushes, she sighs and she shouts. She purifies and purges, travels and transforms. She divides shores, countries, and continents...
...Or does she unite them?

I am wading in the river of time. I am now. History rushes all around me and passes through me, shaping me. Together, River and I are the future of those who stand downstream.
River is a way of seeing and of being. Knowing she was there long before I was born and that she will be there long after I once again turn into earth and rain is a comfort. There is relief in knowing death as transition rather than as finite ending, and in knowing sleep as benevolent practice for that transition.
Sleep is River mirroring night. Sleep teaches us about letting go, as one must, in order to drift into dreaming.

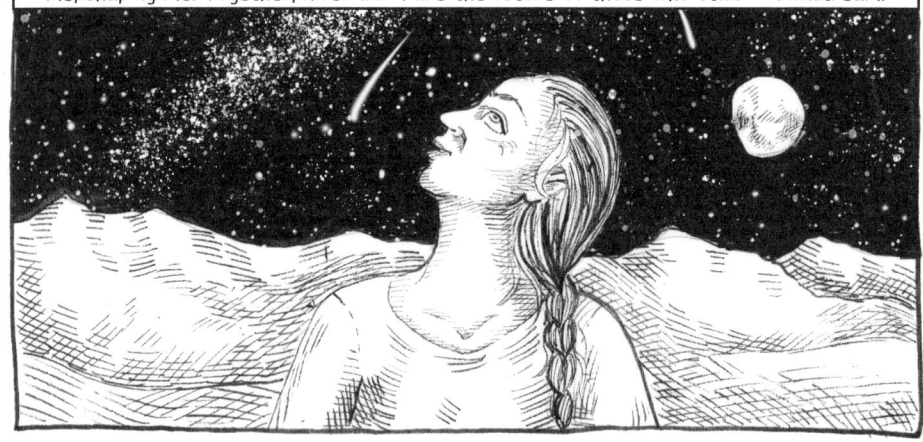

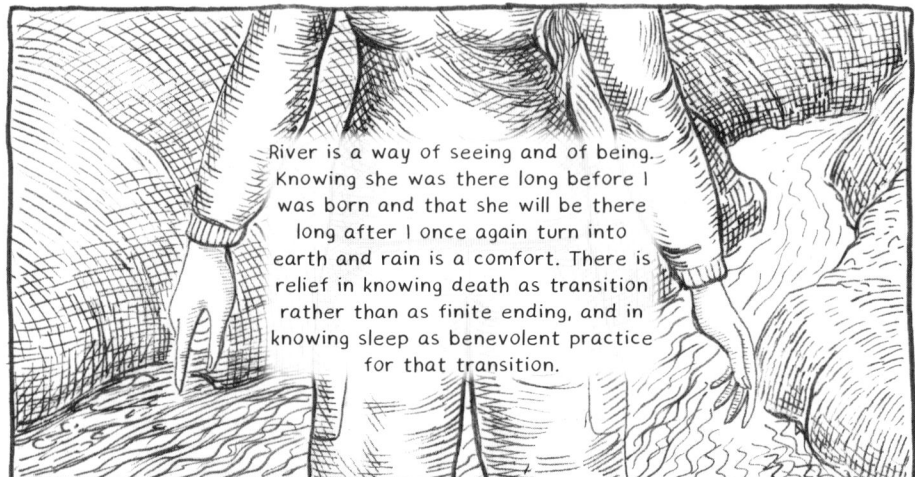

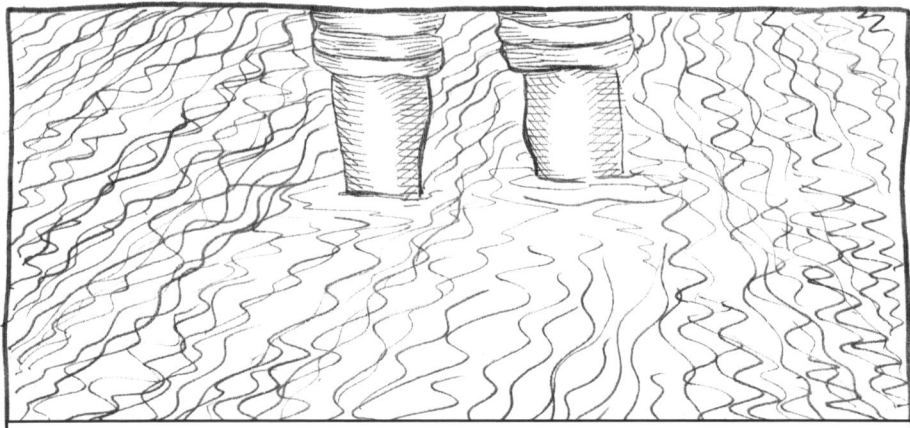

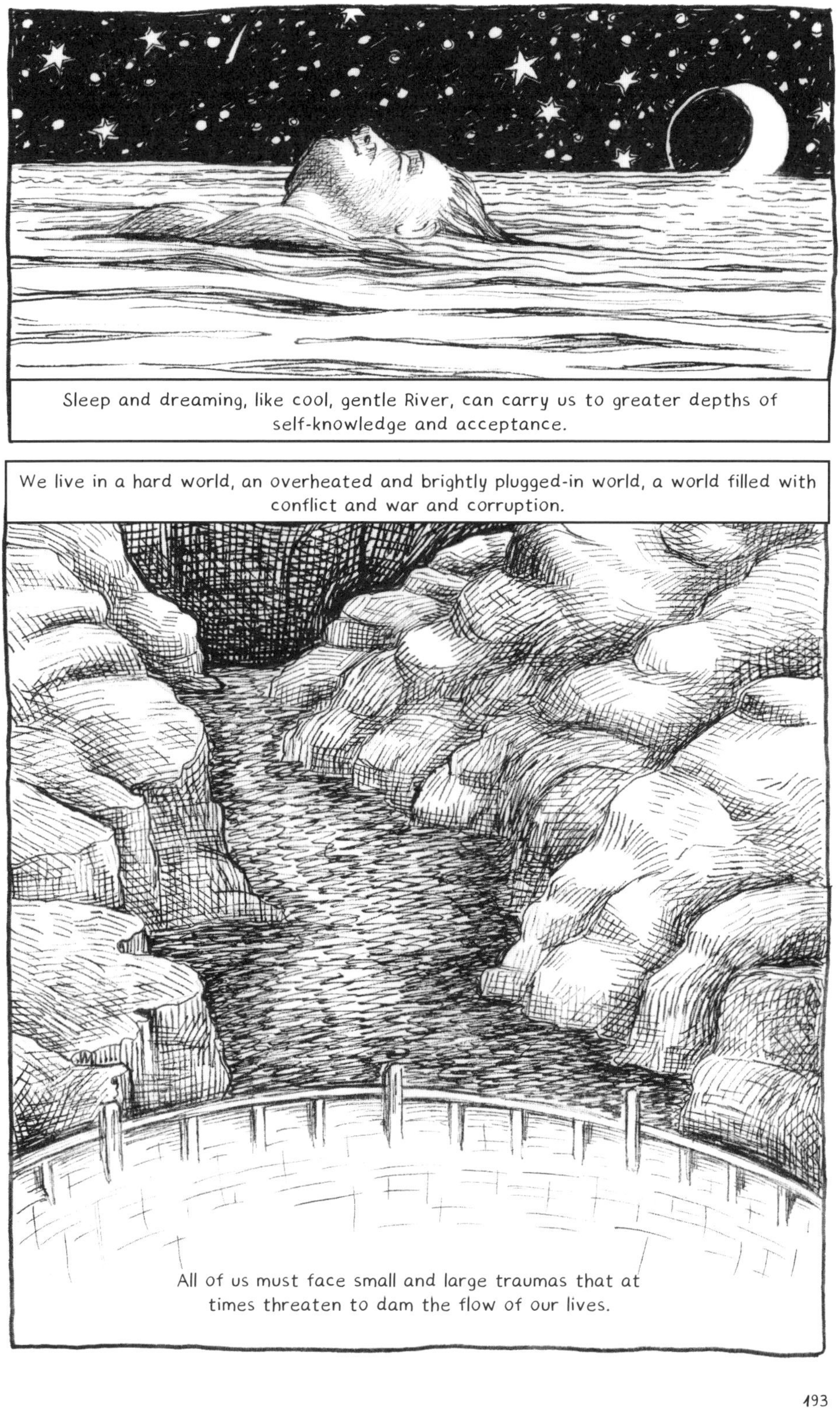
Sleep and dreaming, like cool, gentle River, can carry us to greater depths of self-knowledge and acceptance.
We live in a hard world, an overheated and brightly plugged-in world, a world filled with conflict and war and corruption.
All of us must face small and large traumas that at times threaten to dam the flow of our lives.

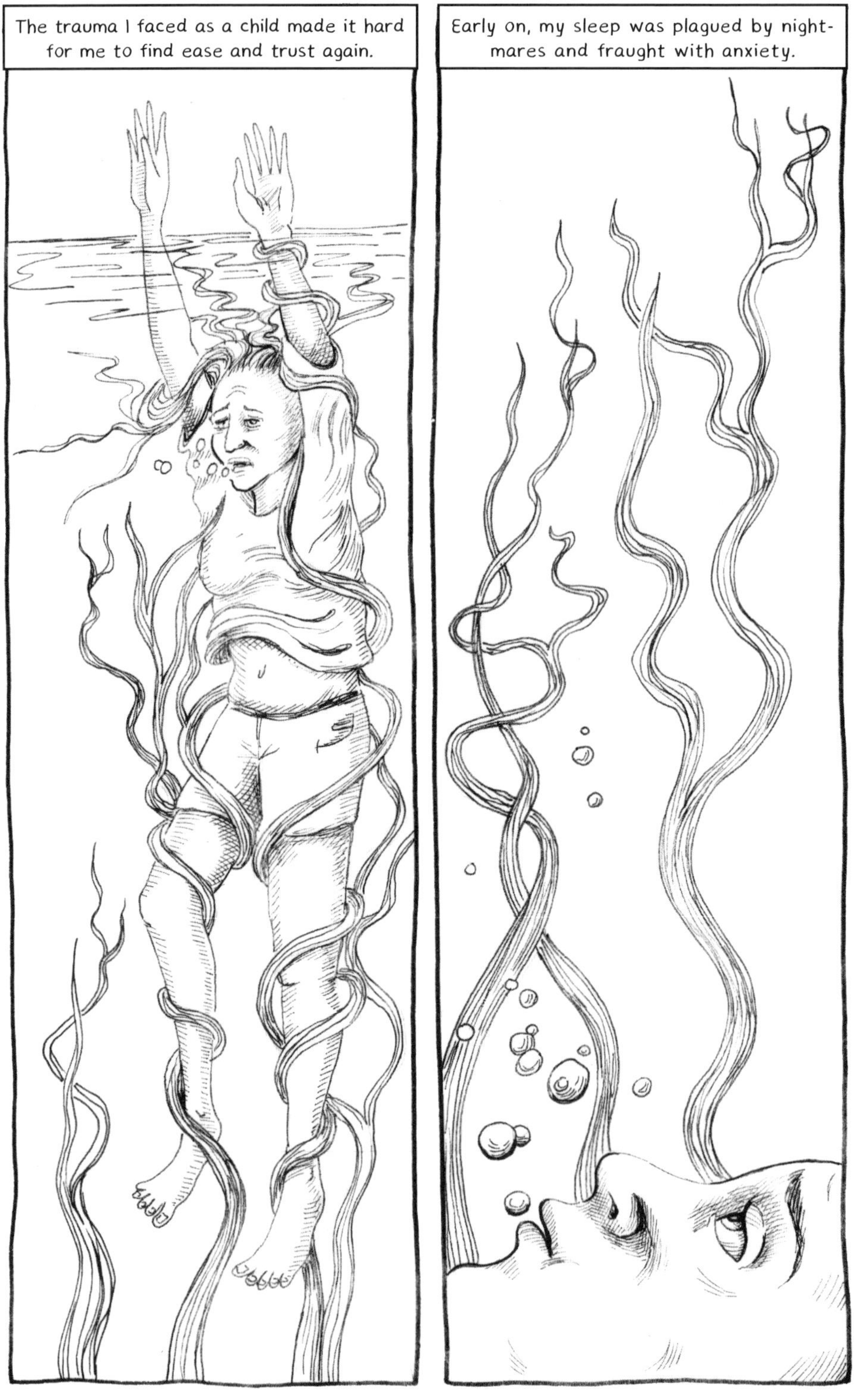
The trauma I faced as a child made it hard for me to find ease and trust again.
Early on, my sleep was plagued by nightmares and fraught with anxiety.

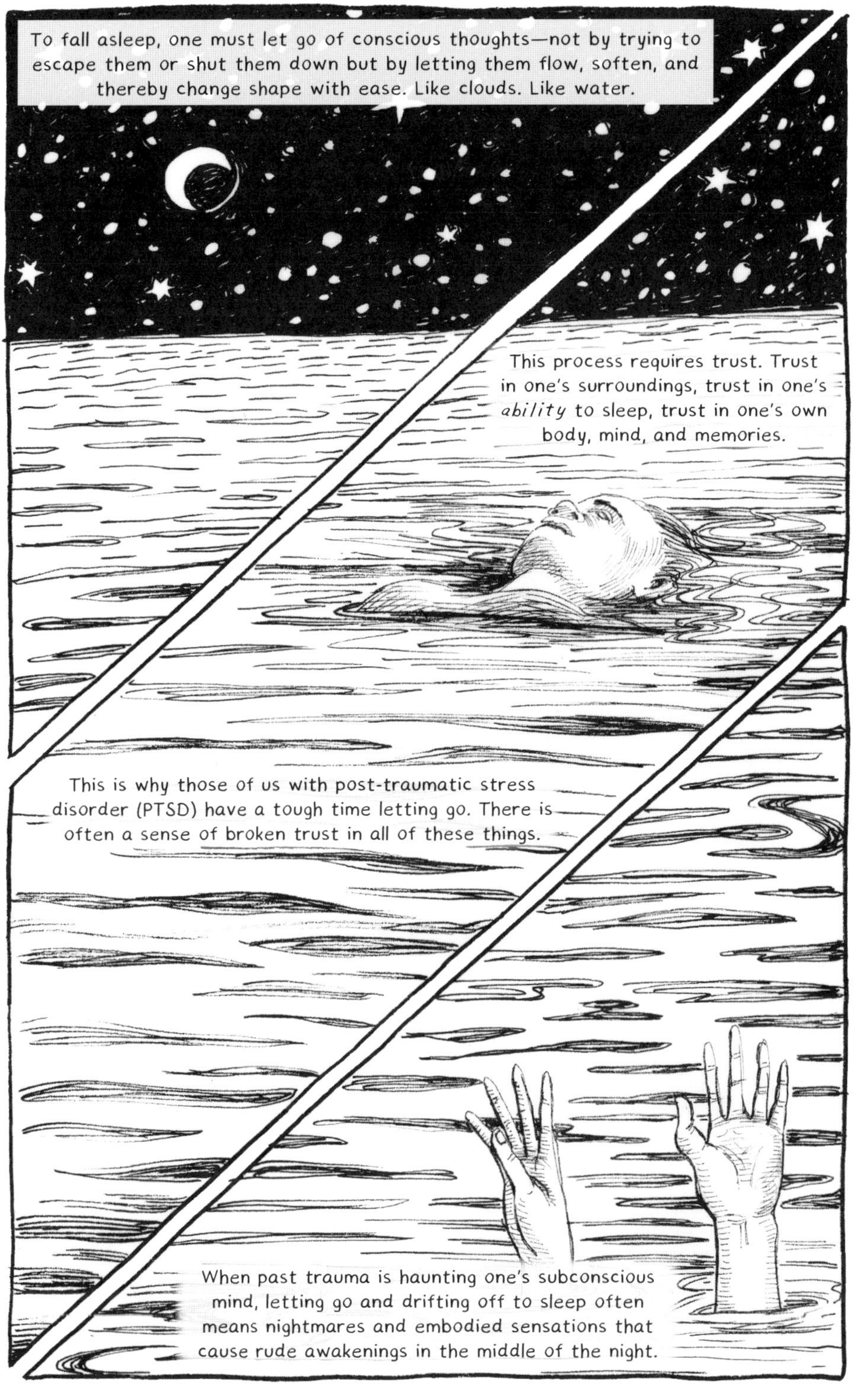

To fall asleep, one must let go of conscious thoughts—not by trying to escape them or shut them down but by letting them flow, soften, and thereby change shape with ease. Like clouds. Like water.
This process requires trust. Trust in one's surroundings, trust in one's *ability* to sleep, trust in one's own body, mind, and memories.
This is why those of us with post-traumatic stress disorder (PTSD) have a tough time letting go. There is often a sense of broken trust in all of these things.
When past trauma is haunting one's subconscious mind, letting go and drifting off to sleep often means nightmares and embodied sensations that cause rude awakenings in the middle of the night.

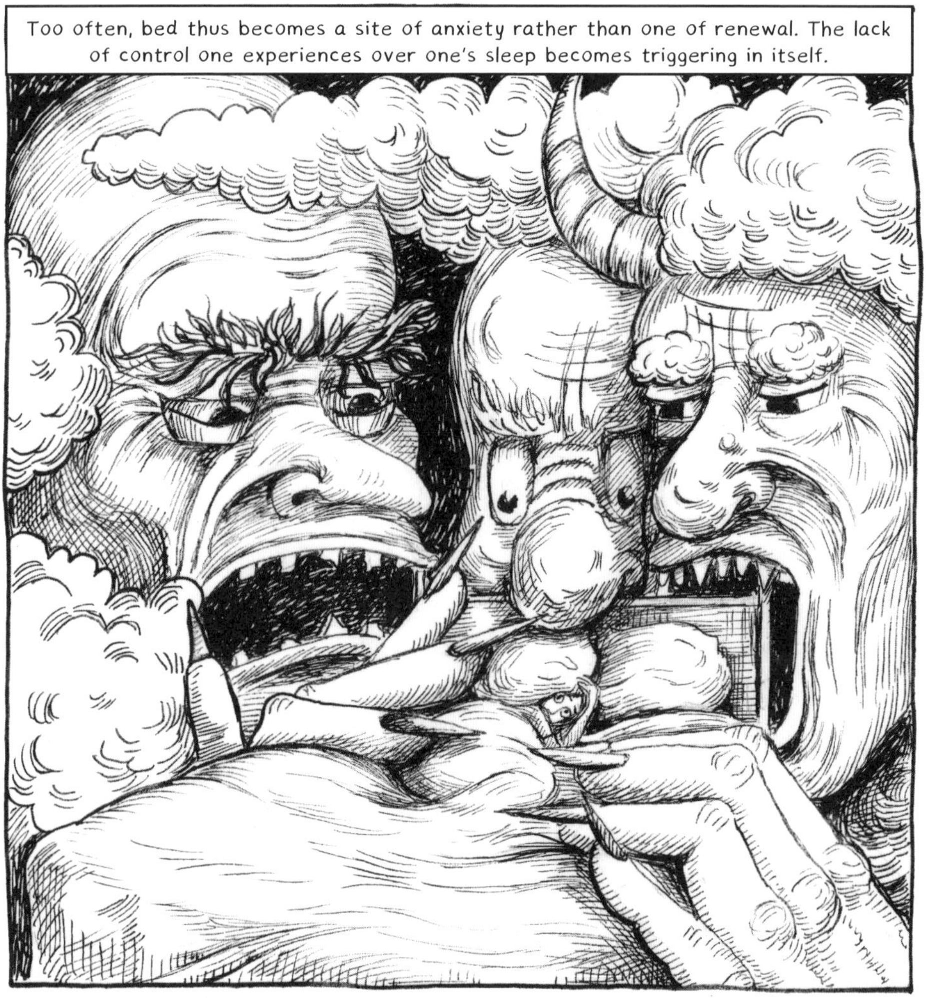
Too often, bed thus becomes a site of anxiety rather than one of renewal. The lack of control one experiences over one's sleep becomes triggering in itself.

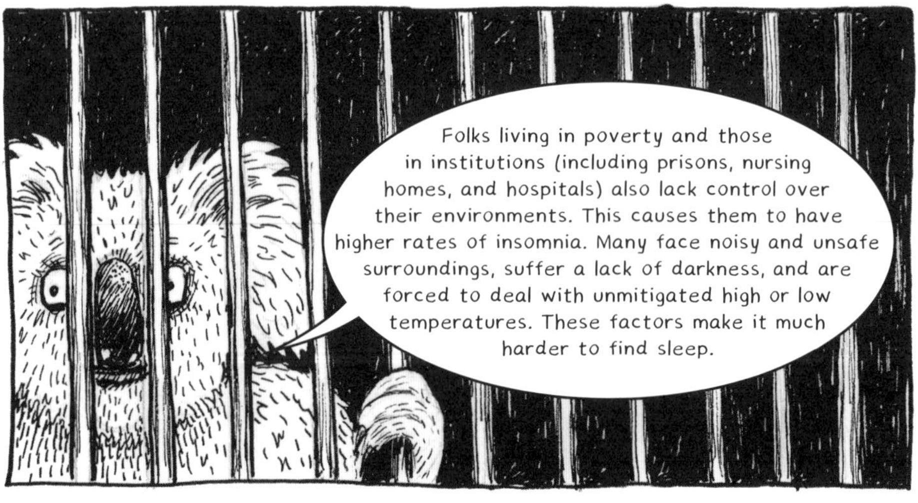
Folks living in poverty and those in institutions (including prisons, nursing homes, and hospitals) also lack control over their environments. This causes them to have higher rates of insomnia. Many face noisy and unsafe surroundings, suffer a lack of darkness, and are forced to deal with unmitigated high or low temperatures. These factors make it much harder to find sleep.

Many insomniacs reach for substances that lessen difficult thoughts and feelings and allow us to make the otherwise seemingly impossible transition to sleep. Things like alcohol, THC, and sleeping pills help us forget the sadness, fear, and anxiety that keep us awake.

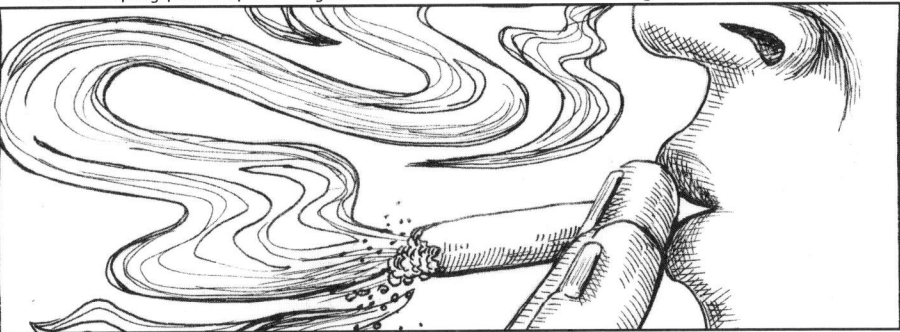

People who suffer from sleep conditions are 5-10 times more likely to also be diagnosed with a substance use disorder than those without insomnia.

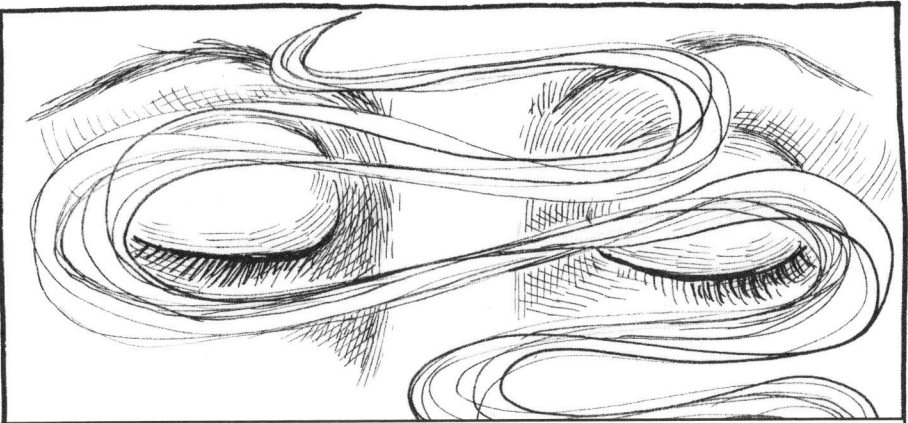

But these substances merely make us unconscious. They wreck our delicate and vital sleep architecture. They rob us of our dreams, both figuratively and, over time, quite literally.

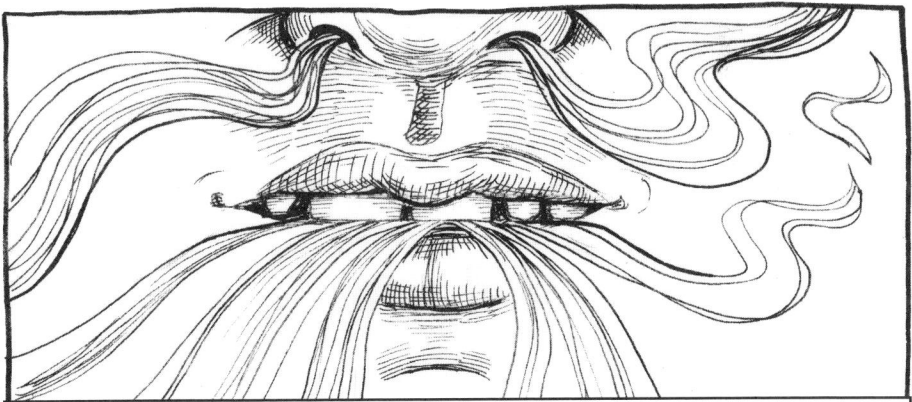

Such shortcuts don't really get us to dreamland. Instead, they leave us adrift in a state of amnesia and rob us of the reparative and revitalizing properties of true sleep and dreaming.

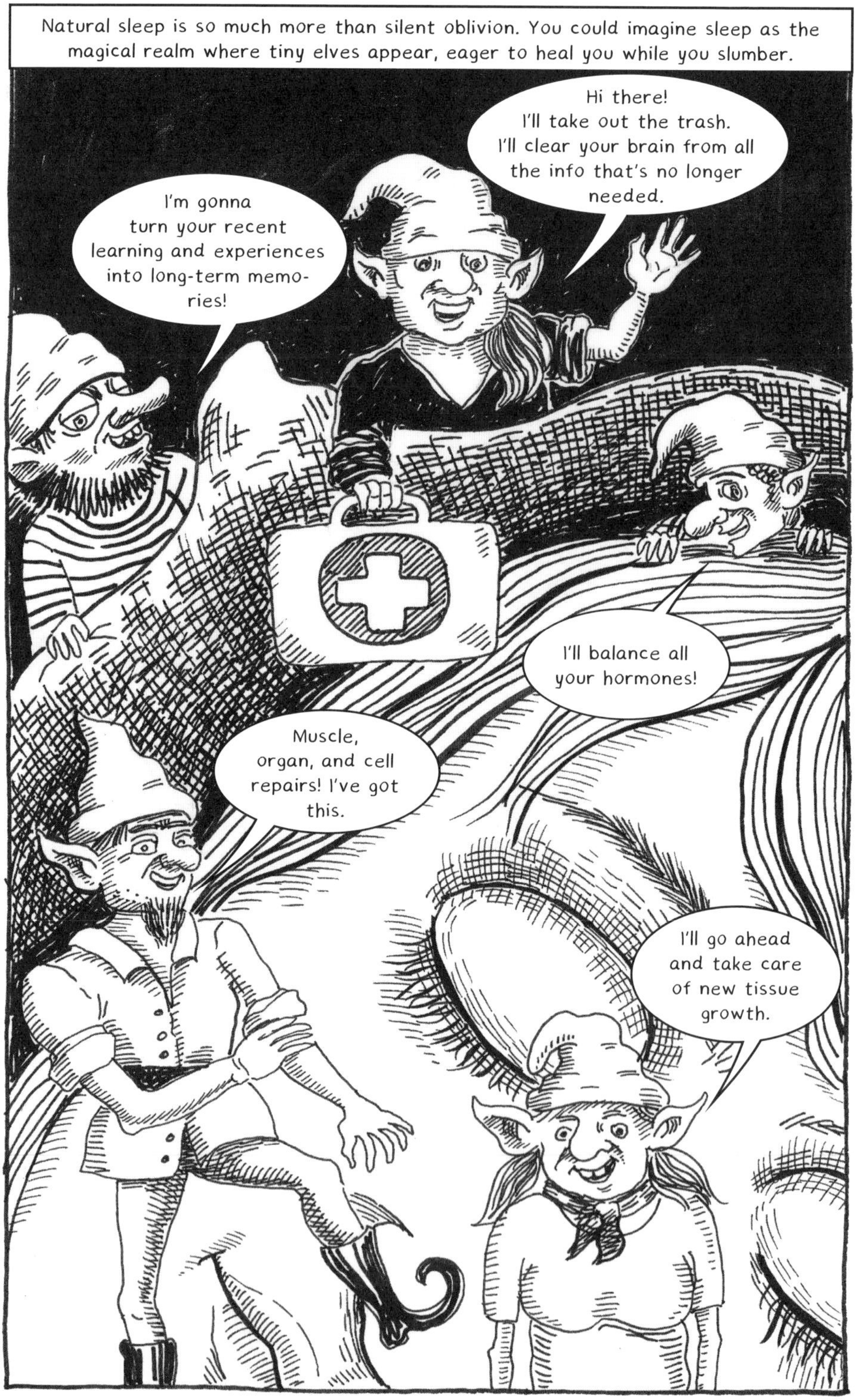
Natural sleep is so much more than silent oblivion. You could imagine sleep as the magical realm where tiny elves appear, eager to heal you while you slumber.
Hi there! I'll take out the trash. I'll clear your brain from all the info that's no longer needed.
I'm gonna turn your recent learning and experiences into long-term memo-ries!
I'll balance all your hormones!
Muscle, organ, and cell repairs! I've got this.
I'll go ahead and take care of new tissue growth.

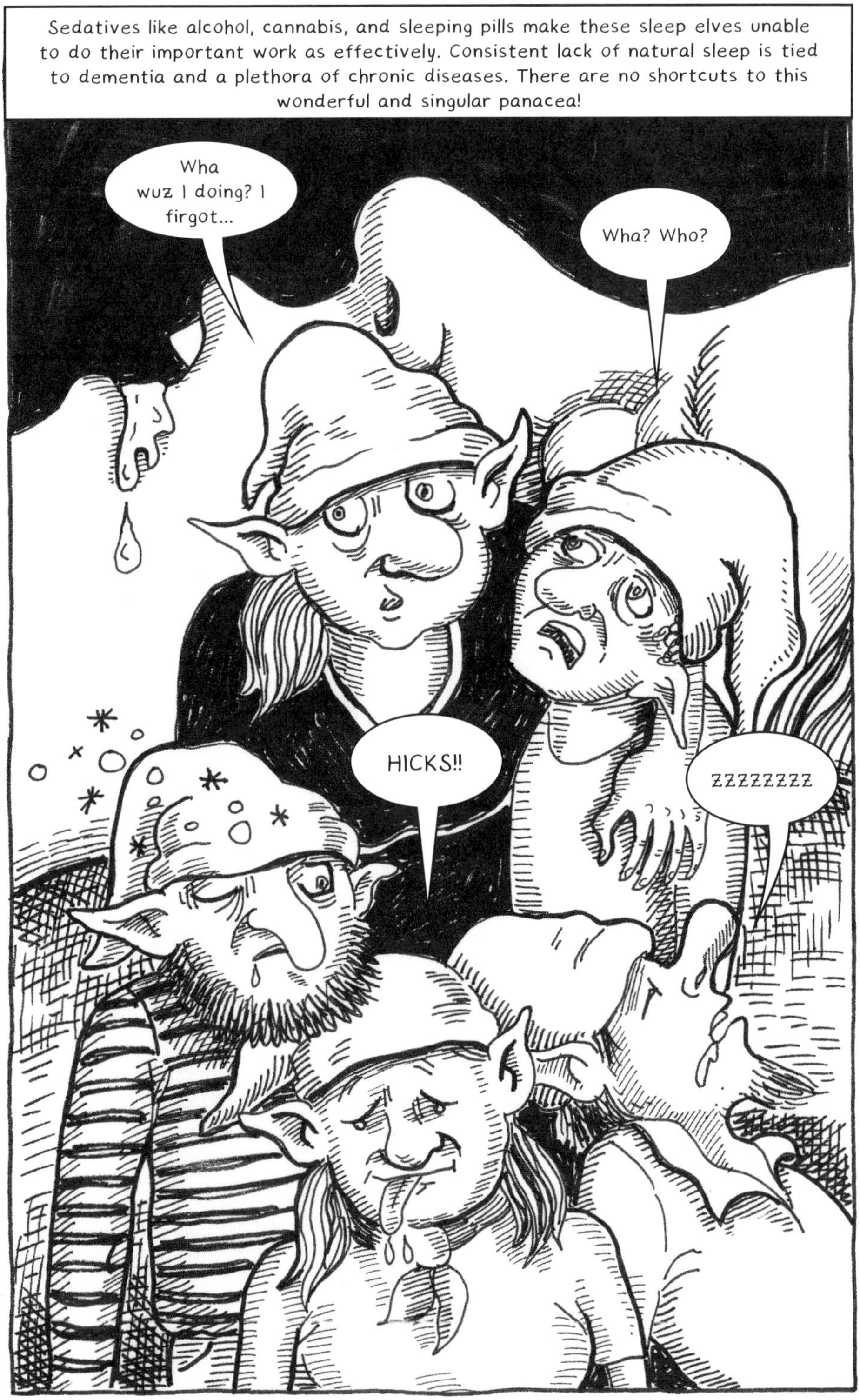
Sedatives like alcohol, cannabis, and sleeping pills make these sleep elves unable to do their important work as effectively. Consistent lack of natural sleep is tied to dementia and a plethora of chronic diseases. There are no shortcuts to this wonderful and singular panacea!
Wha wuz I doing? I firgot...
Wha? Who?
HICKS!!
ZZZZZZZZ

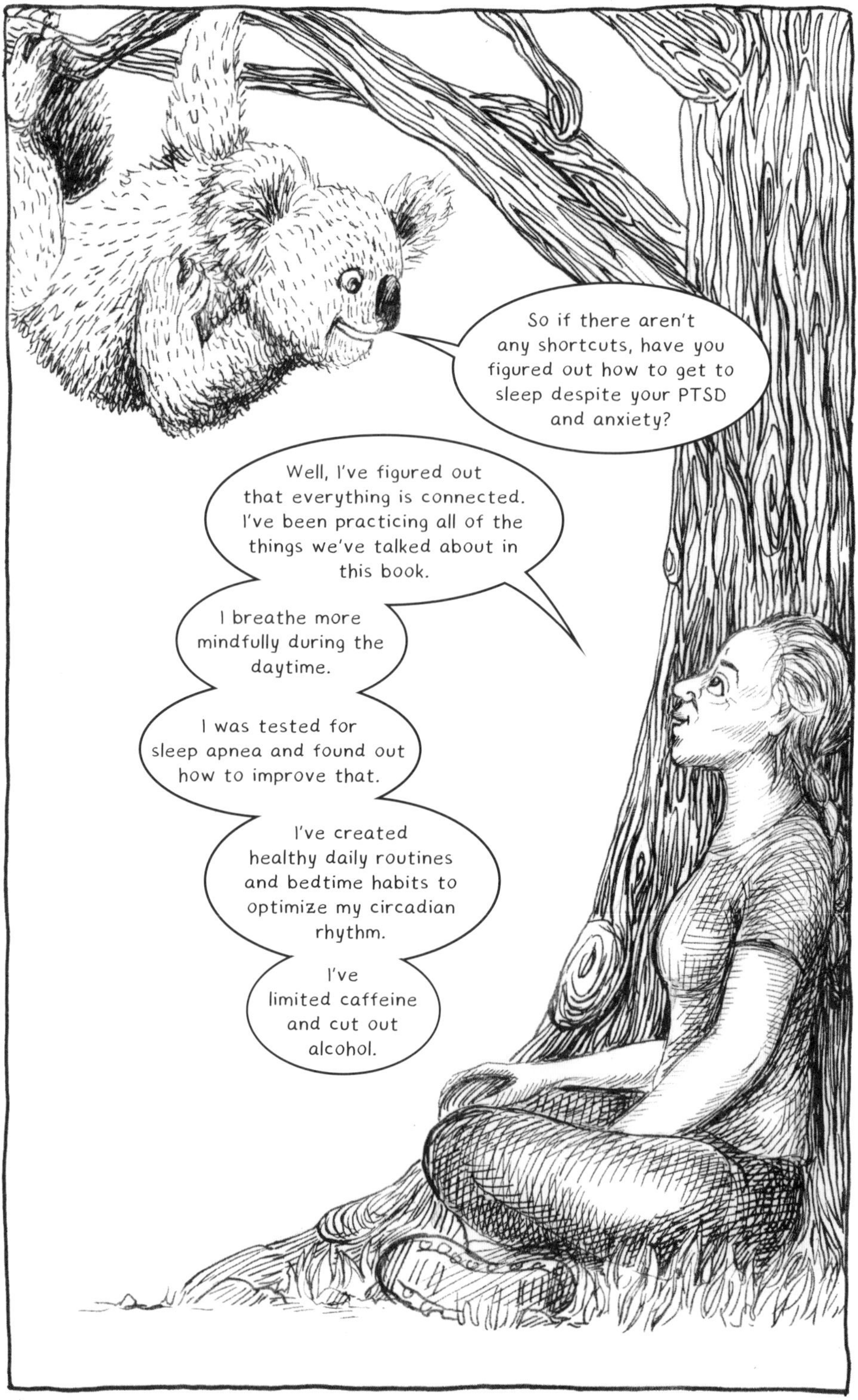
So if there aren't any shortcuts, have you figured out how to get to sleep despite your PTSD and anxiety?
Well, I've figured out that everything is connected. I've been practicing all of the things we've talked about in this book.
I breathe more mindfully during the daytime.
I was tested for sleep apnea and found out how to improve that.
I've created healthy daily routines and bedtime habits to optimize my circadian rhythm.
I've limited caffeine and cut out alcohol.

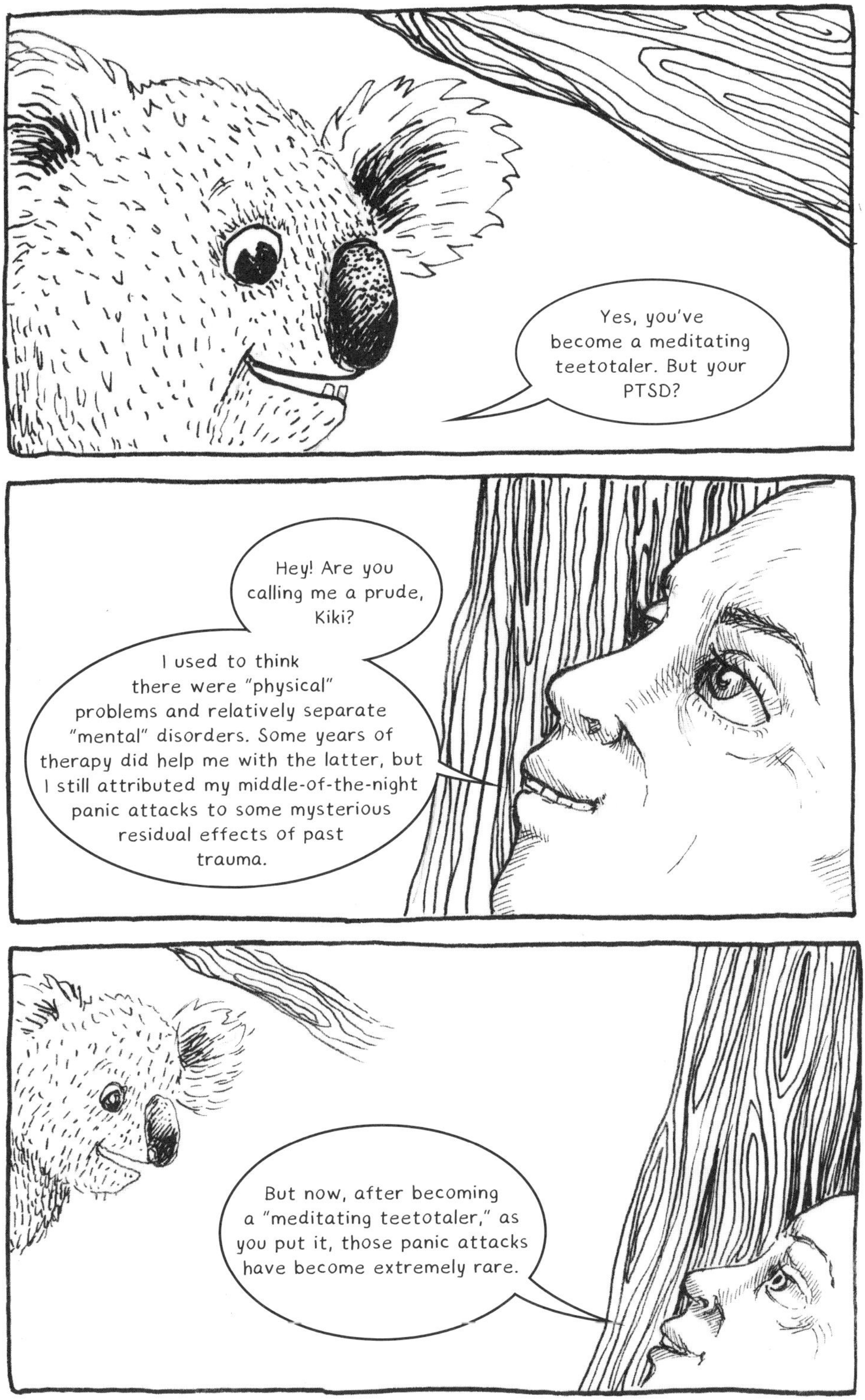
Yes, you've become a meditating teetotaler. But your PTSD?
Hey! Are you calling me a prude, Kiki?
I used to think there were "physical" problems and relatively separate "mental" disorders. Some years of therapy did help me with the latter, but I still attributed my middle-of-the-night panic attacks to some mysterious residual effects of past trauma.
But now, after becoming a "meditating teetotaler," as you put it, those panic attacks have become extremely rare.

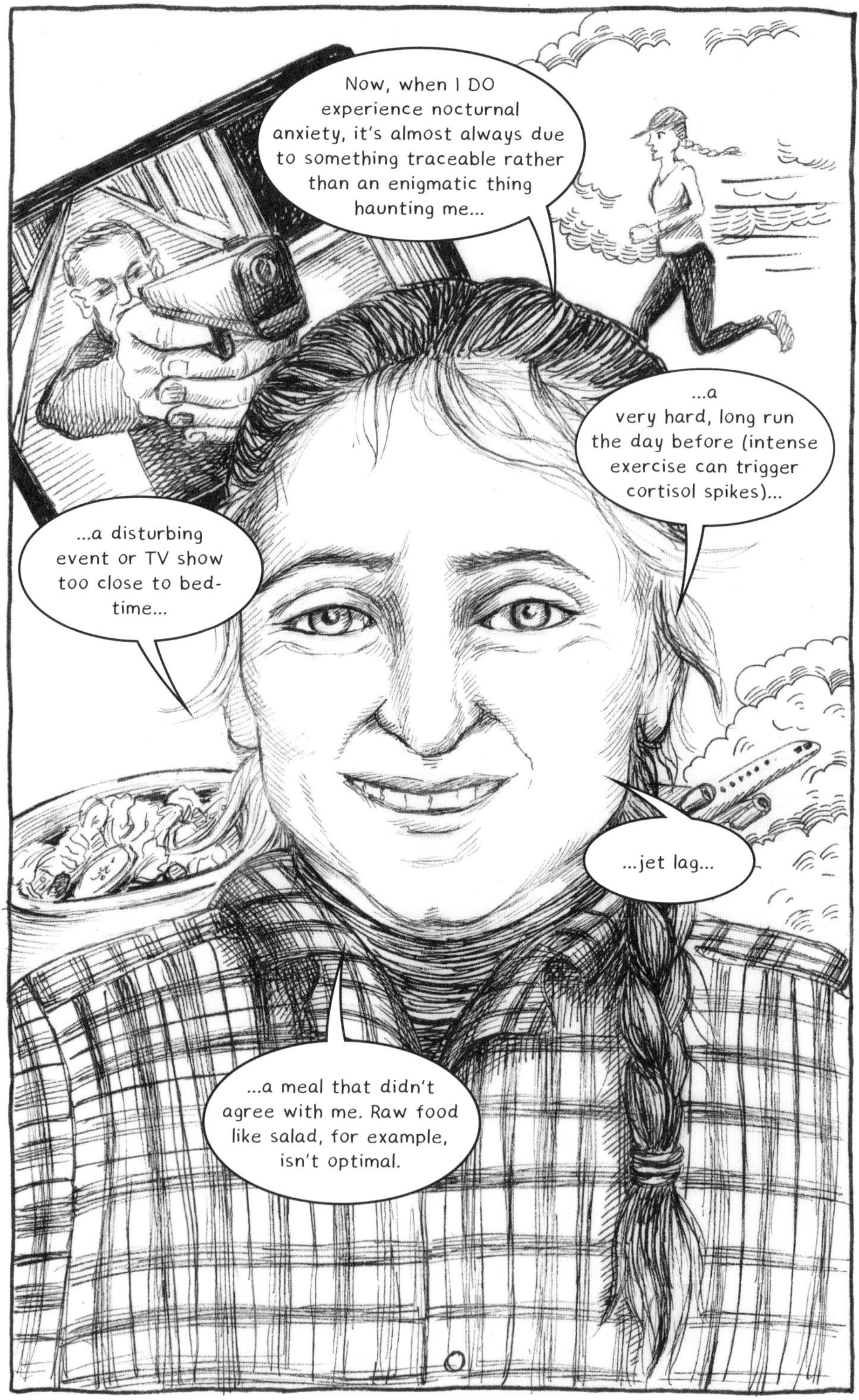
Now, when I DO experience nocturnal anxiety, it's almost always due to something traceable rather than an enigmatic thing haunting me...
...a disturbing event or TV show too close to bed-time...
...a very hard, long run the day before (intense exercise can trigger cortisol spikes)...
...jet lag...
...a meal that didn't agree with me. Raw food like salad, for example, isn't optimal.

Food has a major impact on anxiety and sleep. The connection between gut and brain is so unequivocal that the gut has been referred to as our "second brain." In fact, gut health affects brain health (and vice versa) so powerfully that it doesn't make sense to look at one without also examining the other.

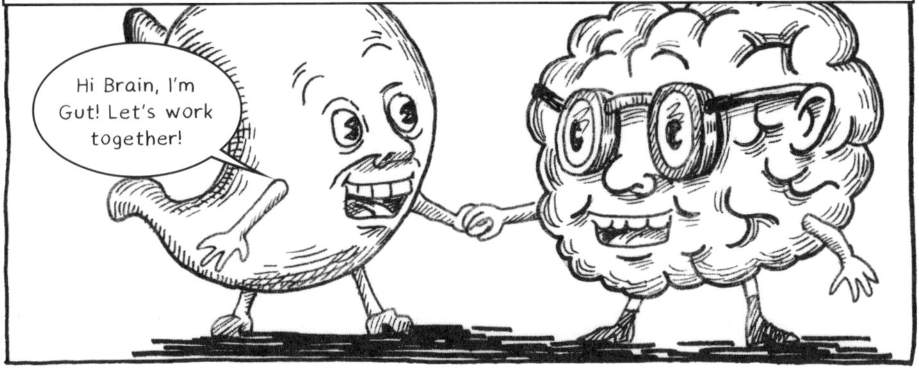
Hi Brain, I'm Gut! Let's work together!

Often, we seem to forget that our brains are part of our bodies.

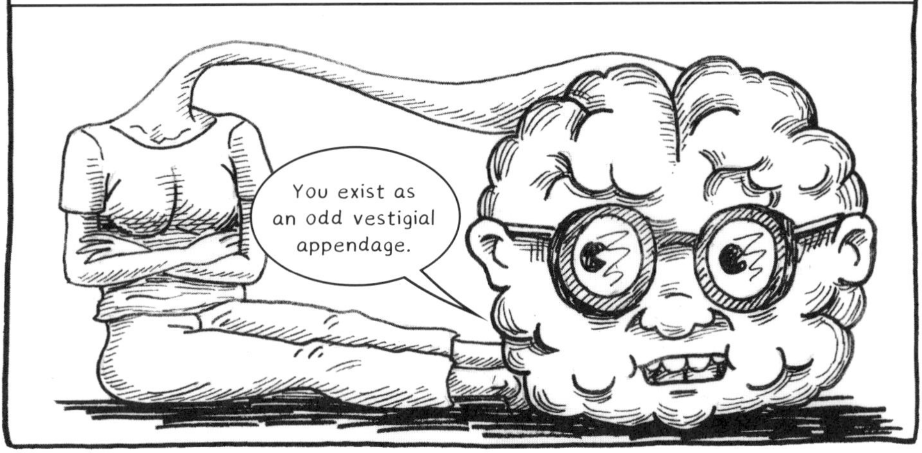
You exist as an odd vestigial appendage.

By eating real food and avoiding corporate rations (products and restaurant foods containing those industrial "vegetable" oils I talked about earlier), we support our gut and our brain health. Those oils negatively alter your cells' metabolic capacity and cause a systemic stress response, like the cortisol awakening response (CAR), too early in the morning.

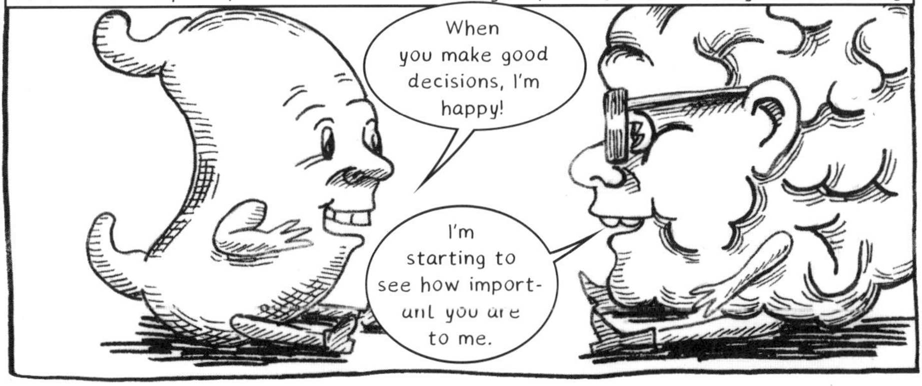
When you make good decisions, I'm happy!
I'm starting to see how important you are to me.

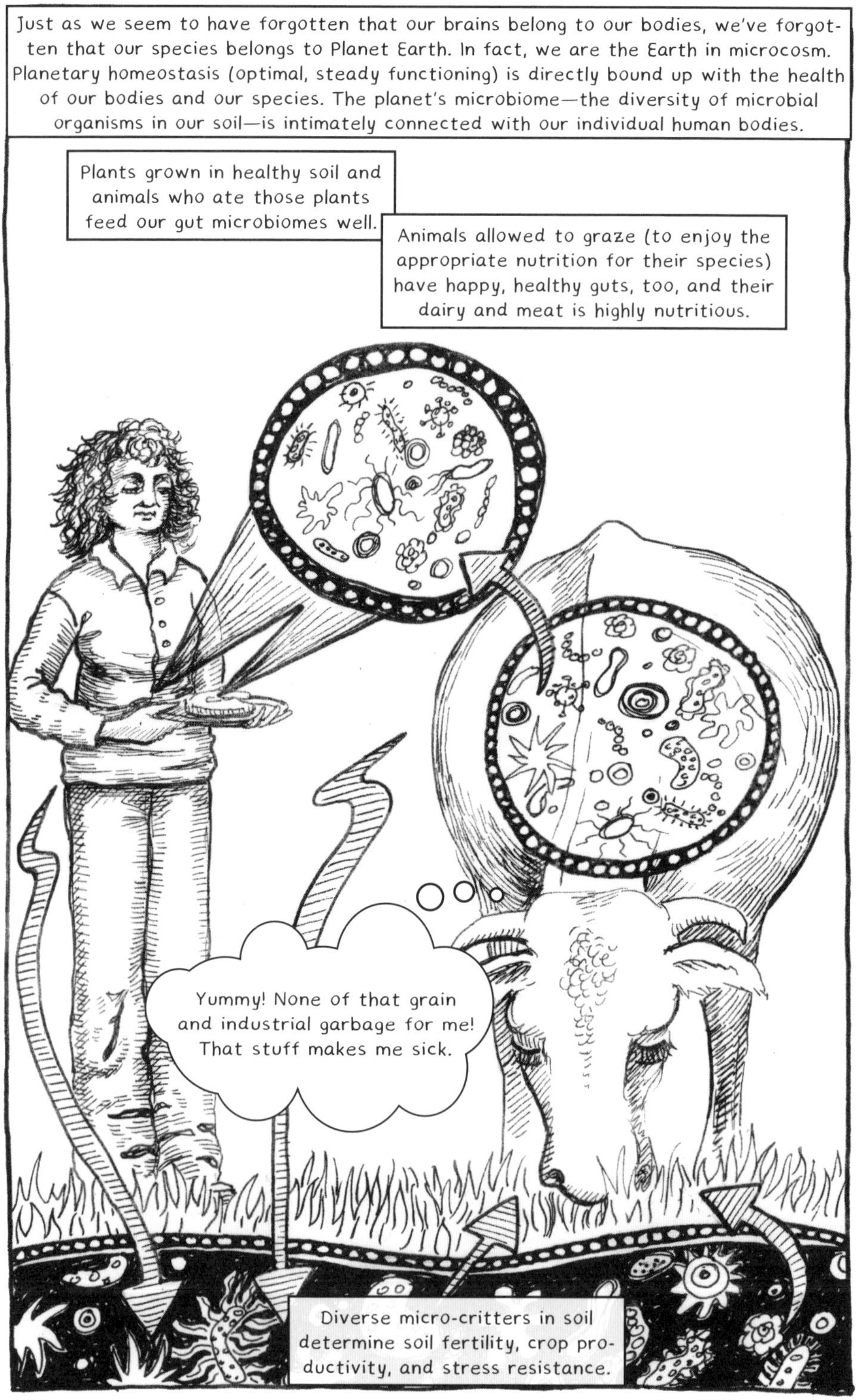
Just as we seem to have forgotten that our brains belong to our bodies, we've forgotten that our species belongs to Planet Earth. In fact, we are the Earth in microcosm. Planetary homeostasis (optimal, steady functioning) is directly bound up with the health of our bodies and our species. The planet's microbiome—the diversity of microbial organisms in our soil—is intimately connected with our individual human bodies.
Plants grown in healthy soil and animals who ate those plants feed our gut microbiomes well.
Animals allowed to graze (to enjoy the appropriate nutrition for their species) have happy, healthy guts, too, and their dairy and meat is highly nutritious.
Yummy! None of that grain and industrial garbage for me! That stuff makes me sick.
Diverse micro-critters in soil determine soil fertility, crop productivity, and stress resistance.

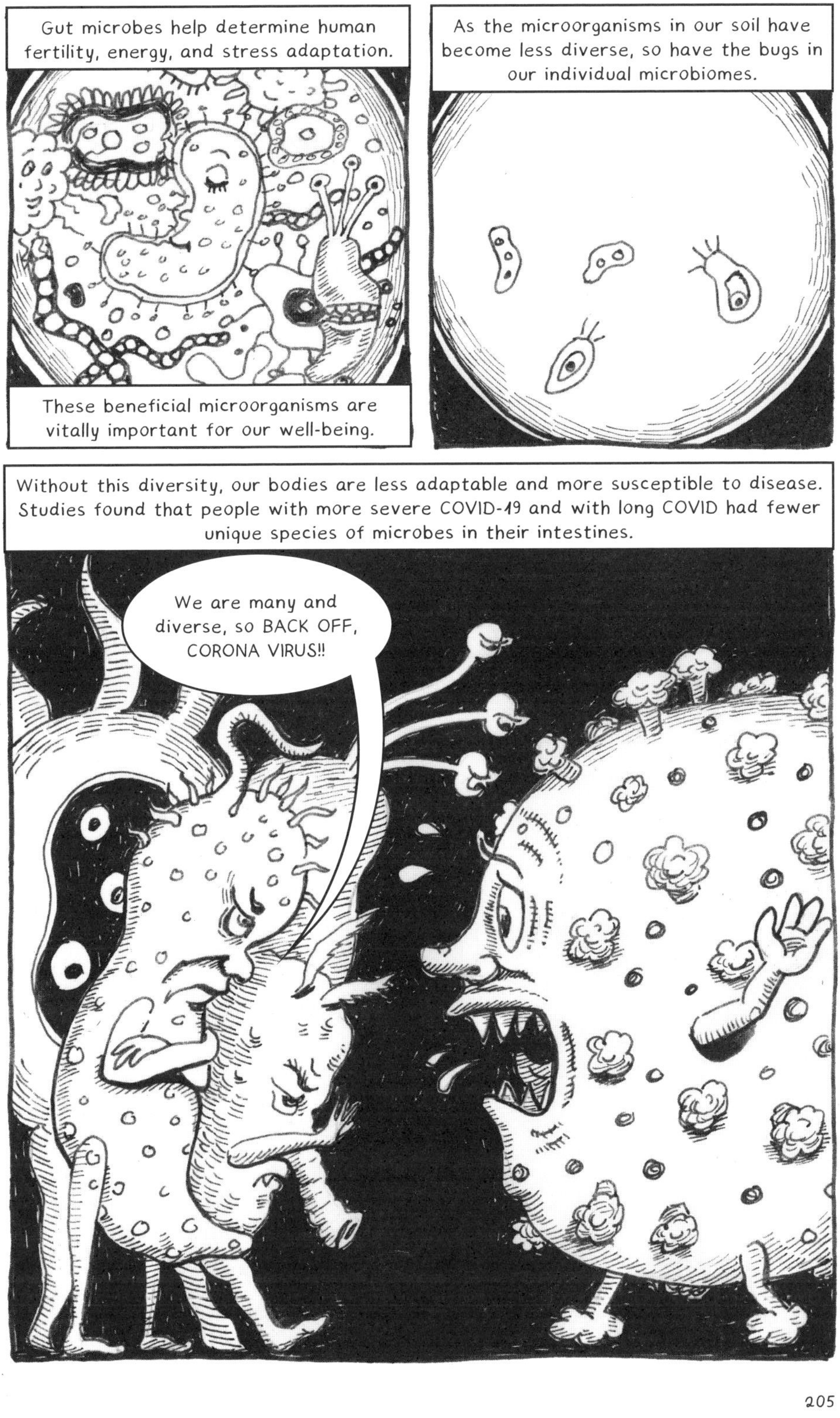

Gut microbes help determine human fertility, energy, and stress adaptation. 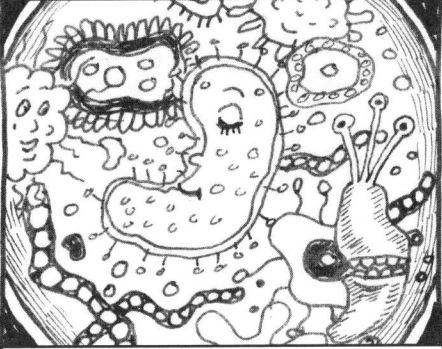 These beneficial microorganisms are vitally important for our well-being.	As the microorganisms in our soil have become less diverse, so have the bugs in our individual microbiomes. 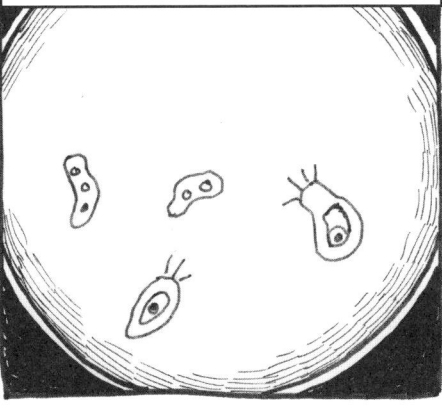

Without this diversity, our bodies are less adaptable and more susceptible to disease. Studies found that people with more severe COVID-19 and with long COVID had fewer unique species of microbes in their intestines.

"We are many and diverse, so BACK OFF, CORONA VIRUS!!"

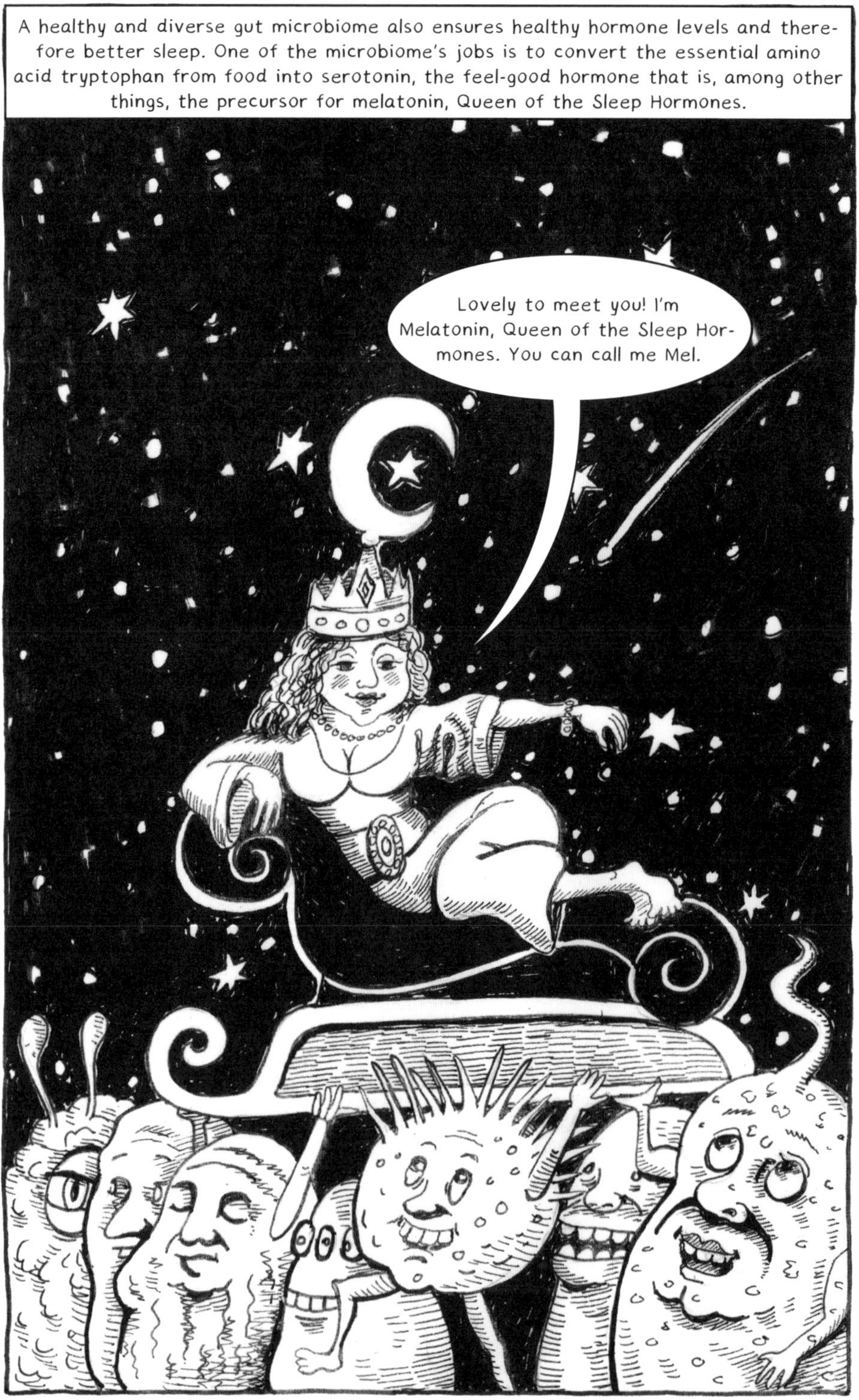
A healthy and diverse gut microbiome also ensures healthy hormone levels and therefore better sleep. One of the microbiome's jobs is to convert the essential amino acid tryptophan from food into serotonin, the feel-good hormone that is, among other things, the precursor for melatonin, Queen of the Sleep Hormones.
Lovely to meet you! I'm Melatonin, Queen of the Sleep Hormones. You can call me Mel.

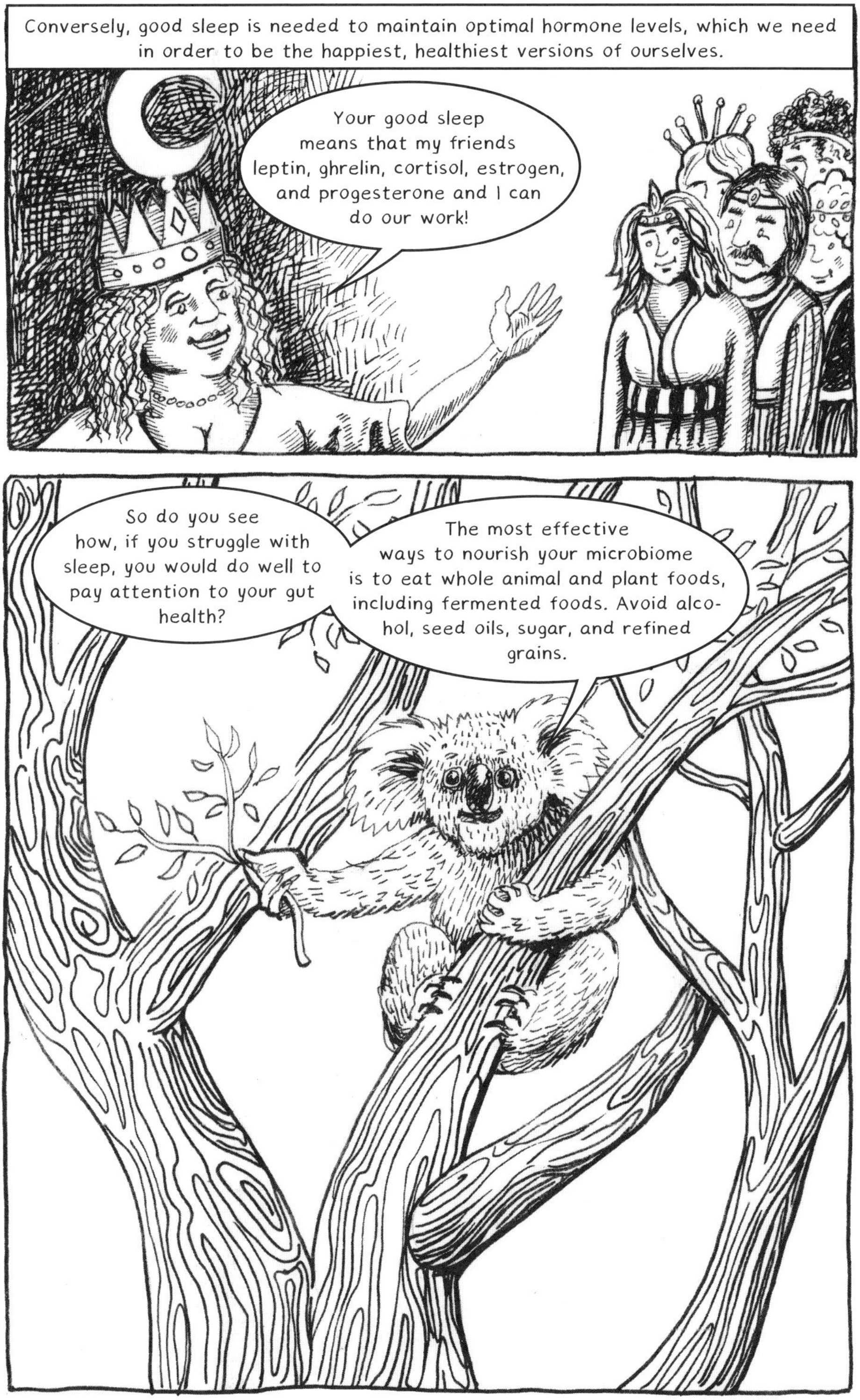
Conversely, good sleep is needed to maintain optimal hormone levels, which we need in order to be the happiest, healthiest versions of ourselves.
Your good sleep means that my friends leptin, ghrelin, cortisol, estrogen, and progesterone and I can do our work!
So do you see how, if you struggle with sleep, you would do well to pay attention to your gut health?
The most effective ways to nourish your microbiome is to eat whole animal and plant foods, including fermented foods. Avoid alcohol, seed oils, sugar, and refined grains.

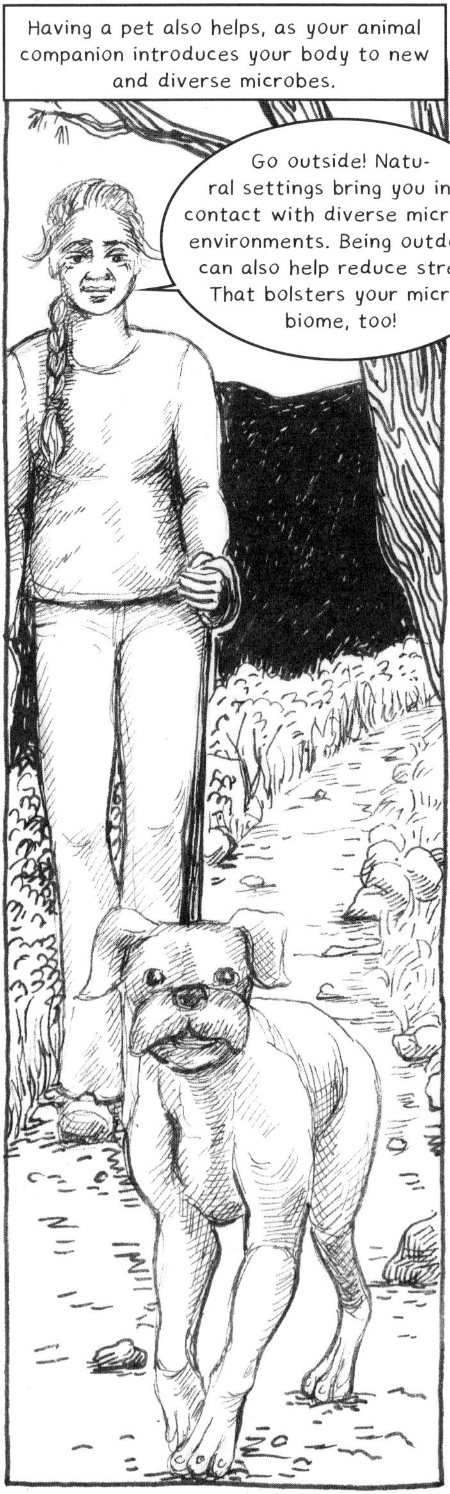
Having a pet also helps, as your animal companion introduces your body to new and diverse microbes.
Go outside! Natural settings bring you into contact with diverse microbial environments. Being outdoors can also help reduce stress. That bolsters your microbiome, too!

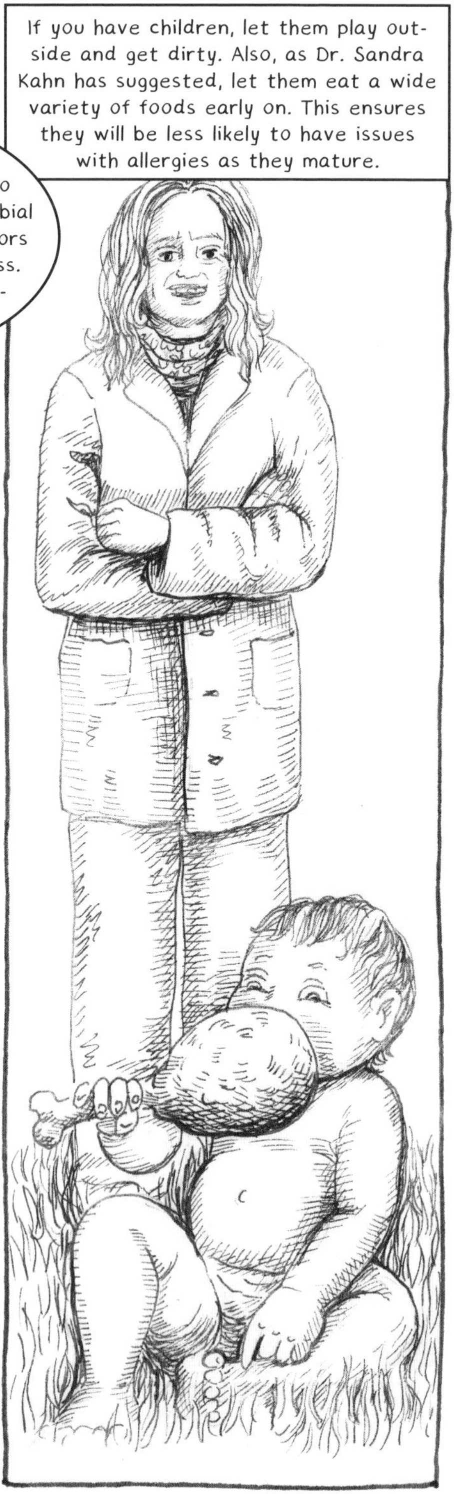
If you have children, let them play outside and get dirty. Also, as Dr. Sandra Kahn has suggested, let them eat a wide variety of foods early on. This ensures they will be less likely to have issues with allergies as they mature.

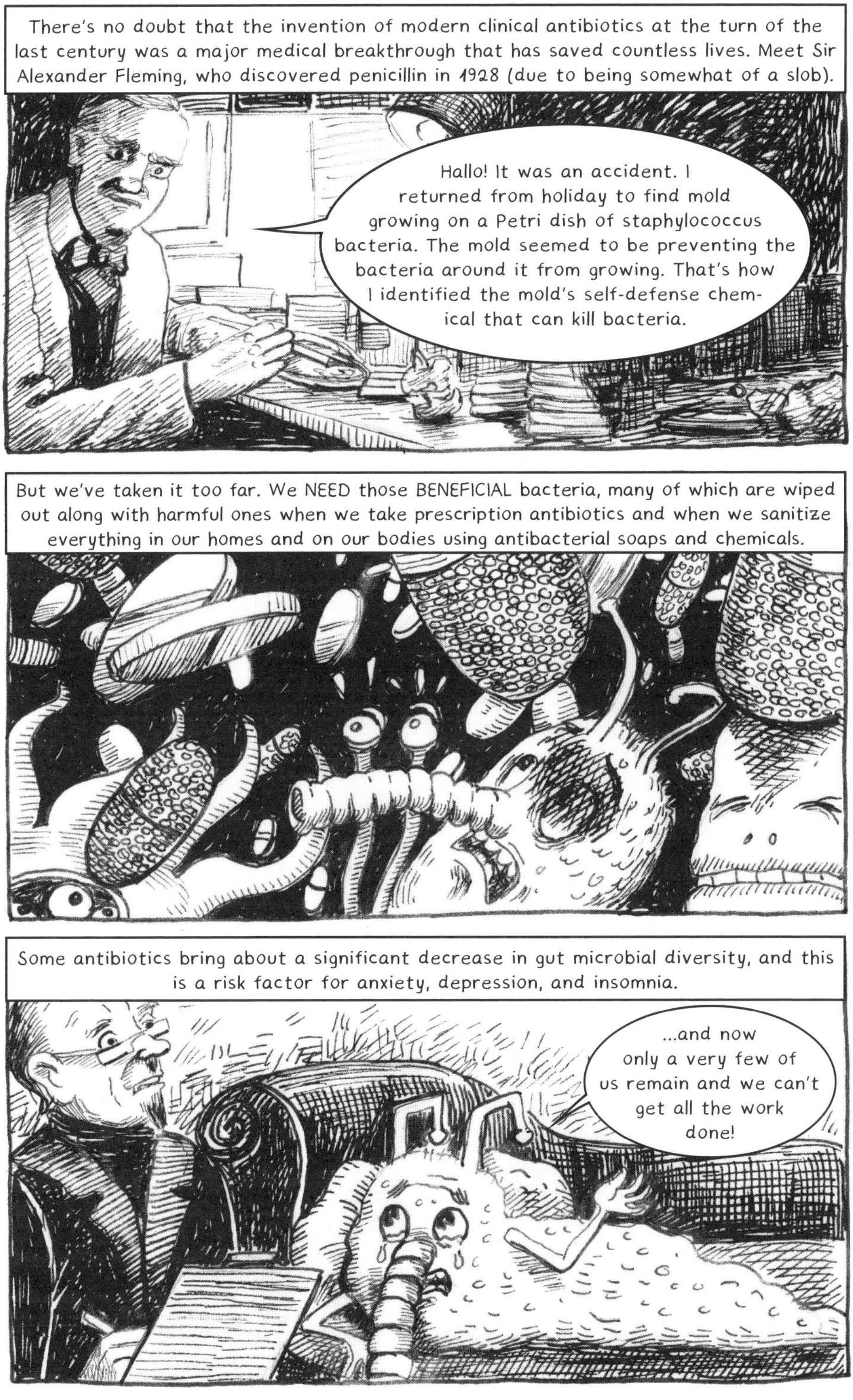
There's no doubt that the invention of modern clinical antibiotics at the turn of the last century was a major medical breakthrough that has saved countless lives. Meet Sir Alexander Fleming, who discovered penicillin in 1928 (due to being somewhat of a slob).
Hallo! It was an accident. I returned from holiday to find mold growing on a Petri dish of staphylococcus bacteria. The mold seemed to be preventing the bacteria around it from growing. That's how I identified the mold's self-defense chemical that can kill bacteria.
But we've taken it too far. We NEED those BENEFICIAL bacteria, many of which are wiped out along with harmful ones when we take prescription antibiotics and when we sanitize everything in our homes and on our bodies using antibacterial soaps and chemicals.
Some antibiotics bring about a significant decrease in gut microbial diversity, and this is a risk factor for anxiety, depression, and insomnia.
...and now only a very few of us remain and we can't get all the work done!

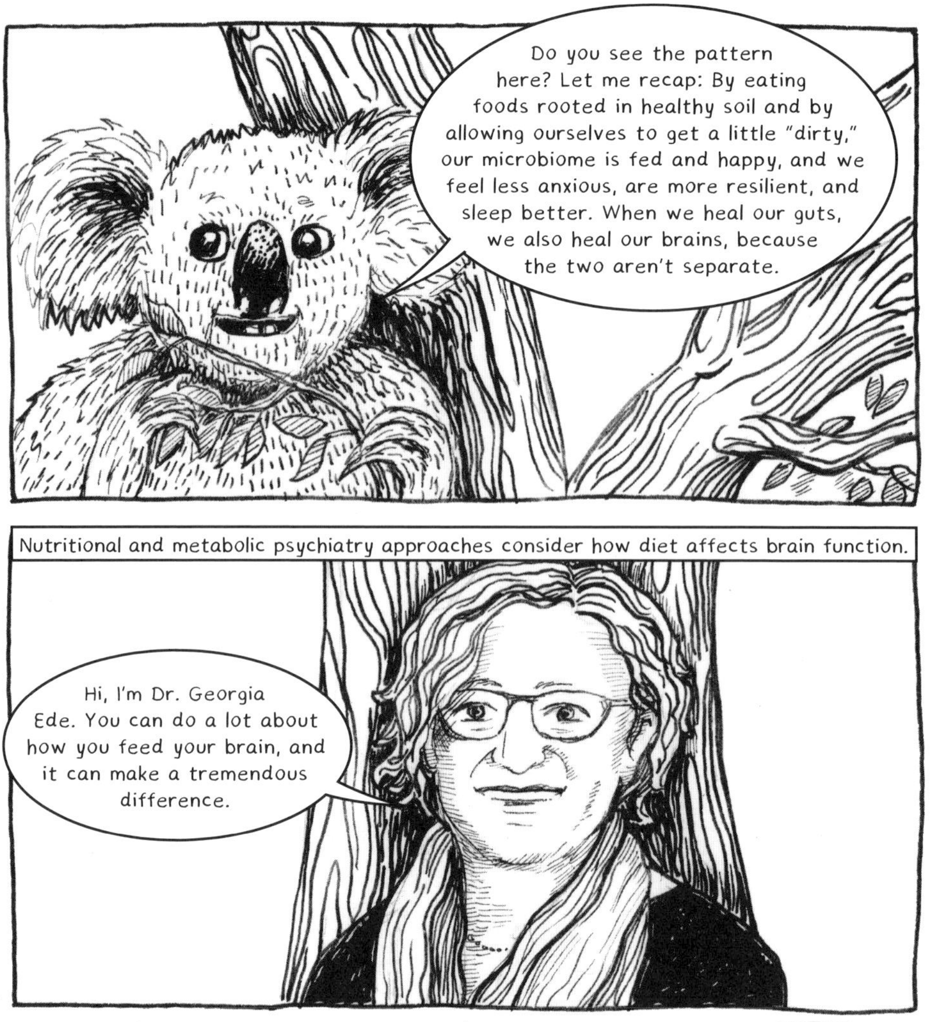
Do you see the pattern here? Let me recap: By eating foods rooted in healthy soil and by allowing ourselves to get a little "dirty," our microbiome is fed and happy, and we feel less anxious, are more resilient, and sleep better. When we heal our guts, we also heal our brains, because the two aren't separate.
Nutritional and metabolic psychiatry approaches consider how diet affects brain function.
Hi, I'm Dr. Georgia Ede. You can do a lot about how you feed your brain, and it can make a tremendous difference.
As I changed what I ate, my "mental" health (or brain health) improved immensely.
Now isn't that the truth! Thank you!

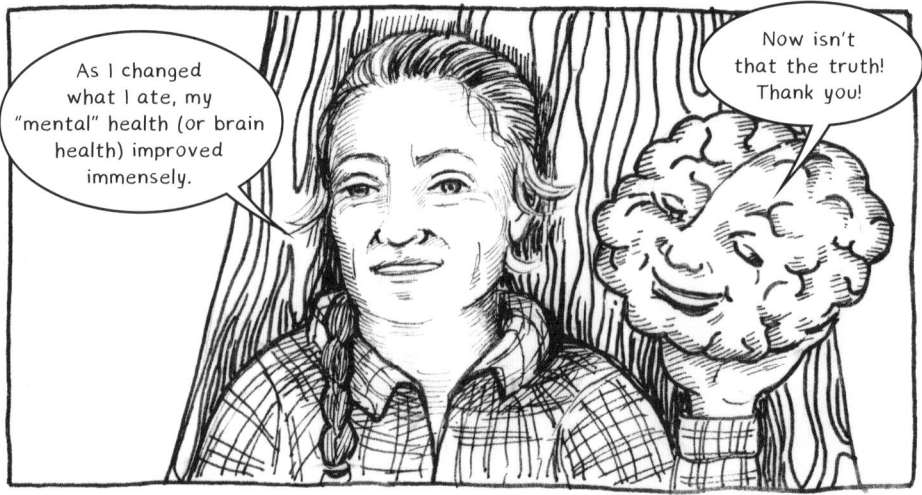

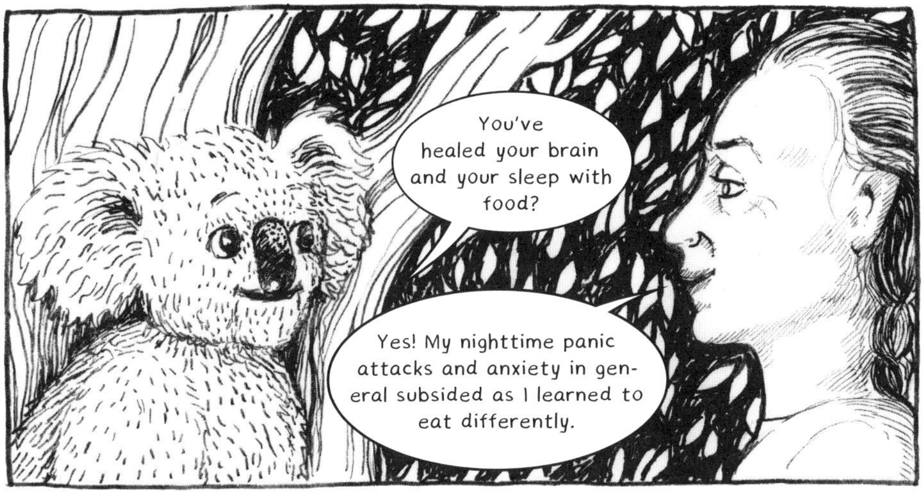
You've healed your brain and your sleep with food?
Yes! My nighttime panic attacks and anxiety in general subsided as I learned to eat differently.

Another approach to shifting your thoughts and feelings at night (and in general!) is by changing your behavior.

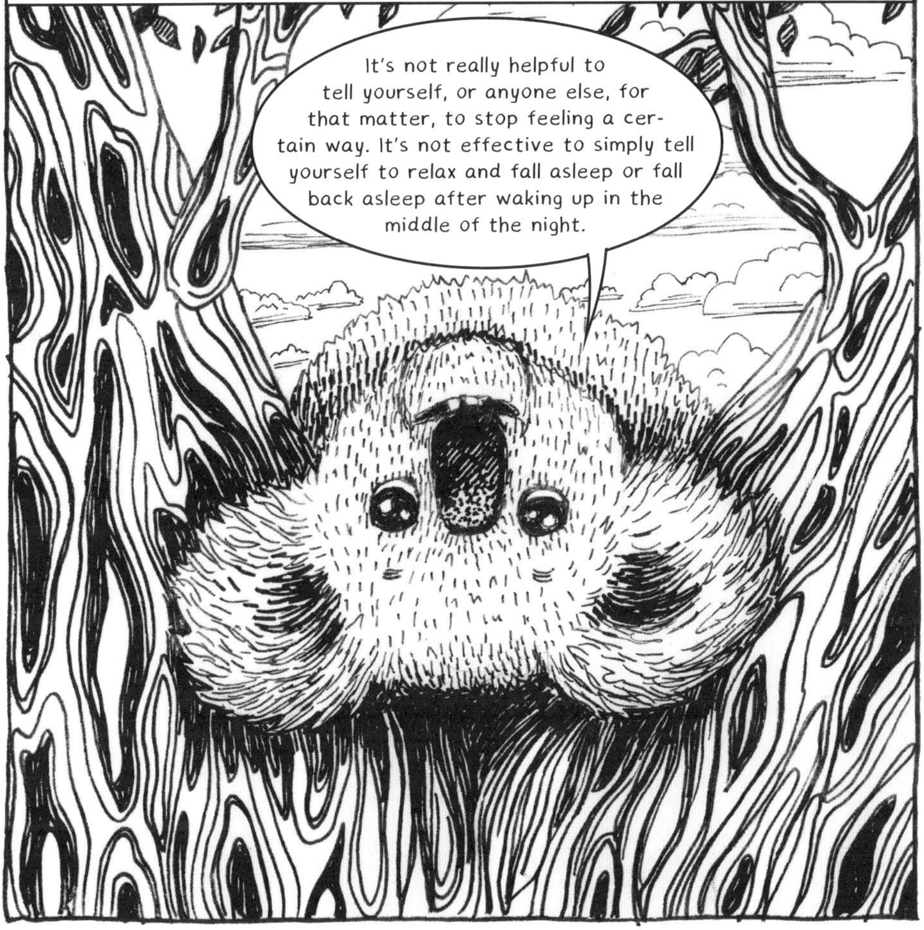
It's not really helpful to tell yourself, or anyone else, for that matter, to stop feeling a certain way. It's not effective to simply tell yourself to relax and fall asleep or fall back asleep after waking up in the middle of the night.

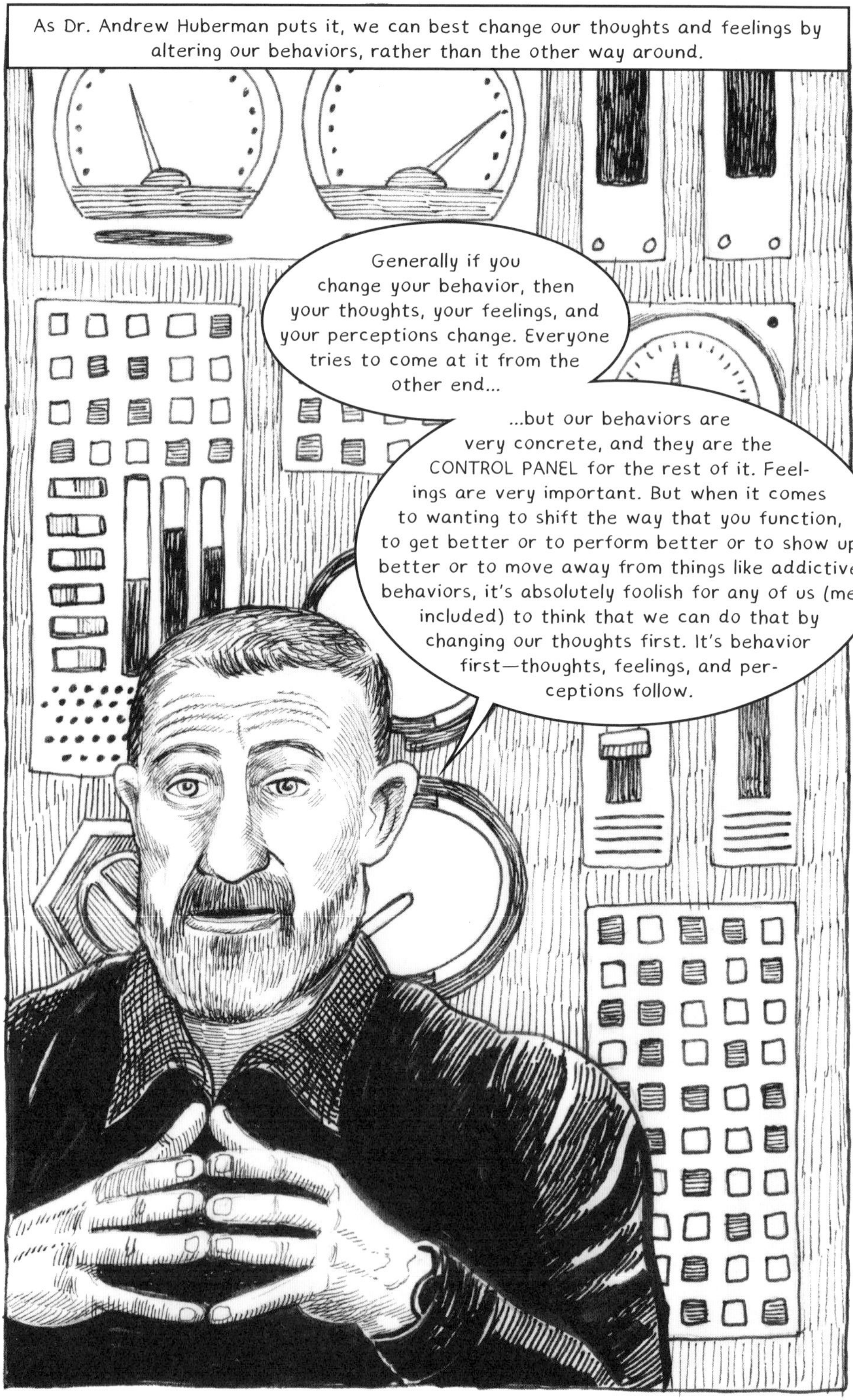
As Dr. Andrew Huberman puts it, we can best change our thoughts and feelings by altering our behaviors, rather than the other way around.
Generally if you change your behavior, then your thoughts, your feelings, and your perceptions change. Everyone tries to come at it from the other end...
...but our behaviors are very concrete, and they are the CONTROL PANEL for the rest of it. Feelings are very important. But when it comes to wanting to shift the way that you function, to get better or to perform better or to show up better or to move away from things like addictive behaviors, it's absolutely foolish for any of us (me included) to think that we can do that by changing our thoughts first. It's behavior first—thoughts, feelings, and perceptions follow.

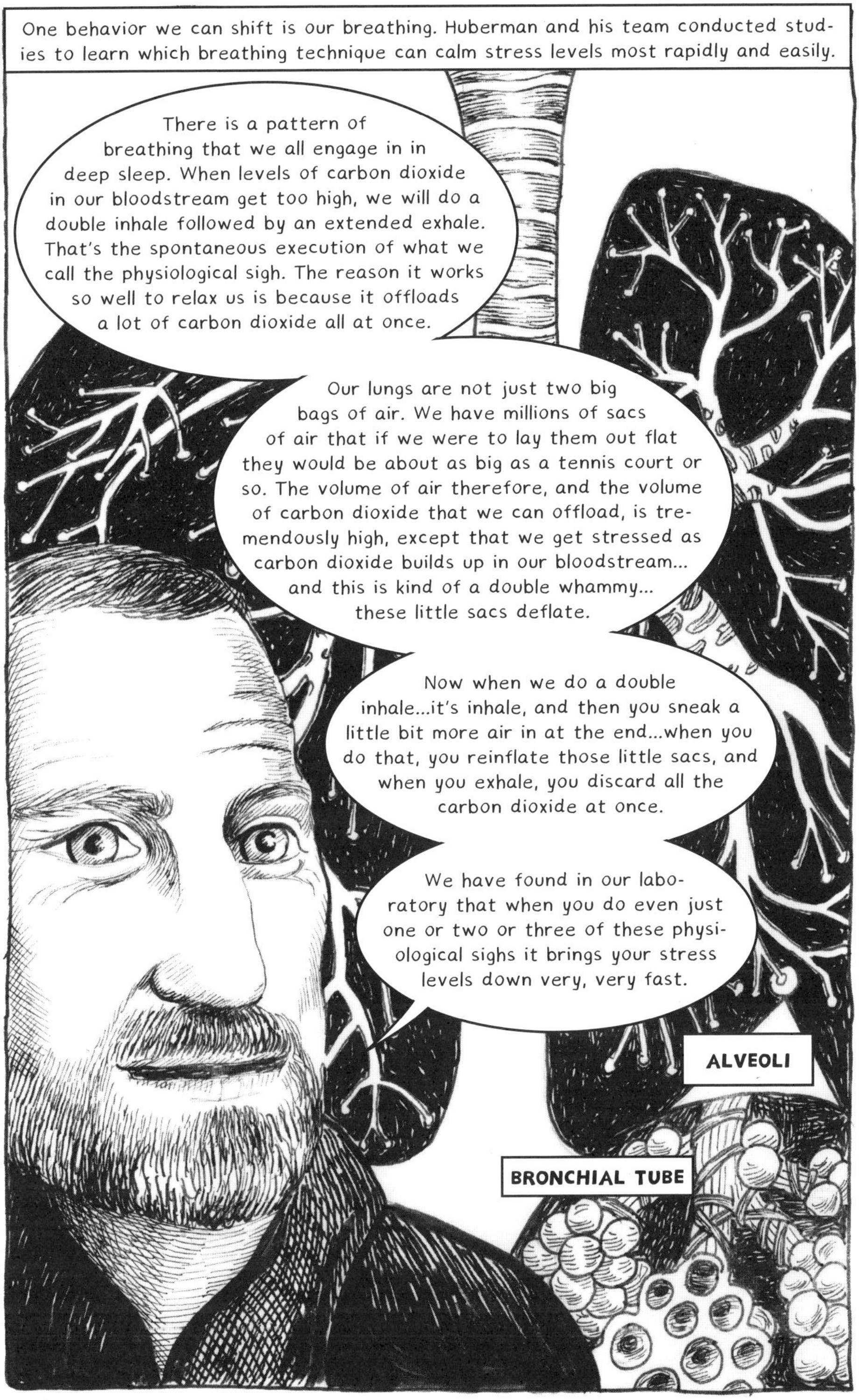

One behavior we can shift is our breathing. Huberman and his team conducted studies to learn which breathing technique can calm stress levels most rapidly and easily.
There is a pattern of breathing that we all engage in in deep sleep. When levels of carbon dioxide in our bloodstream get too high, we will do a double inhale followed by an extended exhale. That's the spontaneous execution of what we call the physiological sigh. The reason it works so well to relax us is because it offloads a lot of carbon dioxide all at once.
Our lungs are not just two big bags of air. We have millions of sacs of air that if we were to lay them out flat they would be about as big as a tennis court or so. The volume of air therefore, and the volume of carbon dioxide that we can offload, is tremendously high, except that we get stressed as carbon dioxide builds up in our bloodstream... and this is kind of a double whammy... these little sacs deflate.
Now when we do a double inhale...it's inhale, and then you sneak a little bit more air in at the end...when you do that, you reinflate those little sacs, and when you exhale, you discard all the carbon dioxide at once.
We have found in our laboratory that when you do even just one or two or three of these physiological sighs it brings your stress levels down very, very fast.
ALVEOLI
BRONCHIAL TUBE

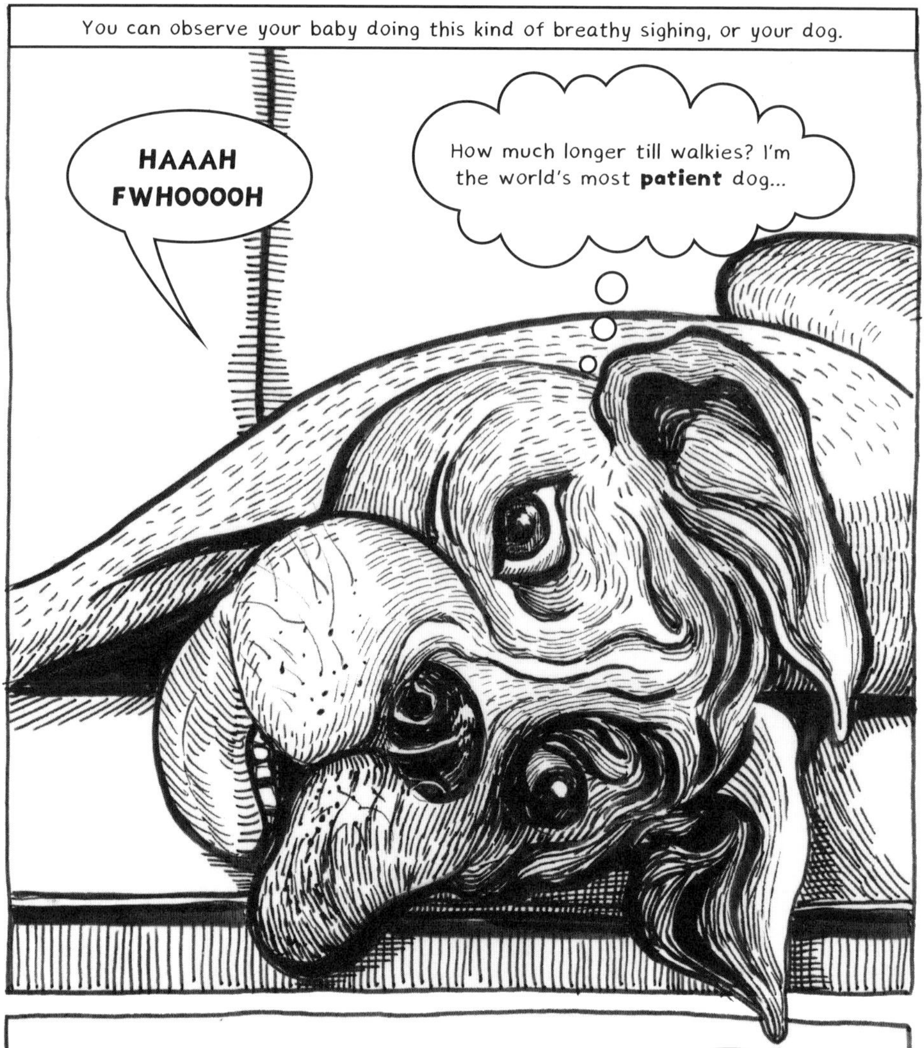

You can observe your baby doing this kind of breathy sighing, or your dog.
HAAAH FWHOOOOH
How much longer till walkies? I'm the world's most **patient** dog...

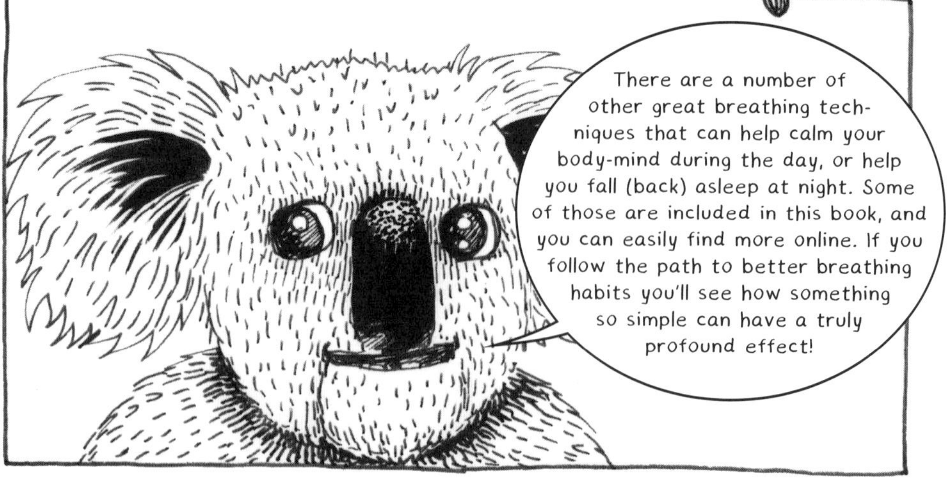

There are a number of other great breathing techniques that can help calm your body-mind during the day, or help you fall (back) asleep at night. Some of those are included in this book, and you can easily find more online. If you follow the path to better breathing habits you'll see how something so simple can have a truly profound effect!

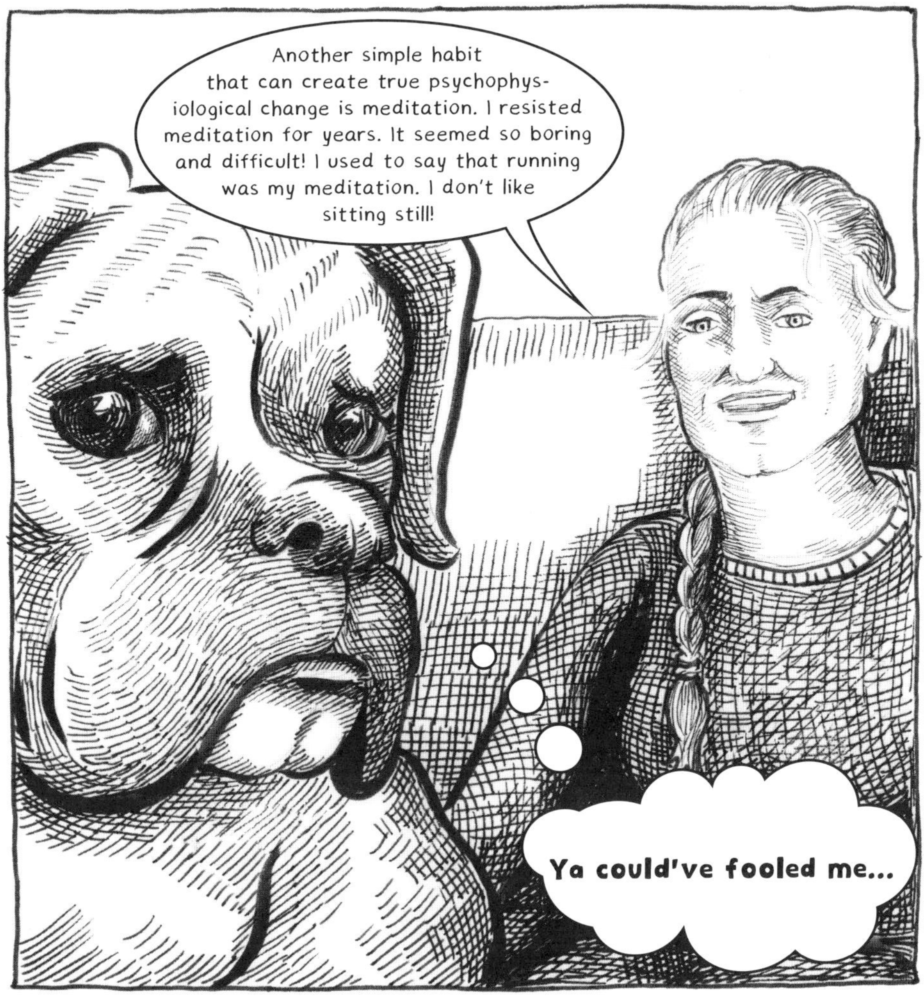
Another simple habit that can create true psychophysiological change is meditation. I resisted meditation for years. It seemed so boring and difficult! I used to say that running was my meditation. I don't like sitting still!
Ya could've fooled me...

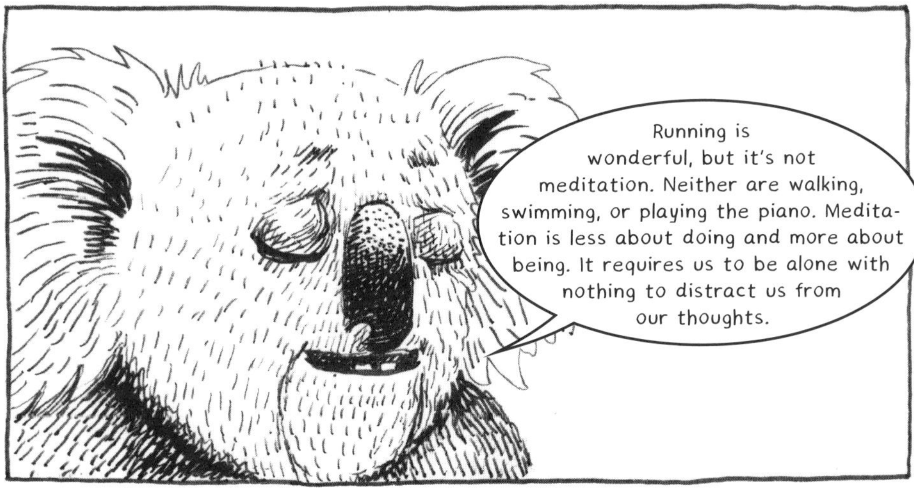
Running is wonderful, but it's not meditation. Neither are walking, swimming, or playing the piano. Meditation is less about doing and more about being. It requires us to be alone with nothing to distract us from our thoughts.

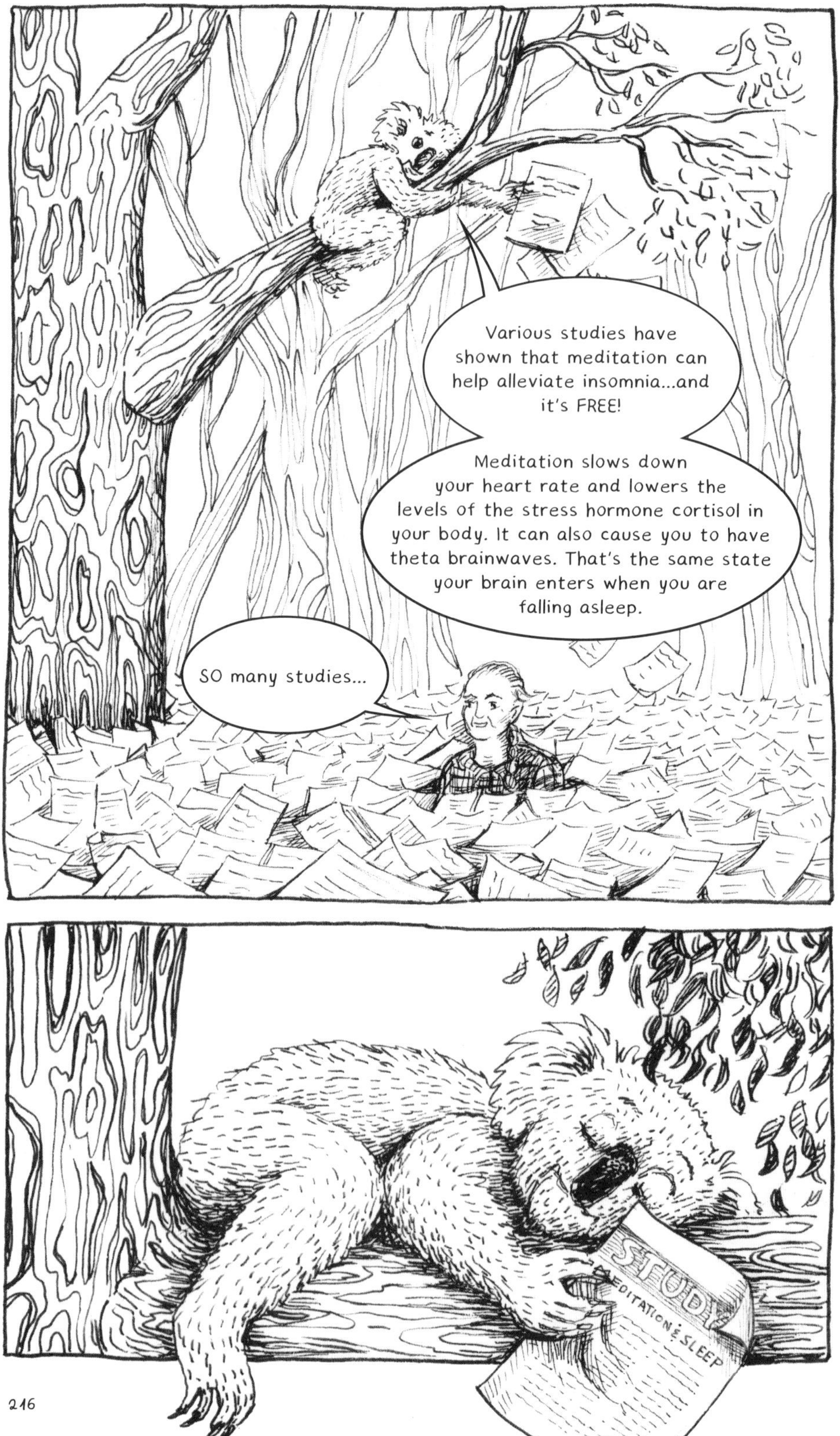
Various studies have shown that meditation can help alleviate insomnia...and it's FREE!
Meditation slows down your heart rate and lowers the levels of the stress hormone cortisol in your body. It can also cause you to have theta brainwaves. That's the same state your brain enters when you are falling asleep.
SO many studies...
STUDY
MEDITATION & SLEEP

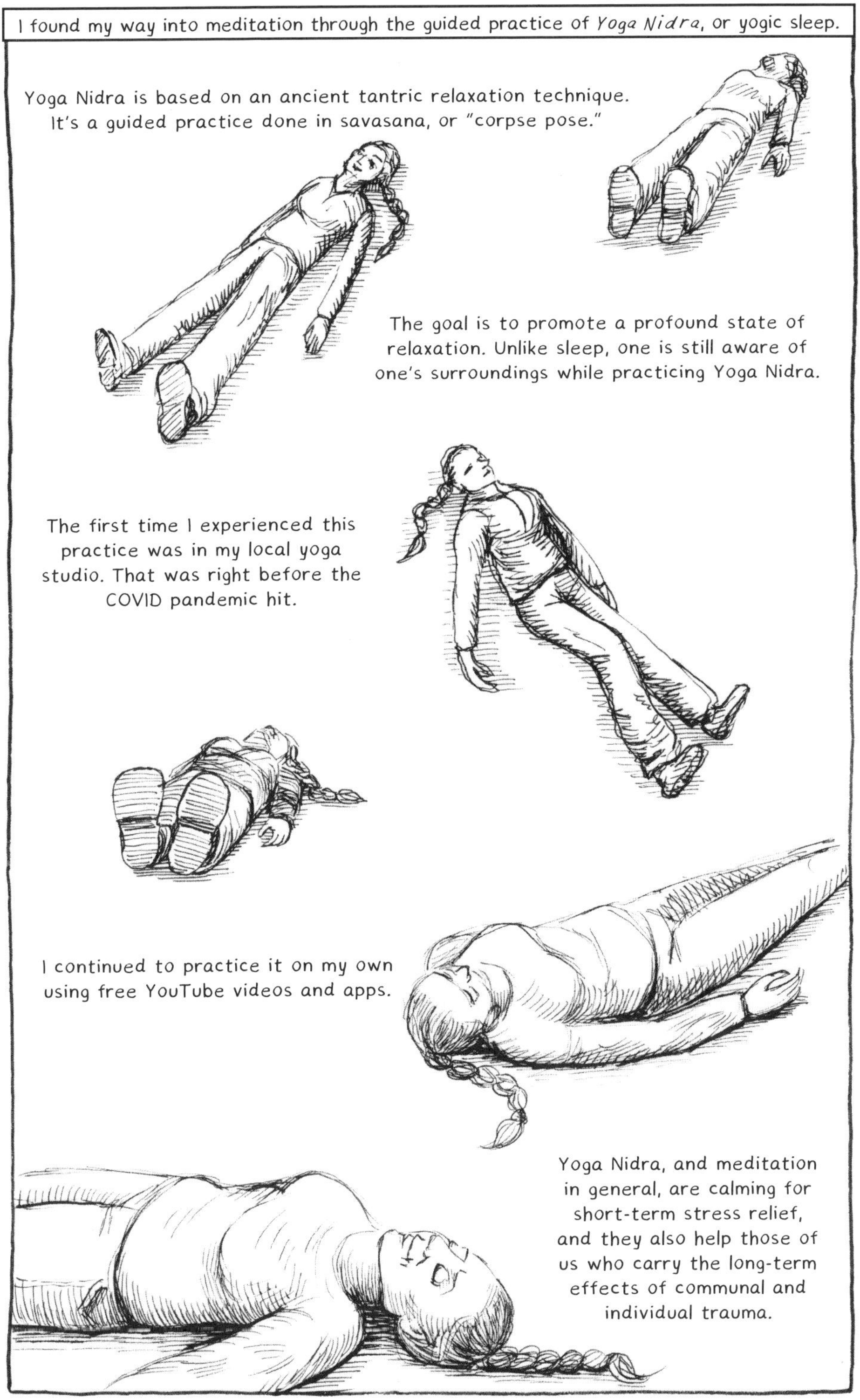

I found my way into meditation through the guided practice of *Yoga Nidra*, or yogic sleep.

Yoga Nidra is based on an ancient tantric relaxation technique. It's a guided practice done in savasana, or "corpse pose."

The goal is to promote a profound state of relaxation. Unlike sleep, one is still aware of one's surroundings while practicing Yoga Nidra.

The first time I experienced this practice was in my local yoga studio. That was right before the COVID pandemic hit.

I continued to practice it on my own using free YouTube videos and apps.

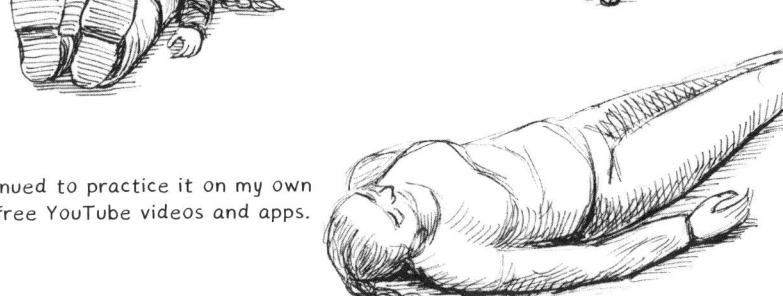

Yoga Nidra, and meditation in general, are calming for short-term stress relief, and they also help those of us who carry the long-term effects of communal and individual trauma.

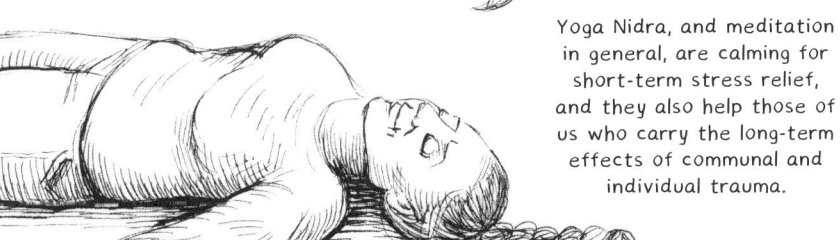

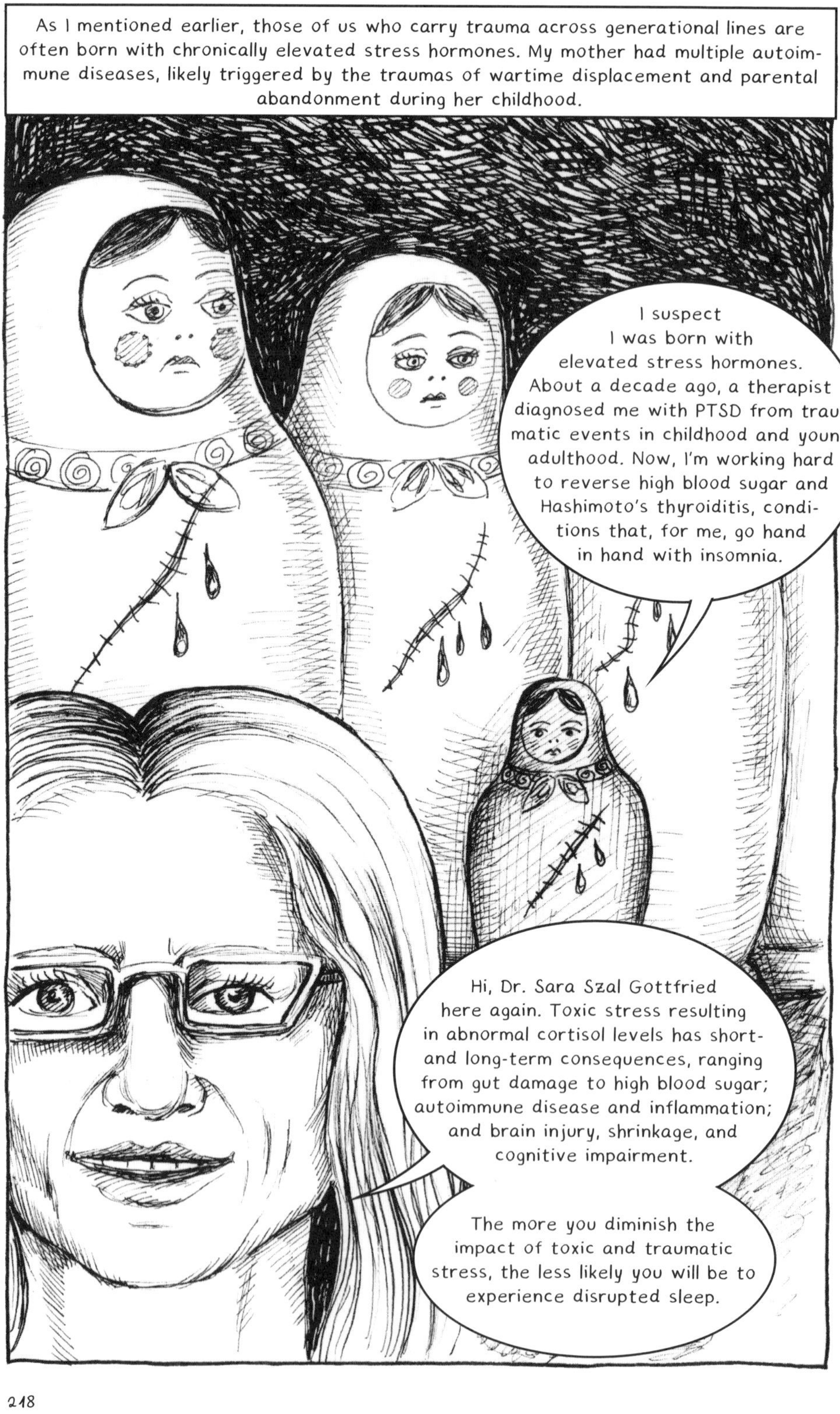
As I mentioned earlier, those of us who carry trauma across generational lines are often born with chronically elevated stress hormones. My mother had multiple autoimmune diseases, likely triggered by the traumas of wartime displacement and parental abandonment during her childhood.
I suspect I was born with elevated stress hormones. About a decade ago, a therapist diagnosed me with PTSD from traumatic events in childhood and young adulthood. Now, I'm working hard to reverse high blood sugar and Hashimoto's thyroiditis, conditions that, for me, go hand in hand with insomnia.
Hi, Dr. Sara Szal Gottfried here again. Toxic stress resulting in abnormal cortisol levels has short- and long-term consequences, ranging from gut damage to high blood sugar; autoimmune disease and inflammation; and brain injury, shrinkage, and cognitive impairment.
The more you diminish the impact of toxic and traumatic stress, the less likely you will be to experience disrupted sleep.

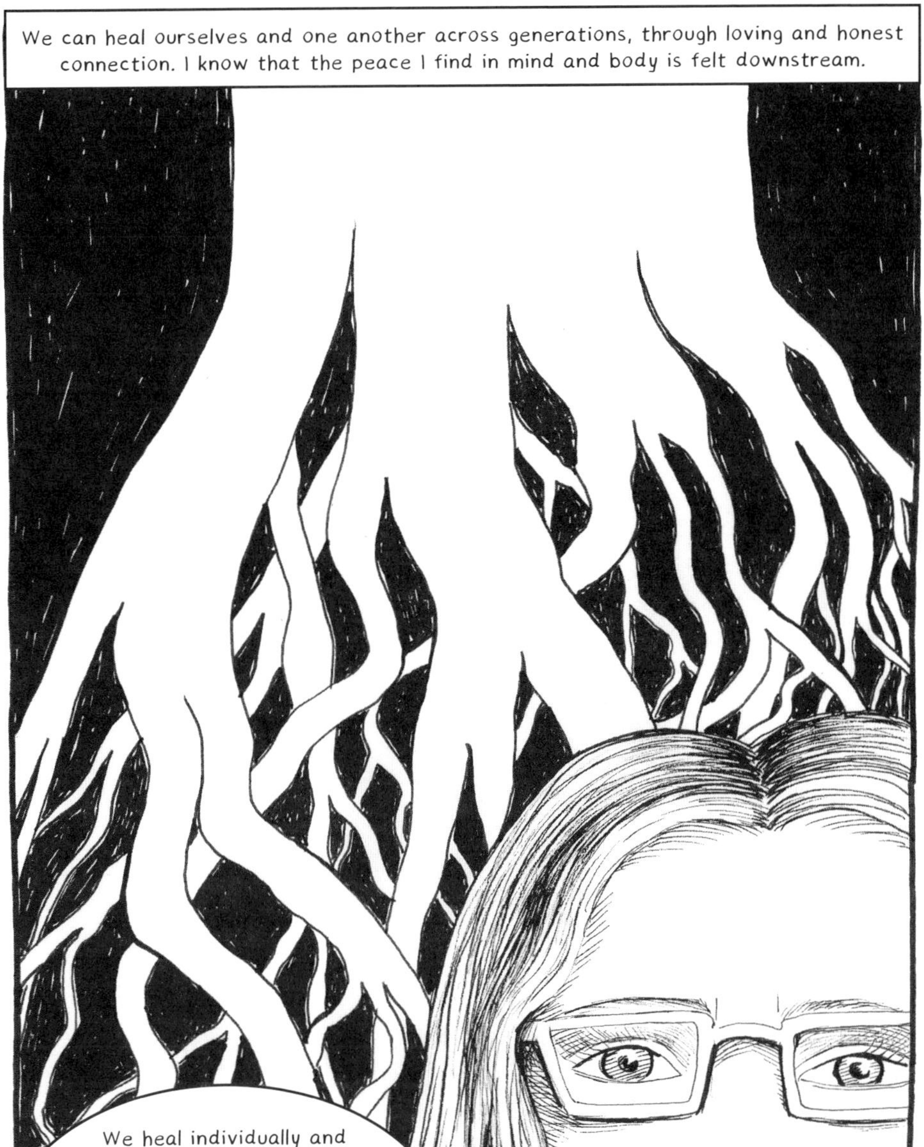
We can heal ourselves and one another across generations, through loving and honest connection. I know that the peace I find in mind and body is felt downstream.
We heal individually and communally. Fortunately, the conduit between the individual and the collective is not only for transmission of trauma, but also for healing from it. As we learn how to regulate the body with healing practices, we can become beacons of regulation for others.

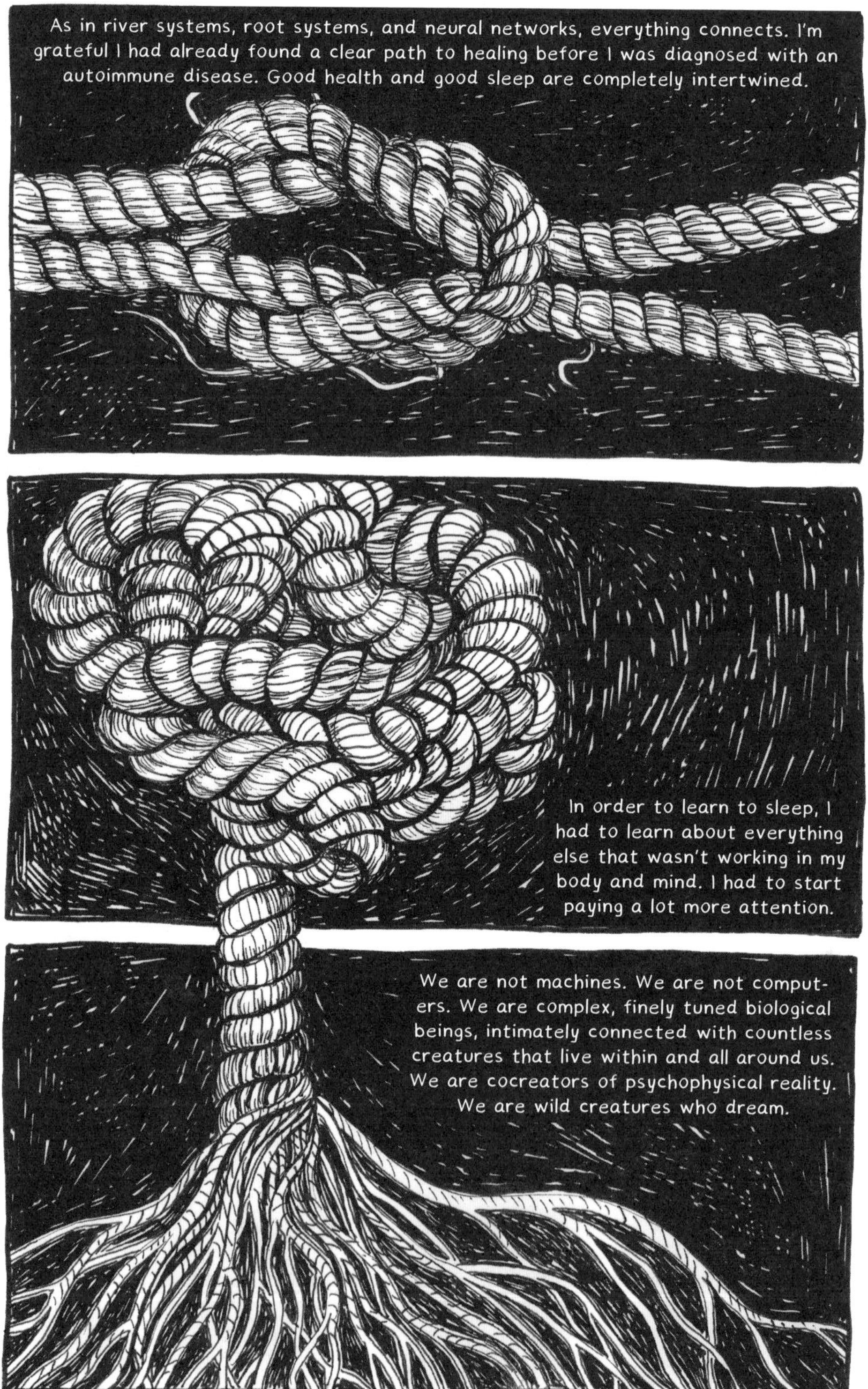
As in river systems, root systems, and neural networks, everything connects. I'm grateful I had already found a clear path to healing before I was diagnosed with an autoimmune disease. Good health and good sleep are completely intertwined.
In order to learn to sleep, I had to learn about everything else that wasn't working in my body and mind. I had to start paying a lot more attention.
We are not machines. We are not computers. We are complex, finely tuned biological beings, intimately connected with countless creatures that live within and all around us. We are cocreators of psychophysical reality. We are wild creatures who dream.

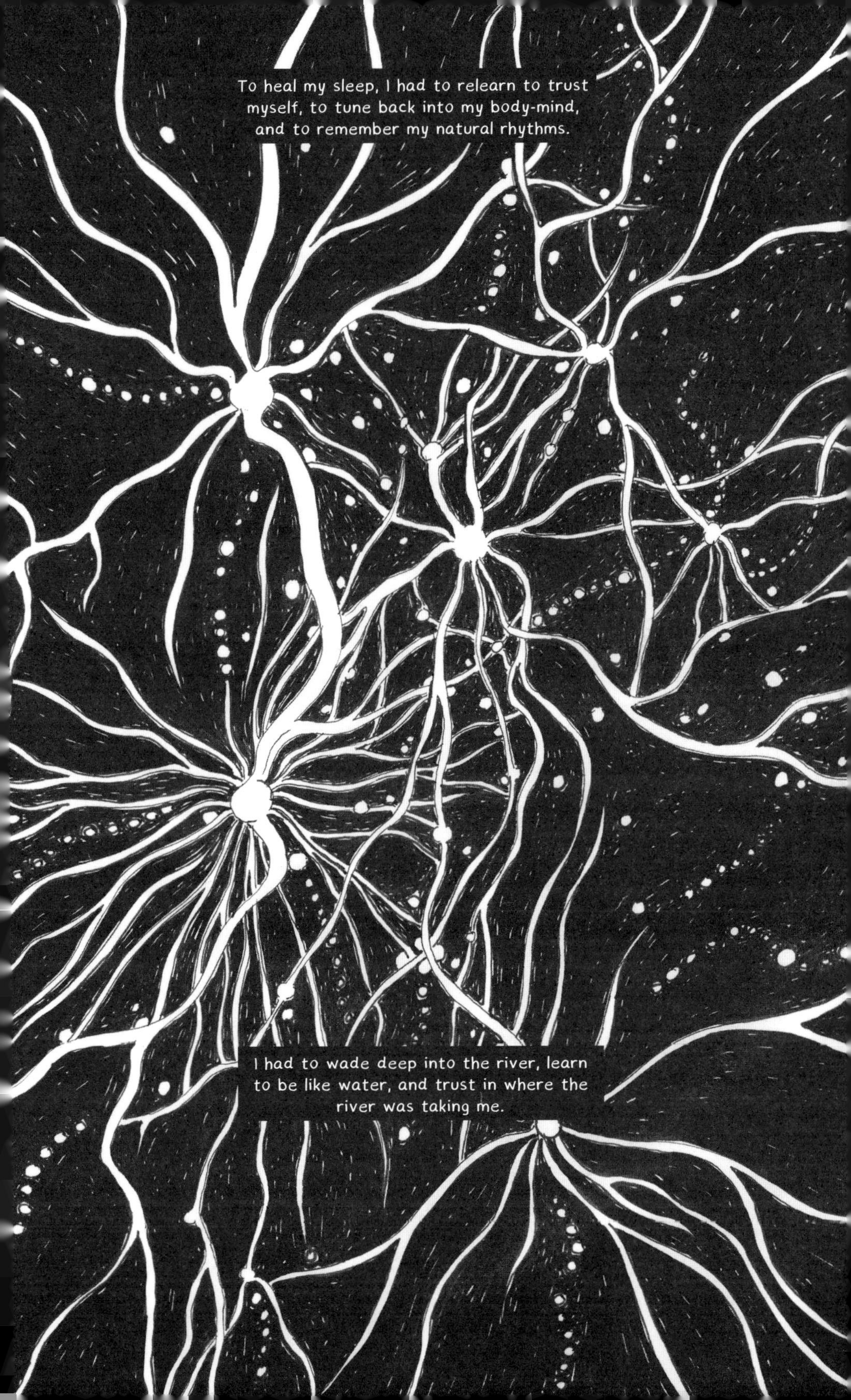
To heal my sleep, I had to relearn to trust myself, to tune back into my body-mind, and to remember my natural rhythms.
I had to wade deep into the river, learn to be like water, and trust in where the river was taking me.

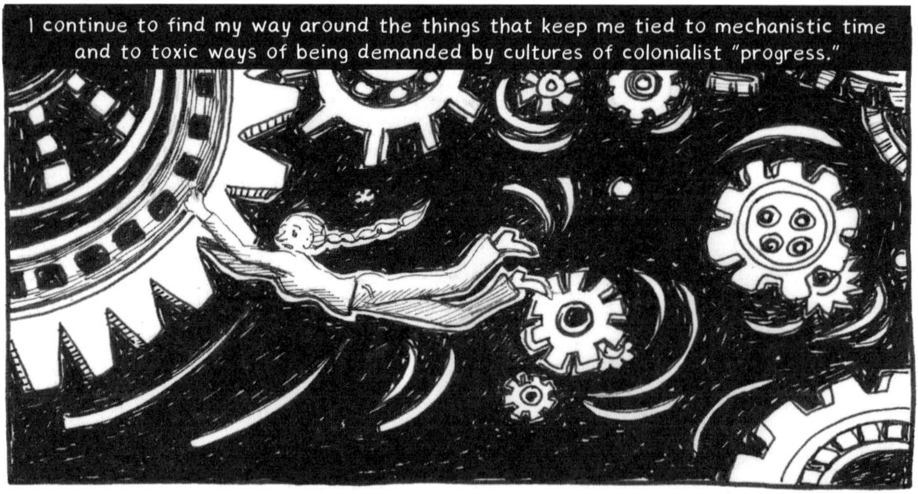
I continue to find my way around the things that keep me tied to mechanistic time and to toxic ways of being demanded by cultures of colonialist "progress."

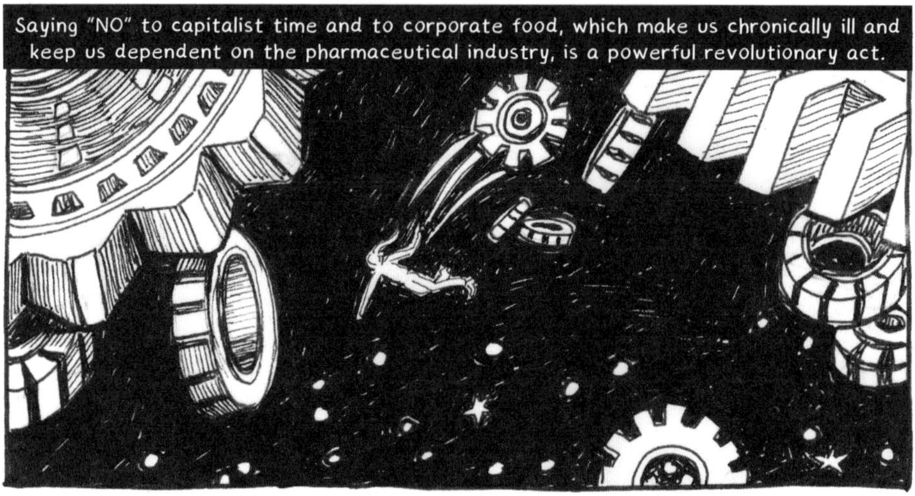
Saying "NO" to capitalist time and to corporate food, which make us chronically ill and keep us dependent on the pharmaceutical industry, is a powerful revolutionary act.

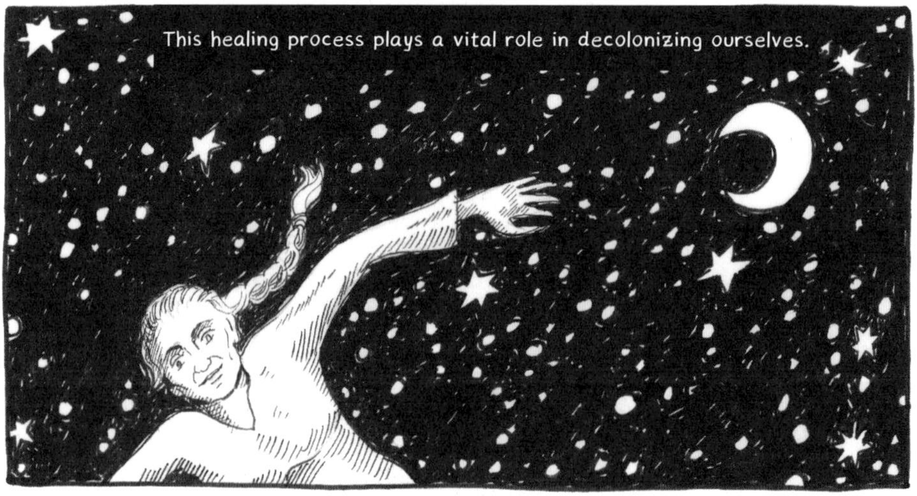
This healing process plays a vital role in decolonizing ourselves.

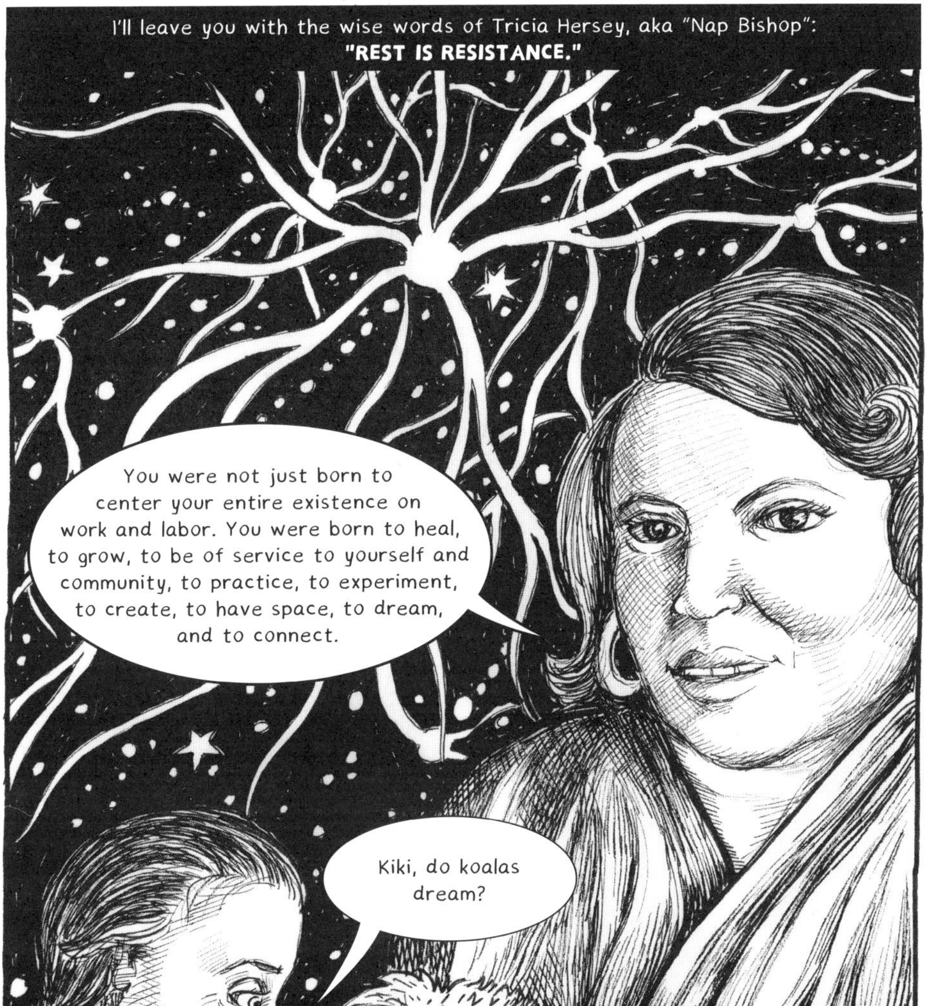
I'll leave you with the wise words of Tricia Hersey, aka "Nap Bishop":
"REST IS RESISTANCE."
You were not just born to center your entire existence on work and labor. You were born to heal, to grow, to be of service to yourself and community, to practice, to experiment, to create, to have space, to dream, and to connect.
Kiki, do koalas dream?
Of course we do. My dreams are also your dreams. My world is also your world...
Building a new life and way of being with healing rest and nourishing foods can't be done all at once. Every self-caring and self-compassionate step of this journey counts. Every step makes a difference. Each one of us makes a difference. Together, we cocreate a new constellation...a different world.

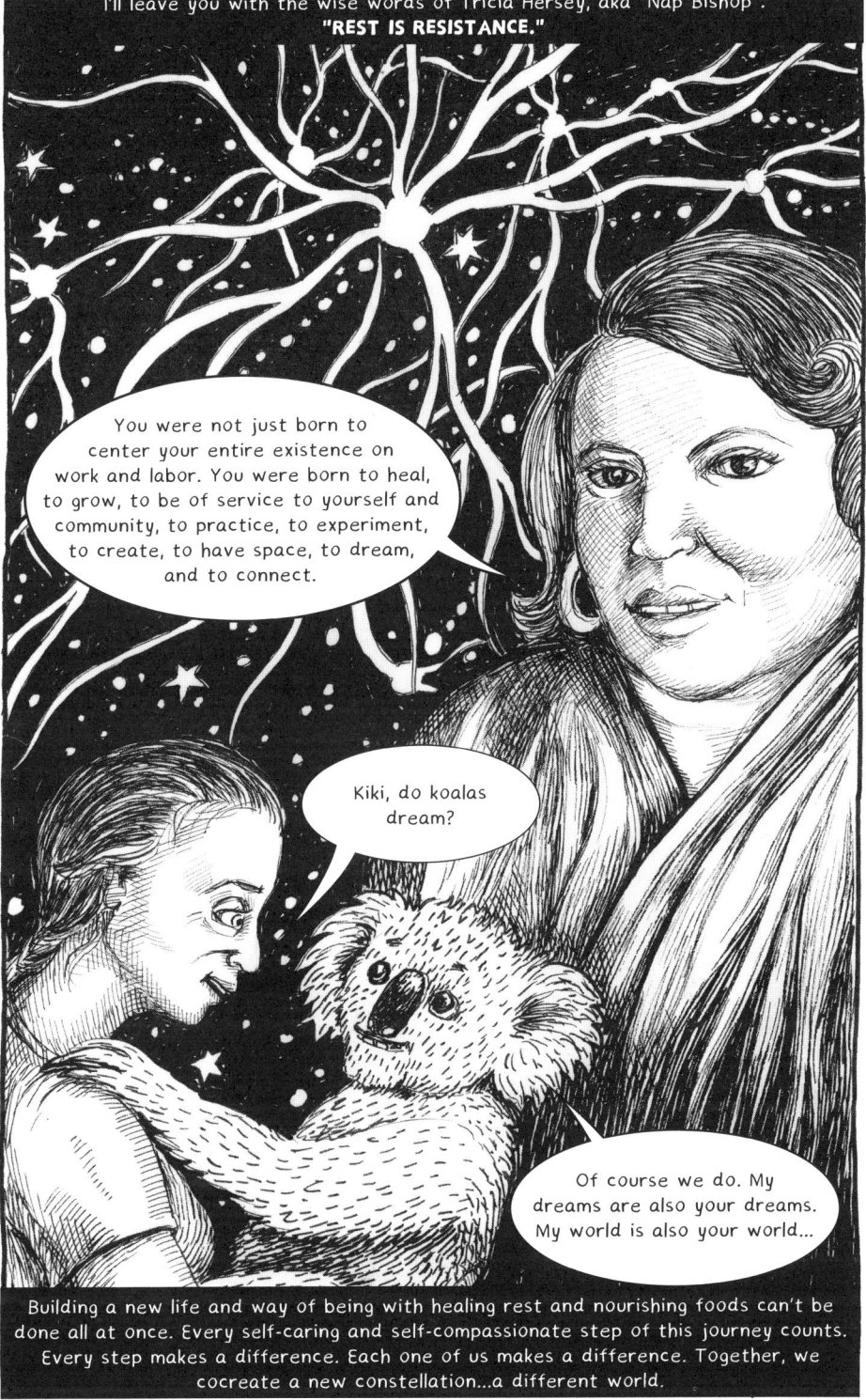

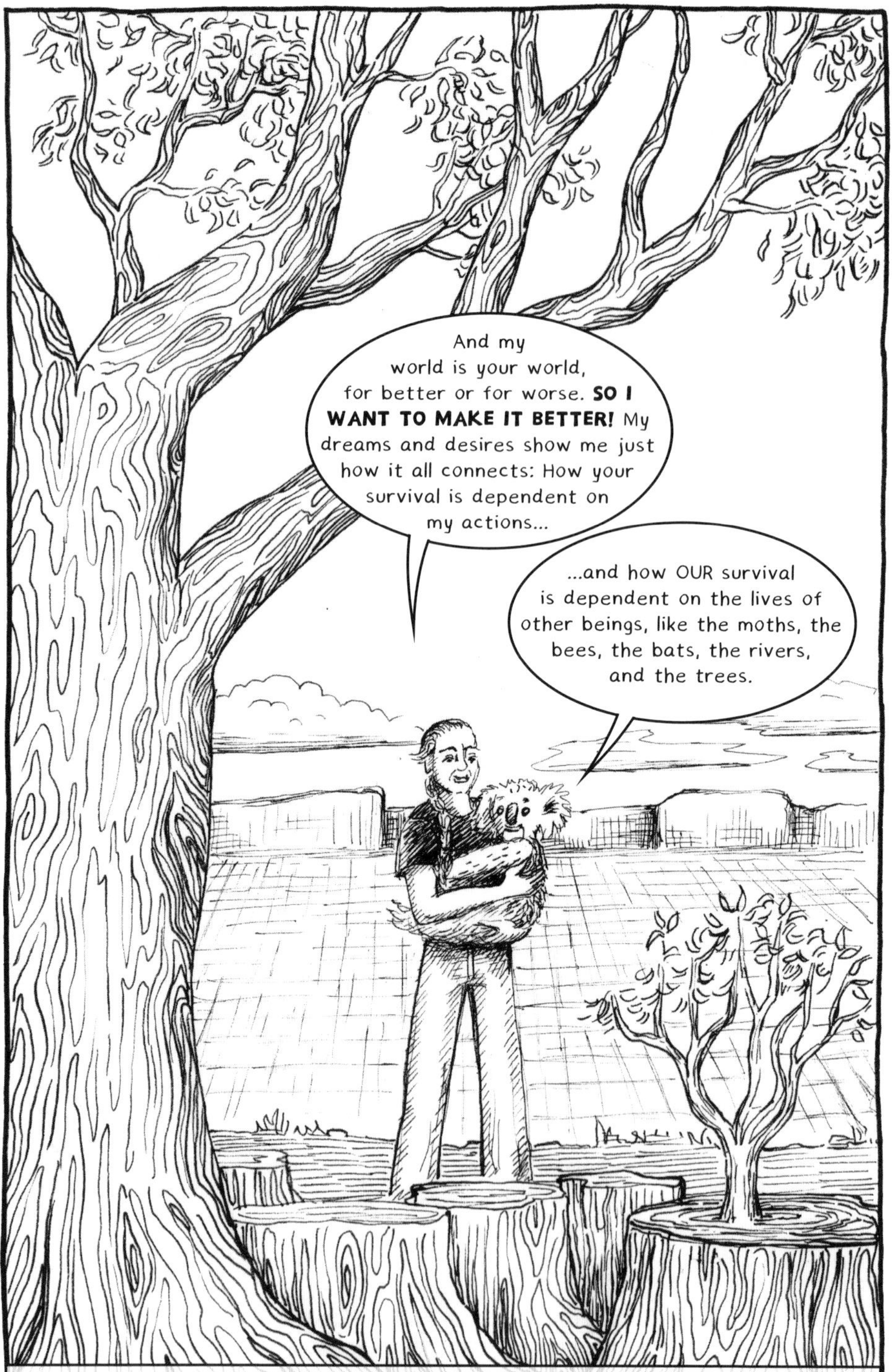
And my world is your world, for better or for worse. **SO I WANT TO MAKE IT BETTER!** My dreams and desires show me just how it all connects: How your survival is dependent on my actions...
...and how OUR survival is dependent on the lives of other beings, like the moths, the bees, the bats, the rivers, and the trees.
Becoming aware of how deeply interconnected it all is and then acting accordingly, that is the process of rewilding ourselves.

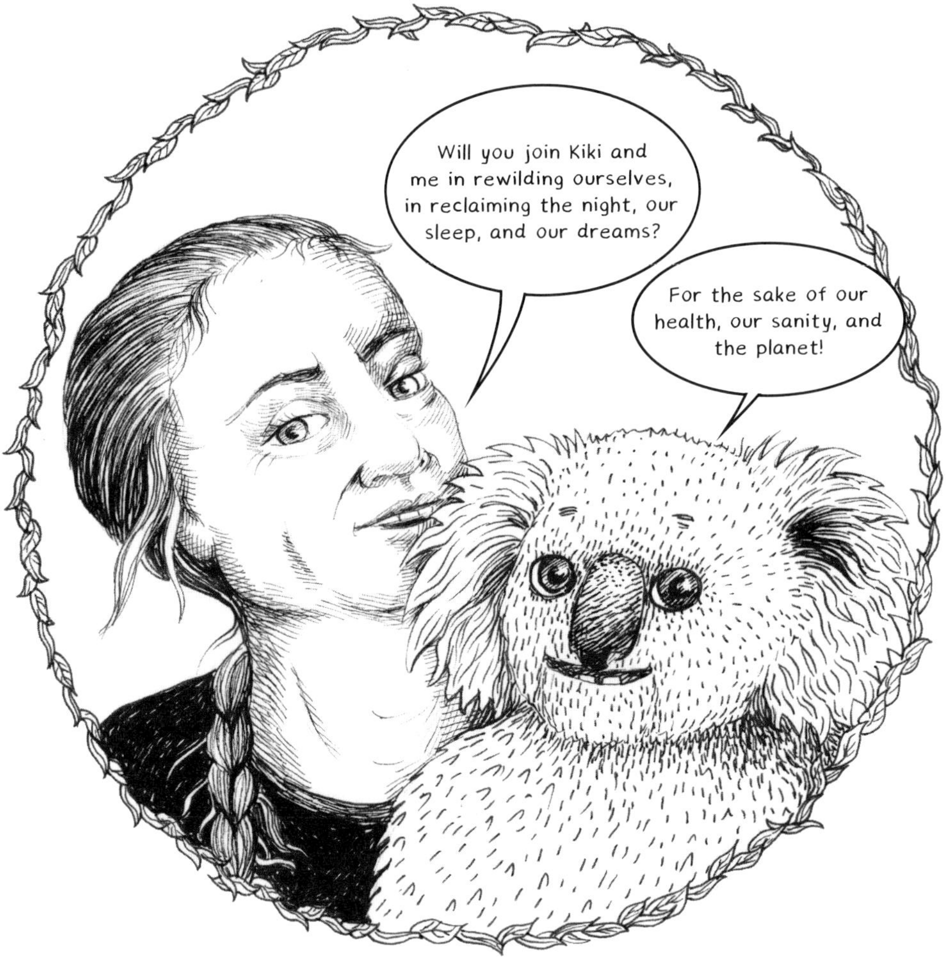
Will you join Kiki and me in rewilding ourselves, in reclaiming the night, our sleep, and our dreams?
For the sake of our health, our sanity, and the planet!

SWEET DREAMS!

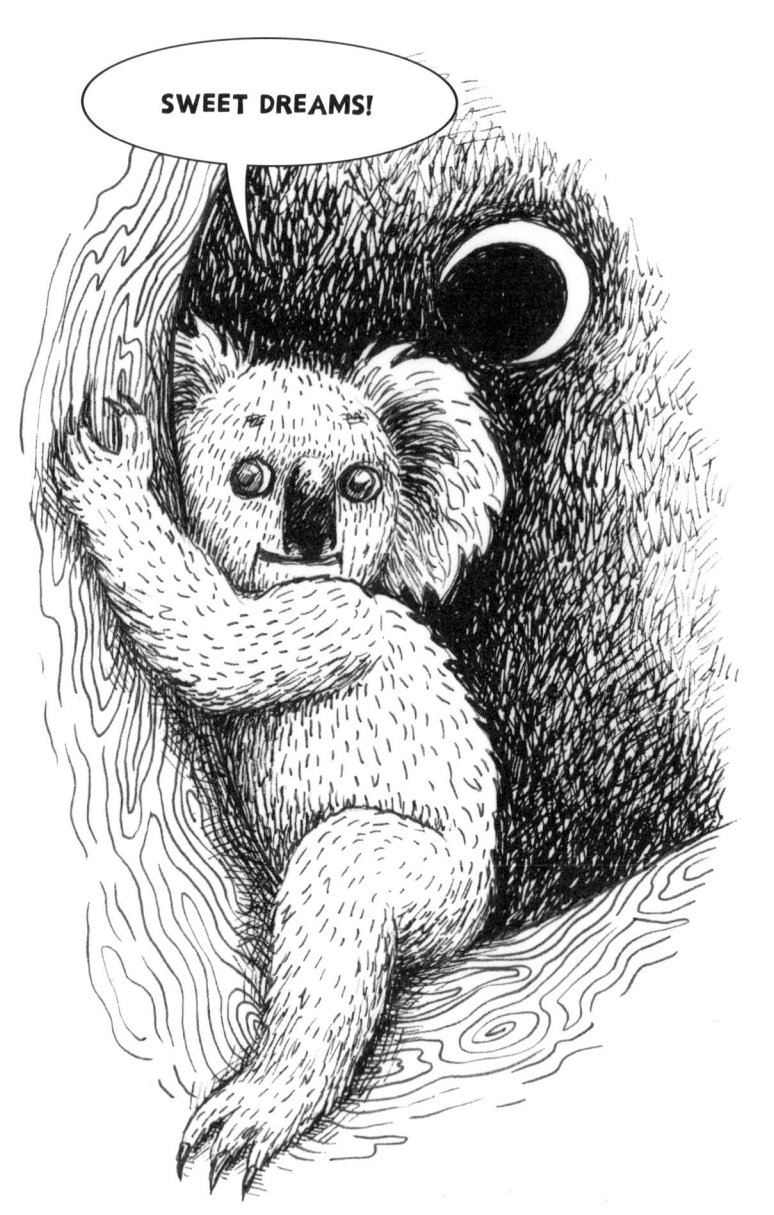

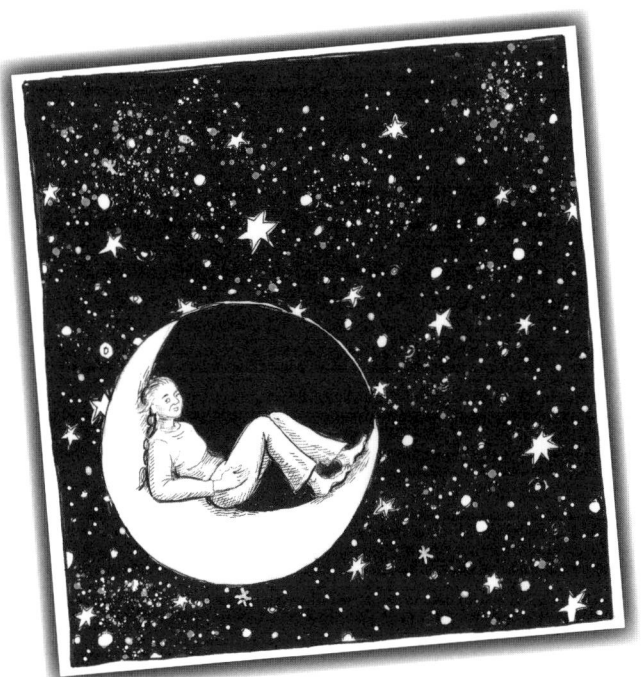

SAMPLE SLEEP LOG

Track your sleep-health habits first thing in the morning.

I went to bed at...

I fell asleep at about...

Number of nighttime awakenings:

Cause(s) of awakening(s):

Total time spent in bed awake:

Total time spent in bed asleep:

Subjective description of sleep:

When did I eat dinner last night?

Did I have any food or drink after dinner?

What did I eat and drink for dinner and before bed?

Did I take any supplements or medications yesterday?

If so, at what time did I take them?

What was my wind-down routine before bed? Did it include...

Limiting blue light exposure

Taking a hot shower or bath

Calming reading

Meditation

Gentle movement

Other

What did I do, eat, or drink yesterday that may have affected my sleep (positively or negatively)?

Caffeine intake/timing:

Alcohol intake/timing:

Exercise, movement:

Time spent outdoors:

Morning outdoor light exposure:

Social interactions (positive or challenging):

Work breaks

Mindfulness

Meditation

Breath work

Other

Morning reflection:

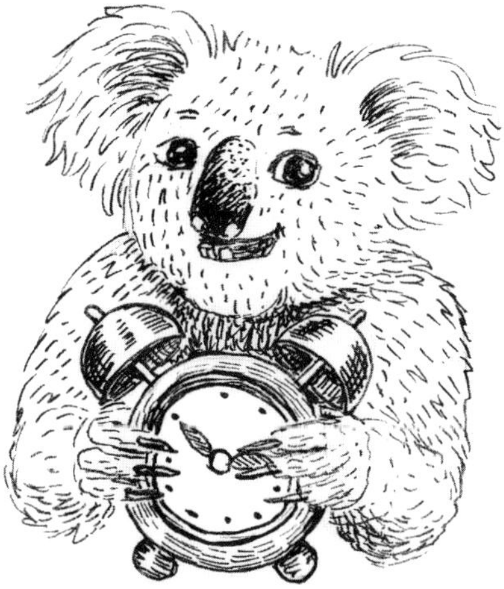

SAMPLE DREAM JOURNAL PAGES
TIPS for dream journaling:

- Write in present tense for more vivid recall.
- Write freely without editing yourself.
- Focus on what you can remember; don't worry if there are gaps. Often, details will emerge as you journal.
- Notice that dreams are highly symbolic. A person, animal, place, or thing often stands in for a concept. For example, a bra might be about support; water often stands in for emotions; vehicles can be about movement from one place to another, hence transformation.
- Take time to parse your dream after you record it. What is your subconscious mind telling you?
- Setting aside time each morning (first thing, before your dreams evaporate!) tells your brain to become more aware of dreams, which makes dream retention much more likely.

For my wife, KimAlix,
whose loving arms have embraced me
through many a sleepless hour.

NOTES

Introduction

Page 7: Learn more about koalas at the Australian Koala Foundation: https://www.savethekoala.com.

Page 17: Find out about the health risks associated with chronic insufficient sleep in Dr. Matthew Walker's groundbreaking book *Why We Sleep: The New Science of Sleep and Dreams* (New York: Penguin Books, 2018). You can also tune into Dr. Matthew Walker's podcast: https://podcasts.apple.com/us/podcast/the-matt-walker-podcast/id1578319649?i=1000692977800.

Part One: Air

Page 36: To learn more about the global prevalence of sleep apnea, see A. V. Benjafield et al., "Estimation of the Global Prevalence and Burden of Obstructive Sleep Apnoea: A Literature-Based Analysis," *The Lancet: Respiratory Medicine* 7, no. 8 (2019): 687–98. https://doi.org/10.1016/S2213-2600(19)30498-5.

Page 38: See J. Shaw, "Head to Toe: David Lieberman Tracks the Evolution of the Human Head," *Harvard Magazine* (January–February 2011), https://www.harvardmagazine.com/2011/01/head-to-toe.

Page 39: S. Kahn and P. R. Ehrlich, *Jaws: The Story of a Hidden Epidemic* (Stanford: Stanford University Press, 2021). Information gleaned from audio version of the book.

Page 41: G. Catlin, *Shut Your Mouth and Save Your Life*, with twenty-nine illustrations from drawings by the author, 4th ed. (London, 1870); J. Nestor, *Breath: The New Science of a Lost Art* (London: Penguin Art, 2020).

Page 42: E. Pratt, Artificial Nipple, No. 4,131. Patented August 4, 1845. https://patents.google.com/patent/US4131A/en.

Page 43: Yes, Queen Victoria allegedly named a cow in the royal stables after her daughter, Alice, who insisted on breastfeeding her child despite her mother's disgust. See J. Cox, "Breast or Bottle Feeding: The Debate Has Its Origins in Victorian Times," *The Conversation*, September 20, 2019, https://theconversation.com/breast-or-bottle-feeding-the-debate-has-its-origins-in-victorian-times-123296. For more on Queen Victoria's awful parenting style, see "Queen Victoria: The Real Story of Her 'Domestic Bliss,'" *BBC*, January 1, 2013, https://www.bbc.com/news/magazine-20782442. A study on how breastfeeding places beneficial orthopedic forces on the jaws: D. C. Page, "Breastfeeding Is Early Functional Jaw Orthopedics (an Introduction)," *Functional Orthodontist* 18, no. 3 (2001): 24–27. From M. Burhenne, "Breastfeeding and Jaw Development: How to Prevent Braces," *Ask the Dentist*, August 25, 2020, https://askthedentist.com/breastfeeding-jaw-development/:

> Breastfeeding supports good jaw development because of the unique way it encourages the tongue to press against the soft palate of the mouth.
>
> Babies use a tongue thrust motion during breastfeeding, pressing the tongue up into the soft palate and down against the front teeth.
>
> During infancy, a baby's soft

palate is soft and "wax-like." Tongue thrust during breastfeeding, swallowing, and talking shapes and expands the soft palate, encouraging proper growth of the upper jaw.

Bottle feeding does not cause the same action, which is why children who are exclusively bottle-fed have a much higher risk of orthodontic issues.

Breastfeeding's impact on jaw growth is also good for the development of a baby's airway. This may help prevent problems with sleep-disordered breathing, such as sleep apnea.

Page 44: More from Dr. Sandra Kahn and colleagues on best practices to encourage optimal jaw development: S. Kahn, P. Ehrlich, M. Feldman, R. Sapolsky, and S. Wong, "The Jaw Epidemic: Recognition, Origins, Cures, and Prevention," *BioScience* 70, no. 9 (September 2020): 759-71, https://doi.org/10.1093/biosci/biaa073.

Page 48: This study shows that didgeridoo playing may have a positive effect on sleep apnea: M. A. Puhan et al., "Didgeridoo Playing as Alternative Treatment for Obstructive Sleep Apnoea Syndrome: Randomised Controlled Trial," *BMJ (Clinical Research Ed.)* 332, no. 7536 (2006): 266-70, https://doi.org/10.1136/bmj.38705.470590.55.

Pages 52-55. Images on these pages were referenced from a video by David Hudson, Aboriginal musician and world-renowned didgeridoo player: https://youtu.be/2IBZ6yPW9WU. See also David Hudson's website, https://www.davidhudson.com.au.

Page 58: For the pronunciation and performance of the *SATANAMA* chant, see https://www.yogapedia.com/definition/10781/sa-ta-na-ma.

Page 65: If you would like to learn more about Linda Stone and healing from email (or screen) apnea, visit her website: https://lindastone.net/category/email-apnea/screen-apnea/. Breathing meditations for the workplace: https://www.psychologytoday.com/us/blog/the-art-of-now/201411/email-apnea. An article with descriptions of a variety of calming breathing techniques: https://www.scientificamerican.com/article/proper-breathing-brings-better-health/.

Page 68: A 21-minute listen where host Allison Aubrey interviews Dr. Matt Walker, who explains how preparing for sleep is a process akin to landing a plane: A. Aubrey, host, "Sleep Better with These Bedtime Rituals," *NPR Life Kit*, December 21, 2022. https://www.npr.org/transcripts/705224709.

Page 74: To learn more about mouth-taping, view "James Nestor on Mouth Taping at Night" on the podcast *Take a Deep Breath*, July 21, 2020, https://youtu.be/4Nxi2kDcZx4?si=Vq57jkO-HqrLnLK9. View the *Andrew Huberman Lab* podcast on proper breathing: Andrew Huberman, "How to Breathe Correctly for Optimal Health, Mood, Learning and Performance," *Huberman Lab Podcast*, February 20, 2023, https://www.youtube.com/watch?v=x4m_PdFbu-s.

Part Two: Fire

Page 91: According to data from the National Institutes of Health, sleep disturbance varies from 16% to 42% before menopause, from 39% to 47% during perimenopause, and from 35% to 60% after menopause.

F. C. Baker, "Optimizing Sleep Across the Menopausal Transition," *Climacteric: The Journal of the International Menopause Society* 26, no. 3 (2023): 198-205, https://doi.org/10.1080/13697137.2023.2173569.

Page 102: According to a July 5, 2022, *TuftsNow* article titled "Only 7% of American Adults Have Good Cardiometabolic Health," author Monica Jimenez states that "researchers evaluated Americans across five components of health: levels of blood pressure, blood sugar, blood cholesterol, adiposity . . . and presence or absence of cardiovascular disease. . . . They found that only 6.8 percent of U.S. adults had optimal levels of all five components as of 2017-2018."

Page 106: Images and canola oil manufacturing process based on "How It's Made Canola Oil," *How It's Made Show*, April 22, 2016, https://www.youtube.com/watch?v=AqxUs66OTy8.

Page 107: Learn more about the story of Procter & Gamble here: "Soap Opera: The Story of Procter & Gamble," *Ohio Memory*, A Collaborative Program of the Ohio History Connection and the State Library of Ohio, July 28, 2017: https://ohiomemory.ohiohistory.org/archives/3392.

Page 108: To learn more about the history of cotton in the US, see "Eli Whitney's Patent for the Cotton Gin," *National Archives*, Educator Resources, https://www.archives.gov/education/lessons/cotton-gin-patent.

Page 109: For more about the history of commercial products derived from cottonseed, see H. Z. Veit, "Eating Cotton: Cottonseed, Crisco, and Consumer Ignorance," *Journal of the Gilded Age and Progressive Era* 18, no. 4 (2019): 397-421.

Page 111: To learn about the seed oil industry and the duping of US consumers, see N. Teicholz, *The Big Fat Surprise: Why Butter, Meat, and Cheese Belong in a Healthy Diet* (New York: Simon & Schuster Paperbacks, 2015).

Page 115: Visit https://drcate.com to find books and articles by biochemist and family physician Dr. Cate Shanahan. Her book *Dark Calories: How Vegetable Oils Destroy Our Health and How We Can Get It Back* (New York: Hachette Go, 2024) outlines in detail the effects of seed oils on human metabolic health.

Page 120: Z. Williams, "Robert Lustig: The Man Who Believes Sugar Is Poison," *The Guardian*, August 24, 2014, https://www.theguardian.com/lifeandstyle/2014/aug/24/robert-lustig-sugar-poison.

Page 121: Cardiologist Dr. Nadir Ali appears on many podcasts and in online lectures, including Dr. Nadir Ali, "Why LDL Cholesterol Goes Up with Low Carb Diet and Is It Bad for Health?," *Low Carb Down Under*, May 3, 2019, https://www.youtube.com/watch?v=qXtdp4BNyOg. David Diamond is a professor in the Departments of Psychology and Molecular Pharmacology and Physiology at the University of South Florida and a research career scientist at the Tampa Veterans Hospital. See "David Diamond— Demonization and Deception in Cholesterol Research," *The IHMC*, September 26, 2015, https://www.youtube.com/watch?v=yX4vBA9bLNk. To learn more about publications by Dr. Sarah Szal Gottfried, visit https://www.saragottfriedmd.com.

e 126: For more detailed information about the invention of calories, see James L. Hargrove, "Does the History of Food Energy Units Suggest a Solution to 'Calorie Confusion'?," *Nutrition Journal* 6, no. 44 (December 17, 2007), https://doi.org/10.1186/1475-2891-6-44.

Page 128: Listen to an *NPR* Morning Edition interview that includes the words of Christopher Barrett, an economist at Cornell University who studies international agriculture and poverty. Dan Charles, "American Farmers Say They Feed the World, But Do They?," September 17, 2013, https://www.npr.org/sections/thesalt/2013/09/17/221376803/american-farmers-say-they-feed-the-world-but-do-they. See also D. R. Montgomery, "3 Big Myths About Modern Agriculture," *Scientific American*, April 5, 2017.

Part Three: Earth

Page 140: See J. Eklöf, *The Darkness Manifesto: On Light Pollution, Night Ecology, and the Ancient Rhythms That Sustain Life* (New York: Scribner, 2022).

Page 150: C. Rutz, M. C. Loretto, A. E. Bates, et al., "COVID-19 Lockdown Allows Researchers to Quantify the Effects of Human Activity on Wildlife," *Nature Ecology and Evolution* 4, nos. 1156–59 (2020). https://doi.org/10.1038/s41559-020-1237-z; Emily Anthes, "Did Nature Heal During the Pandemic 'Anthropause'?," *New York Times*, June 22, 2023, https://www.nytimes.com/2022/07/16/science/pandemic-nature-anthropause.html.

Page 153: M. A. Jackson and M. Bollinger, "Section 1: How Blue Light Affects the Eye and Body / Chapter 4," *How to Save Your Eyes in the Digital Age: The Handbook for Eye Care and Electronics*, https://eyesafe.com/chapter-4/.

Page 154: E. Finucane et al., "Does Reading a Book in Bed Make a Difference to Sleep in Comparison to Not Reading a Book in Bed? The People's Trial—an Online, Pragmatic, Randomized Trial," *Trials* 22, no. 873 (December 4, 2021), https://doi.org/10.1186/s13063-021-05831-3.

Page 159: *Ha'a'aahjigo dighádídeeshwot*, I will run to the East, from B. Shorty, *Navajo Word of the Day*, March 5, 2015, https://navajowotd.com/word/running/. "Toward the Rising Sun," *Trail Runner Magazine*, April 26, 2017, https://www.trailrunnermag.com/people/profiles-people/toward-the-rising-sun/.

Page 161: "The Five Daily Prayer Times and Why We Observe Them," muslimhands.org.uk, March 28, 2019.

Pages 175–90: Cognitive behavioral therapy for insomnia (CBT-I) is the preferred method for regulating sleep-wake cycles and promoting maximally restorative sleep without medication. There are a number of very good resources online, including this sampling:

> Sleepwell: An excellent not-for-profit resource site maintained by Dalhousie University in Nova Scotia, Canada. https://mysleepwell.ca/cbti/.
>
> Sleep Foundation: A group that was once a part of the nonprofit National Sleep Foundation. The Sleep Foundation publishes topical information. https://www.sleepfoundation.org/insomnia/treatment/cognitive

-behavioral-therapy-insomnia.

The National Sleep Foundation, founded in 1990, is committed to advancing excellence in sleep health theory, research, and practice. They are committed to sleep information and advocacy. https://www.thensf.org.

Free CBT-I is a website dedicated to providing free information about cognitive behavioral therapy for insomnia. They provide information in English, Korean, Spanish, Italian, and Chinese. https://freecbti.com.

Sleep Health Foundation. The Sleep Health Foundation (SHF) was established in 2009 as a not-for-profit health promotion charity with a vision to improve peoples' lives through better sleep. SHF was founded from within the Australasian Sleep Association (ASA), the nation's peak scientific body representing clinicians, scientists, and researchers in the broad area of sleep, with its active support. https://www.sleephealthfoundation.org.au/sleep-disorders/cognitive-behavioural-therapy-for-insomnia-cbt-i.

Part Four: Water

Page 199: Statistics about the correlation between insomnia and substance abuse taken from addictioncenter.com. Addiction Center states that their content is created by a team of researchers and journalists. The topics are chosen based on informational interviews with recovering addicts and treatment professionals to provide valuable information. They claim that all articles are fact-based and sourced from relevant publications, government agencies, and medical journals. https://www.addictioncenter.com/dual-diagnosis/insomnia/. Cannabidiol (CBD) is one notable exception to substances people reach for in an effort to sleep better. More research needs to be done on this. See M. Walker, "Sleep and CBD," *The Matt Walker Podcast*, episode 77, July 1, 2024, https://podcasts.apple.com/us/podcast/the-matt-walker-podcast/id1578349649?i=1000660765009.

Page 212: Learn more about the nutrition-brain-mental health connection in Dr. Georgia Ede's groundbreaking book *Change Your Diet, Change Your Mind: A Food-First Plan to Optimize Your Mental Health* (New York: Balance, 2024).

Pages 214–15: A. Huberman, "How to Breathe Correctly for Optimal Health, Mood, Learning and Performance," *Huberman Lab Podcast*, February 20, 2023, 220–21; Dr. S. Szal Gottfried, *Autoimmune Cure: Healing the Trauma and Other Triggers That Have Turned Your Body Against You* (London: Harper Collins, 2025), 17, 139, 189, 190.

Page 225: T. Hersey, *Rest Is Resistance: A Manifesto* (New York: Little, Brown Spark, 2022).

Page 228: A beautiful gratitude meditation: https://soundcloud.com/one-world-academy/gratitude-meditationenglish.

ACKNOWLEDGMENTS

My sincerest gratitude to my dear friend and publisher, Kendra Boileau, and to the brilliant publishing team at Graphic Mundi who helped us bring this book into the world.

I want to express my heartfelt gratitude to the health caregivers and researchers who work with diligence, deep intelligence, and compassion to shed light on stubborn chronic health conditions borne of our ultra-processed, overstimulated, and overheated world. Thanks to Dr. Sara Szal Gottfried, whose books put me on the path to healing from stubborn hormone imbalances. I owe a debt of gratitude to Matt Walker, PhD, whose book and podcast have been my North Star in navigating the fascinating world of sleep science, and to Ruben Naiman, whose beautiful writing about sleep graces my bedside table. Thanks also to Dr. Cate Shanahan for her urgent work to let the world know how dangerous industrial oils are for our metabolic health; to Dr. Jack Lustig, Dr. Nadir Ali, Nina Teicholz, PhD, and David Diamond, PhD, for guiding me through the fog of dietary mythologies. Thanks to Andrew Huberman for his excellent podcast; to Dr. Georgia Ede and Dr. Daniel Amen for their innovative work to break down the barriers between physical and mental health modalities; to Dr. David Lieberman for putting contemporary health issues into evolutionary perspective; to James Nestor for calling our attention to the importance of breathing better; to Dr. Sandra Kahn for her vital perspective on jaw development; to Linda Stone for making me aware of email apnea; and to Drs. Chesnea and Anderson for reminding me to exhale! I owe much gratitude to many other researchers and experts, some mentioned in this book and others whose voices via audiobooks and podcasts kept me company and informed me during countless hours of inking the art. A special thanks also to David Hudson, who inspired me with his gorgeous and haunting mastery of the time-honored didgeridoo.

I am grateful to the doctors and health care providers who persist in untangling the mysteries of my body-mind, who listen and invest real time and interest in their patients' struggles.